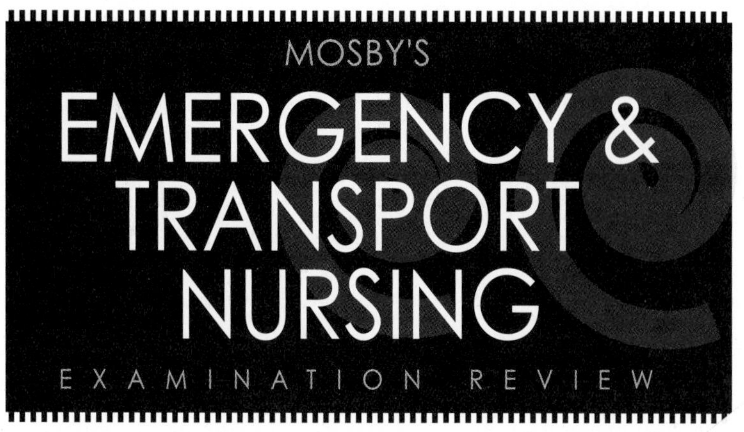
MOSBY'S
EMERGENCY &
TRANSPORT
NURSING
EXAMINATION REVIEW

FOURTH edition

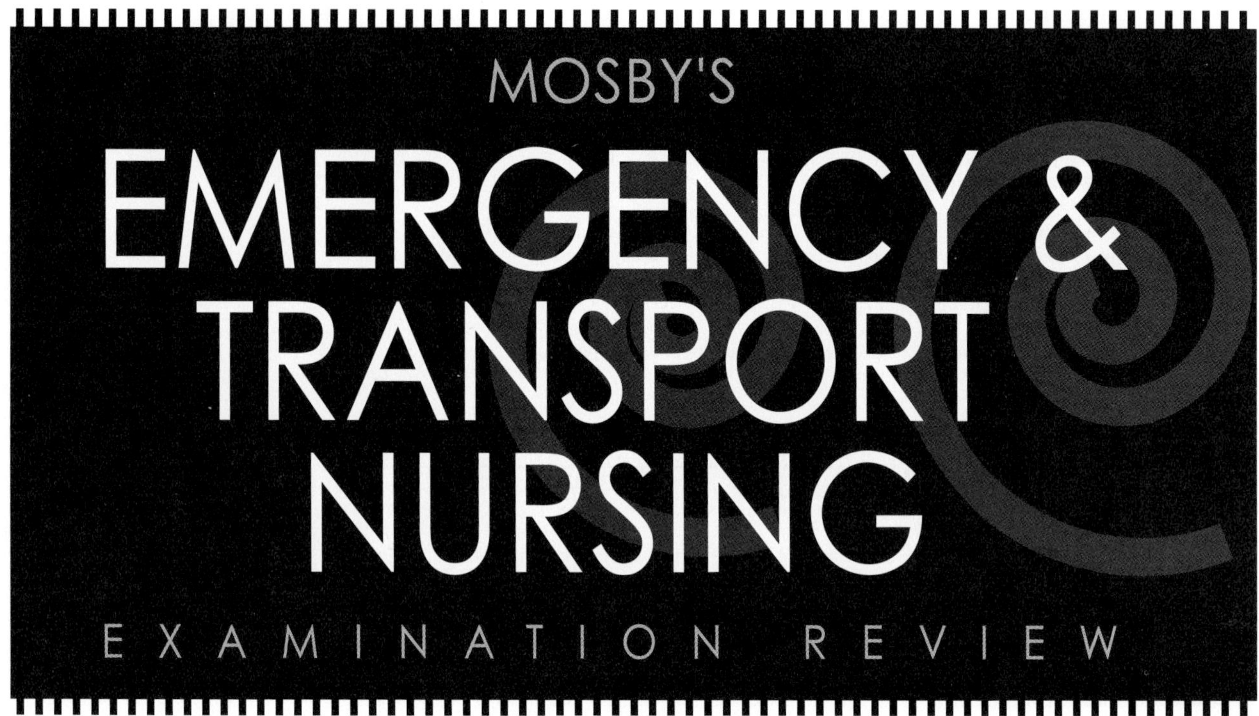

Reneé Semonin Holleran

Nurse Manager
Adult Transport Services
IHC Life Flight
Salt Lake City, Utah

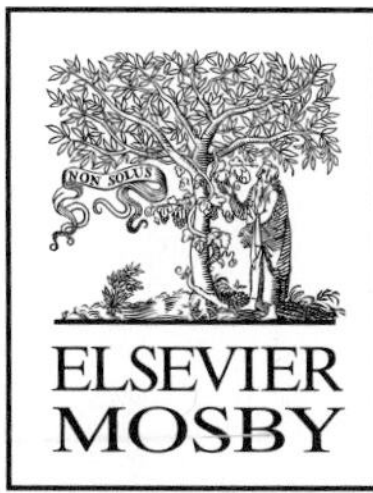

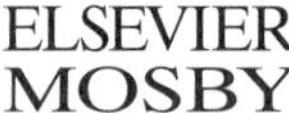

11830 Westline Industrial Drive
St. Louis, MO 63146

MOSBY'S EMERGENCY & TRANSPORT NURSING EXAMINATION REVIEW ISBN 0-323-03137-4

Notice

Emergency and transport nursing is an ever-changing field. Standard safety precautions must be followed, but as new research and clinical experience broaden our knowledge, changes in treatment and drug therapy may become necessary or appropriate. Readers are advised to check the most current product information provided by the manufacturer of each drug to be administered to verify the recommended dose, the method and duration of administration, and contraindications. It is the responsibility of the licensed prescriber, relying on experience and knowledge of the patient, to determine dosages and the best treatment for each individual patient. Neither the publisher nor the author assumes any liability for any injury and/or damage to persons or property arising from this publication.

Previous editions copyrighted 2001, 1996, 1992
CEN® is a federally registered trade mark of the BCEN in the United States.

International Standard Book Number 0-323-03137-4

Acquisitions Editor: *Susie Epstein*
Developmental Editor: *Jean Fornango*
Publishing Services Manager: *John Rogers*
Project Manager: *Doug Turner*
Senior Designer: *Kathi Gosche*

Printed in the United States of America

Last digit is the print number: 9 8 7 6 5 4 3 2 1

Dedication

The fourth edition of this book is dedicated as always to my family
—Micke, Erin, Sara, and my mom—
for all their patience and support.

It is also dedicated to my Air Care family, who will always be in my heart.
I hope this book helps nurses and others to see that emergency and
transport nursing is the way of my life.

Contributors

Donna York Clark, RN, SM, CFRN, CCRN
Director, DHART
Dartmouth-Hitchcock Medical Center
Lebanon, New Hampshire

Jonathan D. Gryniuk, FP-C, CCEMT-P, NREMT-P, RRT
Past President
National Flight Paramedics Association;
Flight Paramedic
Life Net of New York
Albany, New York

Sally Houliston, RCpN, BN, CFN (NZ), PG Cert Critical Care
Transport Clinical Team Leader
Hawkes Bay District Health Board
New Zealand

Jill Johnson, RN, MSN, CCRN, CEN, CFRN
Director of Clinical & Educational Services
Flight Nurse
Kentucky Aeromedical Team
Lexington, Kentucky

Gerardine Malone, RN, BSN, MS RHP
Staff Development Coordinator
Department of Health
Glenelg East, Australia

Jean A. Proehl, RN, MS, CEN, CCRN
Emergency Clinical Nursing Specialist
Dartmouth-Hitchcock Medical Center
Lebanon, New Hampshire

Michael Rouse, RN, MCN, CRNA
Former Flight Nurse
University Air Care
University of Cincinnati Hospital
Cincinnati, Ohio

Greg Schano, RN, CCRN, CMTE, EMTP, RT(R)
Medical Transport Quality Specialts
The Health Alliance Medical Transport Services
Cincinnati, Ohio

Nancy F. VonRotz, RN, MSN, FNP
Flight Nurse
University Air Care
University of Cincinnati Paramedic Program
Cinicinnati, Ohio;
Nurse Manager
Emergency Department
Clinton Memorial Hospital
Wilmington, Ohio

Reviewers

Lisa B. Valente, RN
Staff Nurse
Emergency Department
Massachusetts General Hospital
Boston, Massachusetts

Russell Wilshaw, RN, MS, CEN
Trauma Coordinator
Emergency Department
Utah Valley Regional Medical Center
Provo, Utah

THE CERTIFICATION IN EMERGENCY NURSING AND CERTIFICATION IN FLIGHT NURSING EXAMINATIONS

Purpose of Certification

Certification is a process whereby qualifications are validated and the knowledge required for practice in a defined functional or clinical area of nursing is measured. The purpose of both the Certification in Emergency Nursing (CEN®) and Certification in Flight Nursing (CFRN) examinations is to provide a method of measuring competency in the attainment and application of emergency and transport nursing.

Why do nurses and other professionals seek certification? The information that comes with both the certification for emerency nurses and transport nurses states that the value of certification includes:[1,2]

- Assurance to the general public that the nurse is competent and current in his or her practice
- Personal satisfaction through confidence and personal growth
- Validation of emergency and transport nursing expertise
- Monetary differentials
- Employment opportunities
- Markerting tool
- Professional recognition

A recent study published in *Nursing Outlook* confirmed this same perspetive by certified perioperative nurses.[3] Factor analysis found that over 61% of the variance was explained by three factors related to why nurses became certified: personal value, recognition by others, and professional practice.

Attaining certification in one's professional practice demonstrates dedication and a desire to be at the pinnacle of one's practice. Following this section is a discussion of the Flight Paramedic Certification (FP-C) and how to complete this certification.

History of the CEN® and the CFRN Examinations

The Board of Certification first offered the emergency nursing certification examination in July 1980 for Emergency Nursing. The registered nurse who passes this test is designated as a certified emergency nurse, or CEN®.

The certification examination for flight nursing was first offered in July 1993. This examination was created through collaboration between the National Flight Nurses Association, now known as the Air and Surface Transport Nurses Association (ASTNA), and the Board of Certification for Emergency Nursing. The registered nurse who passes this test is designated as a certified flight nurse, or CFRN.

CEN® and CFRN are primarily available through computer-based testing. Although this may pose a challenge to some, the advantages include the ability to offer the tests in more locations and more frequently than was done in the past. However, due to the challenges that have occurred over the years with the use of computer-based testing, both the Emergency Nurses Association (ENA) and the ASTNA have offered paper-and-pencil testing at some of their national meetings. The examinations are also offered internationally, and the list of countries in which the examinations are offered continues to grow.

Components of the Examinations

Each of the examinations has established "test blueprints" over the years. Using core curriculum, textbooks, journals, and other resources, questions are written by item writers and modified for the examination. The questions are then tested as well for validity and reliability. Currently, questions for the CEN® exam come from some of the following areas:

- Cardiovascular emergencies
- Gastrointestinal emergencies

- Obstetrical, genitourinary, and gynecological emergencies
- Maxillofacial and ocular emergencies
- Neurological emergencies
- Orthopedic and wound management emergencies
- Psycho/social emergencies
- Respiratory emergencies
- Patient care management

The CFRN examination includes questions based on the effects of transport. The current core curriculum for transport nursing is being revised and should be available at the beginning of 2005. The contents of the core will contain the following:

- History of transport nursing
- Standards of transport nursing
- Transport physiology
- Transport assessment and triage
- Transport planning and patient preparation
- Airway management
- Respiratory transport
- Cardiovascular transport
- Mechanically assisted cardiovascular-assisted transport
- Shock transport
- Multiple trauma transport
- Musculoskeletal transport
- Surface trauma transport
- Maxillofacial, anterior neck, and eye transport
- Medical emergency transport
- Abdominal transport
- Neurological transport
- Genitourinary and gynecological transport
- Obstetric transport
- Neonatal transport
- Pediatric transport
- Toxicological emergency transport
- Burn transport
- Environmental emergency transport
- Basics of radiological interpretation for transport
- Air operations
- Ground operations
- Crew resource management
- Search and rescue
- Scene management/extrication
- Program management
- Emergency medical services systems
- Communications
- Critical incident stress management
- Disaster management
- Military transport nursing
- Transport nurse education
- Community education/outreach
- Legal issues in transport
- Research in transport

Preparing for the Examinations

There are several ways to prepare for the CEN® or CFRN examination. The following test-taking strategies may help you to improve your test-taking skills and increase your test scores.

Before the Examination

First, obtain information about the CEN® or CFRN examination at either the ENA or ASTNA web sites. Both associations also provide hard copies of the information required to take the examinations. The information will point out how to register for the exams, the cost of the exams, and testing locations.

ENA and ASTNA members receive a discount on the examination fee. One of the other important benefits of membership in these associations is the availability of journals, conferences, and resources that can help you prepare for both examinations and remain up to date on all information and changes that affect our practice. Information about membership is available on both associations' web sites.

Next, prepare for the examination a few months before the test date. Set aside an hour or two a few days each week to review the major content areas of the examination. Review *Mosby's Emergency and Transport Nursing Review*, the *Emergency Nursing Core Curriculum*, and the *Transport Nurse Core Curriculum*. Additional suggested review resources are listed at the end of this section.

Consider taking a CEN® or CFRN examination review course and ask yourself the following questions:

- Will this course actually help me to pass the examination?
- Who are the faculty?
- Are the faculty members CEN®s or CFRNs?
- What are the objectives of the course?
- Is the course accredited?

Most of these courses help you to identify your learning needs. They are not a substitute for studying. Talk to your nursing colleagues who are CEN®s or CFRNs. Ask what worked for them in preparing for the examination and if they have any suggestions.

Review information in courses that are requirements for most emergency and transport nurses such as Advanced Cardiac Life Support (ACLS), Pediatric Advanced Life Support (PALS), Trauma Nursing Core Course (TNCC), Emergency Nursing

Pediatric Course (ENPC), and Transport Nurse Advanced Trauma Course (TNATC) (see Chapter 1 for suggestions for additional courses).

Concentrate on those areas that you have identified as areas of weakness. If, for example, your knowledge or understanding of arterial blood gases (ABGs) is lacking, concentrate on this subject for a few days. Read a chapter on respiratory physiology from a pathophysiology text. Copy and read articles on ABGs. Practice ABG interpretation on each of your patients who have arterial blood gases drawn. Discuss your findings with another nurse or physician. Applying principles to the clinical setting is the best way for most nurses to learn. Remember, the key here is not only to study but also to keep your studying clinically focused.

It may help to keep your review materials handy, especially at work, so that you can review material during slower times in the emergency department or transport down time. Current emergency nursing journals (e.g., *Journal of Emergency Nursing* and *Annals of Emergency Medicine)* and transport journals (e.g., *Air Medical Journal)* are rich sources of information.

It may also help to keep a simple log on how much time you spend reviewing (even if it is only 10 minutes between appointments). After a while you may be surprised to see how much unscheduled time you have accumulated in studying. This also helps to boost self-confidence.

Another useful way to review information in preparation for the CEN® or CFRN examination is to use the Internet and some of the web-based education offered. In addition, many medical and nursing journals are available on-line. The Centers for Disease Control and Prevention provide guidelines, research, and pertinent bulletins on-line. Both the ENA and the ASTNA have web sites as previously noted. Nicoll, editor of *Computers in Nursing*,[4] has written a particularly useful guide to getting started using the Internet. "Surfing the Web" also provides you with the opportunity to practice your computer skills.

One more point about spending time preparing for the CEN® or CFRN examination: because each examination is based on current emergency and transport nursing practice, it is important that you think about how many hours you have worked in the emergency department or how much transport time you have accrued. Full-time employment works out to be about 2080 hours per year; part-time employment is about 1040 hours per year. The best way to prepare yourself for this examination is to have at least 2 years of current emergency or flight or transport nursing experience, so you may have already spent thousands of hours in preparation. You may know more than you think; but nonetheless, be prepared.

If you have not tested well in the past, or if you have not taken a test in several years, consider taking the practice test from other review books. The current edition of this book provides you with an opportunity to practice taking the test on a computer. If you have limited exposure to computer testing, it is a good idea to practice "clicking." *The CEN® and CFRN examinations will now allow you to skip questions and return to them. Again, if you are not familiar with doing that on a computer, practice!*

Finally, get a good night's sleep the night before the test. Do not drink alcohol or take unnecessary medications to help you sleep because they may affect your performance the following day. Eat a good but light breakfast to "feed your brain" as well as your stomach.

During the Examination

As you begin to take the test, remember to relax. Anxiety will prevent you from doing a good job. Do not let brief and needless anxiety affect your knowledge of emergency or transport nursing. Your skills are tested every day with human lives; sitting down to take an examination is the easy part of an emergency or transport nurse's job.

Remember a cardinal rule for test taking: always keep the first answer you choose. Do not go back and change an answer unless you are certain the new one is correct. Do not overlook key words such as *early*, *late*, *except*, *not*, *immediate*, or *nursing intervention*. There is usually no pattern to the answers on a test. Do not select *B* simply because you have not answered *B* for the last 10 questions.

Beware of answer choices that contain qualifiers such as *always*, *never*, *all*, or *every*. These are blanket terms, and we know that in nursing nothing is ever 100% certain. Answers that contain these words can usually, but not always, be considered incorrect.[5]

What if you come to a question that confuses you? It cannot be overemphasized how clinically oriented these examinations are. Imagine yourself in that particular clinical situation. What would you do? You may be surprised at how automatically some answers to confusing questions will come to you if you put yourself in a clinical setting. And remember, who is better at sorting out confusion than an emergency or transport nurse?

If you come to a question that you cannot answer, return to it later. The new examination will allow you to skip a question and return to it. However, it might be a good idea to write down the number of the question skipped because you no longer have a written examination in front of you, and the screens will change. Perhaps another question on the test may give you a clue to the correct answer. Narrow your choices to a question by eliminating the obviously wrong answers. Each test is now composed of 175 questions, and you will receive your score at the test site.

Finally, we wish you well. It is a big commitment to work toward becoming a CEN® or CFRN. Congratulations on putting forth the effort. We hope that these suggestions will make taking the examination a more positive experience. The time you invest in studying will pay off. Good luck!

Reneé Semonin Holleran
Terry Mathew Foster

REFERENCES

1. CEN examination information from www.ena.org. Accessed July 4, 2004.
2. CFRN examination information from www.astna.org. Accessed July 4, 2004.
3. Gaberson KB, Schroeter K, Killen AR, Valentine WA: The perceived value of certification by certified perioperative nurses, *Nursing Outlook* 51(6):272–6, 2003.
4. Nicoll LH: *Nurses' guide to the Internet*, Philadelphia, 1998, Lippincott.
5. CEN® and CFRN news, *J Emerg Nurs* 26(1):37A, 2000.

STUDY REFERENCES

Association of Air Medical Services: *Guidelines for air medical crew members*, Alexandria, VA, 2004, Author.

Arndt K, editor: *Standards for critical care and specialty rotor-wing transport*, Denver, CO, 2003, ASTNA.

James SE, editor: *Standards for critical care and specialty ground transport*, Denver, CO, 2002, ASTNA.

Marx J, senior editor: *Rosen's emergency medicine: concepts and clinical practice*, St Louis, 2002, Mosby.

Newberry L, editor: *Sheehy's emergency nursing*, ed 5, St Louis, 2003, Mosby.

Proehl J, editor: *Emergency nursing procedures*, ed 3, Philadelphia, 2004, WB Saunders.

Semonin Holleran R, editor: *Air and surface patient transport: principles and practice*, ed 3, St Louis, 2003, Mosby.

Preparing for the Certified Flight Paramedic (FP-C) Examination

In 2000 the National Flight Paramedics Association released the Certified Flight Paramedic (FP-C) examination. Since its inception, this examination has gone through several evolutions and is now overseen by a board of directors separate from the National Flight Paramedics Association. Oversight of the certification is now controlled by the Board for Critical Care Transport Paramedic Certification (BCCTPC). The FP-C examination process was the culmination of several years of planning, development, and evaluation of flight paramedic practice. While the examination was created independently of any nursing influences, it has become widely apparent that parallels exist with the CFRN and CEN® examinations. Interviews with examinees who have successfully completed one or both of these nursing examinations and the FP-C examination reveals that despite the philosophical differences between paramedic and nursing practices, the information required of these individuals to function in the emergency care and transport environments is nearly identical. With that understanding, one can surmise that any study reference that was created to assist in preparation for these nursing certifications can be of value in preparing for the FP-C examination.

Paramedic practice in the United States varies, depending upon locale and sponsoring agency. While some air medical programs perform missions incorporating a standard of care consistent with Advanced Life Support protocols, others utilize an expanded scope of practice consistent with critical care transport guidelines. One of the primary goals in developing a standardized examination process for flight paramedics focused specifically on minimizing these regional and program variances. The FP-C examination was created with the understanding that the majority of flight paramedics practice with an expanded critical care scope of practice. Therefore, in preparation for the Certified Flight Paramedic examination, the examinee must focus attention on areas of paramedic practice that may exceed their own regional, state, or program's standard of practice. Further, whether or not a paramedic may be allowed to perform a specific skill or utilize a specific device or medication, the paramedic should still have an understanding of the skills, devices, or medications that are utilized by their nursing or other specialty counterparts in order to act as effective patient advocates. An example of this is the understanding of intra-aortic balloon pump (IABP) devices. In some transport programs, the flight paramedic may not have any responsibilities in managing IABP devices. This responsibility may be left to the transport nurse, respiratory care practitioner, or a perfusionist, depending upon the practice of the managing transport program. However, given the high risk potential for a poor patient outcome that may occur with mismanagement of this device, the Certified Flight Paramedic should have an understanding of the basic physiology and use of the IABP.

In utilizing "review" materials in preparation for the FP-C examination, the examinee needs to remember that these resources are meant to act as study aids for information that has already been learned. Following the release of the FP-C examination, the National Flight Paramedics Association released a position paper entitled, "The Role of the Certified Flight Paramedic (FP-C) as a Critical Care Provider and the Required Education." This document outlines general areas of education and suggested minimum hours of study in each content area to prepare the paramedic for critical care practice and successful completion of the FP-C examination. The outlined educational areas are in addition to the areas of study in the standard Department of Transportation Emergency Medical Technician-Paramedic curriculum. Failure to obtain this additional education greatly diminishes the likelihood that the candidate will successfully complete the examination process. A variety of avenues are available for obtaining this additional education. Many flight programs complete comprehensive didactic and clinical education within these study areas upon hire of the flight paramedic. Commercially available critical care paramedic education programs may also meet these basic educational requirements. Finally, self-study utilizing references such as this text to identify areas of educational weakness should assist greatly in obtaining what is considered by many to be the pinnacle of paramedic practice, the FP-C designation.

Jonathan Gryniuk, FP-C, CCEMT-P, NREMT-P
Flight Paramedic
Life Net of New York;
Past President
National Flight Paramedics Association

Preface

It is hard to believe that this is the fourth edition of this book. It began as a CEN® review book and now it includes transport questions that can be used for both the CFRN and FP-C examinations. One important thing that I must emphasize is that this is a review book based on my experience as an emergency and a transport nurse and one who has had the opportunity to learn how to write test questions. I have no affiliation with the Board of Certification (BCEN), though I feel very strongly that all nurses should belong to their professional associations (ENA and ASTNA for example).

I would like to thank all of my contributors, who despite my nagging remain good friends. Also, thanks to the guidance and patience of Suzi Epstein who never lost faith in me despite the "moving" changes I have experienced over the last year.

This edition has expanded to include questions for emergency and transport nursing as well as for those who are preparing to take the flight paramedic certification exam. However, the text and questions can also serve as method to review core emergency and transport nursing principles, whether the examinations are taken or not.

As always, we welcome your comments and suggestions for improvement.

Contents

PART **ONE**

Practice and Patient Care Issues

CHAPTER 1

Emergency and Transport Nursing Education

REVIEW OUTLINE

I. Emergency nursing education
   A. Knowledge in
      1. Pediatrics
      2. Obstetrics
      3. Medicine
      4. Cardiology
      5. Trauma
      6. Oncology
      7. Infectious diseases
      8. Psychosocial issues
      9. General patient management
      10. Safety issues (personal, environmental)
      11. Emerging trends in emergency medicine and emergency nursing
      12. Legal issues
      13. Ethical issues
      14. Pain management
      15. Pharmacology
   B. Collaborative care with other health care providers
   C. Crisis intervention and stress management skills
   D. Demonstrated competency in knowledge of equipment used in the emergency department
   E. Prehospital care environment
   F. Disaster preparation and response
   G. Weapons of mass destruction
   H. Management of violence
   I. Reimbursement issues, managed care, health care reform
   J. Legal and ethical issues
   K. Triage
   L. Patient and family education
   M. Patient education principles: adult, child, and community
   N. Illness and injury prevention strategies
   O. Professional behaviors
      1. Autonomy
      2. Critical thinking
      3. Leadership
      4. Delegation
      5. Collaborative roles
   P. Emergency nursing standards
   Q. Advanced practice roles
      1. Advanced practice nurse (APN)
      2. Clinical nurse specialist (CNS)
      3. Nurse practitioner (NP)

II. Emergency nursing skills and competencies
   A. Performance of a primary survey and initiation of critical interventions
      1. Airway assessment and management (cervical spine immobilization in the injured patient)
      2. Breathing and ventilation assessment and management
      3. Circulation assessment and management
      4. Neurological assessment and management
      5. Exposure management
         a. Temperature
         b. Evidence collection
      6. Vital signs assessment and management
   B. Performance of a secondary survey
      1. Obtain a patient history
         a. Chief complaint
         b. Mechanism of injury
         c. Medical history
         d. AMPLE history
            (1) Allergies
            (2) Medication
            (3) Past medical history
            (4) Last food or drink, time of

(5) Events and environment related to injury
e. CIAMPEDS
(1) Chief complaint
(2) Immunizations and isolation
(3) Allergies
(4) Medications
(5) Past health history
(6) Events preceding the problem
(7) Diet and elimination
(8) Symptoms associated with the problem
2. Review of the systems using inspection, palpation, auscultation, and percussion as indicated
a. Neurological
b. Cardiovascular
c. Pulmonary
d. Gastrointestinal
e. Musculoskeletal
f. Integumentary
g. Genitourinary
h. Psychosocial
i. Family
3. Diagnostic
a. Laboratory values
b. Electrocardiogram
c. Gastric lavage
d. Whole blood glucose monitoring
4. Equipment management
a. Airway equipment
b. Ventilation equipment
c. Circulation equipment
d. Cervical spine immobilization
e. Basic life support (BLS) equipment
f. Advanced life support (ALS) equipment
g. Age-specific equipment (e.g., pediatric)
h. Illness-specific or injury-specific equipment (e.g., casts, splints, cervical traction)

III. Educational resources
A. Trauma Nursing Core Course (TNCC)[1]
B. Emergency Nursing Pediatric Course (ENPC)[2]
C. Emergency Nursing Core Curriculum[3]
D. Standards of Emergency Nursing Practice[4]
E. Course in Advanced Trauma Nursing-II: a Conceptual Approach to Injury and Illness (CATN-II)[5]
F. Core Curriculum for Pediatric Emergency Nursing[6]
G. Emergency Nurses Association orientation program
1. Acid-base imbalances
2. Assessment and priority setting
3. Cardiovascular emergencies
4. Drug dosage calculations
5. Dysrhythmia recognition
6. Ear, nose, and throat emergencies
7. Environmental emergencies
8. Fluid and electrolyte imbalances
9. Gastrointestinal and genitourinary emergencies
10. General medical emergencies
11. Infectious diseases
12. Multiple trauma
13. Musculoskeletal emergencies
14. Neurological emergencies
15. Obstetrical and gynecological emergencies
16. Ocular emergencies
17. Oncological emergencies
18. Organ and tissue procurement
19. Pain management and sedation procedures
20. Psychiatric emergencies
21. Respiratory medical emergencies
22. Special patient population: geriatric
23. Special patient population: pediatric
24. Surface trauma
25. Toxicology
26. Violence, abuse, and forensic evidence
27. Disaster, hazmat preparedness, and weapons of mass destruction
28. Emergency department operations
29. Emergency medical services systems
30. Legal issues
31. Professional approaches
H. Emergency nursing procedures[7]
1. Examples
a. Basic airway management
b. Advanced airway management
c. Defibrillation
d. External pacing
e. Arterial pressure monitoring
f. Gastric lavage
2. Triage
3. Evidence collection

IV. Transport nursing education
A. Knowledge in
1. Basic Life Support (BLS)
2. Advanced Life Support (ALS)
3. Neonatal Advanced Life Support (NALS)

4. Pediatric Advanced Life Support (PALS)
5. Trauma (Transport Nurse Advanced Trauma Course [TNATC])[8]
6. Safety (aircraft, scene, personnel)
7. Survival skills and competencies
8. Medical
9. Infectious diseases
10. Obstetrical
11. Altitude and flight physiology
12. Transport equipment

B. Communication
C. Public relations
D. Legal and ethical issues
E. Outreach education
F. Collaborative care
G. Prehospital care environment

V. Transport nursing skills and competencies[9-11]

A. Airway management
1. Basic airway management
2. Advanced airway management
3. Rapid sequence intubation
4. Difficult airway management
5. Failed airway management

B. Ventilation management
1. Needle decompression
2. Chest tube insertion

C. Circulation management
1. Pericardiocentesis
2. Central line insertion
3. Venous cutdown
4. External and transvenous pacing
5. Defibrillation
6. Escharotomy
7. Intraaortic balloon pump
8. Blood and blood products administration

D. Medication management and administration
E. Fetal monitoring
F. Emergent delivery
G. Extrication management and safety
H. Triage
I. Disaster response
J. Weapons of mass destruction and effects: nuclear, biological, and chemical

VI. Educational resources

A. TNATC[8]
B. Basic Trauma Life Support (BTLS)
C. Neonatal Resuscitation Certification Program
D. Prehospital Trauma Life Support (PHTLS)
E. Trauma Nurse Specialist (TNS)
F. Mobile Intensive Care Nurse (MICN)
G. Standards of Rotor-wing Transport[9]
H. Standards for Critical Care and Specialty Ground Transport[10]
I. Transport Nursing Core Curriculum[11]

The practice of emergency and transport nursing requires that nurses possess knowledge in all areas of patient care that they may encounter. Emergency and transport nurses provide care for neonatal, pediatric, adult, emergencies, as well as geriatric, medical, surgical, traumatic, oncological, infectious disease, and psychological emergencies. The patients may be suffering from minor to life-threatening emergencies. The question then becomes: how does one prepare for everything?

One of the most vital sources of education is experience. It is difficult to procure the knowledge that experience can teach. The more one is exposed to different types of patient care situations, the more comfortable and educated one becomes. The ability to become competent in one's practice is enhanced with experience and continuing education.

The nursing process is the model on which nursing care is based. Using the concepts of assessment, diagnosis, outcome identification, planning, implementation, and evaluation, the emergency and flight or transport nurse can plan care for individuals and groups of patients. Nurses care for the "whole" patient, including the family and environment with which the patient interacts. This process is what makes nurses different from the other health care professionals with whom we work, such as medical and prehospital care providers.

Emergency and transport nursing practice requires a team or collaborative approach to patient care. Depending on the nurses' skill levels and their job descriptions, they may be responsible for additional advanced patient care interventions, such as endotracheal intubation or chest decompression.

Both emergency and transport nurses function in various roles in their practice, including direct patient care, research, education, management, consultation, advocacy, and administration. These roles require additional education and preparation in order to function with care and competence.

Emergency and transport nurses need to demonstrate that they are competent practitioners. Competence involves an integration of knowledge and technical skills, while applying the principles of the nursing practice.[12,13] Competence is also a measure of one's professional growth, and it can be measured against accepted standards. Confusion arises as to what describes a competent emergency or transport nurse. Nursing practice varies from state to state, and emergency and transport nursing practice is definitely influenced by the types of patients for whom care is provided. For example, some emergency departments now routinely care for patients with invasive lines and intracranial pressure monitors, and some transport nurses are permitted to create surgical airways and insert central lines.

Transport nursing involves care in the field and in transport vehicles, such as helicopters, fixed-wing aircraft, and ground ambulances. This requires additional training and education to ensure both patient and crew safety. Johnson, Childress, and Herron[14] found that 44, or 88%, of the states in the United States have no nursing-oriented credentialing process for registered nurses who practice in the prehospital care environment. Some states require that nurses obtain additional certifications, such as emergency medical technician (EMT) or emergency medical technician-paramedic (EMT-P), before they can function in the prehospital environment.[14]

Another important role for emergency transport nurses involves providing education for patients and the communities that they serve. The Joint Commission on Accreditation of Healthcare Organizations (JCAHO) and the American Hospital Association's Patient's Bill of Rights address the need for patients and their families to be provided with information about their health care problems and how to manage them. Developing and providing educational programs for patient, family, and health care providers—including prehospital care providers—is an important responsibility of the practice of emergency and transport nursing.[15-17]

Both the Standards of Emergency Nursing Practice[4] and the transport standards that include all modes of transport (air and ground)[9-11] provide some guidelines for preparation and continuing education. The above outline contains a catalog of skills, courses, and reference books that may be helpful for educational preparation. As with life, it will continually change and grow, and as practicing emergency and transport nurses we must be open to the changes that are an integral part of our practice.

References

1. Emergency Nurses Association: *Trauma nursing core course,* Des Plaines, IL, 2000, Emergency Nurses Association.
2. Emergency Nurses Association: *Emergency nursing pediatric course,* Des Plaines, IL, 2004, Emergency Nurses Association.
3. Jordan KS: *Emergency nursing core curriculum,* Philadelphia, 2000, WB Saunders.
4. Emergency Nurses Association: *Standards of emergency nursing practice,* ed 4, St Louis, 1999, Mosby.
5. Emergency Nurses Association: *Course in advanced trauma nursing-II: a conceptual approach to injury and illness,* Des Plaines, IL, 2003, Emergency Nurses Association.
6. Thomas DJ, Bernardo LM, Herman B: *Core curriculum for pediatric emergency nursing,* Boston, 2003, Jones and Bartlett.
7. Proehl J: *Emergency nursing procedures,* ed 3, Philadelphia, 2004, WB Saunders.
8. Air and Surface Transport Nurses Association: *Transport nurse advanced trauma course,* Denver, 2002, Air and Surface Transport Nurses Association.
9. Arndt K: *Standards for critical care and specialty rotor-wing report,* Lexington, KY, 2003, Myers Printing.
10. James S: *Standards for critical care and specialty ground transport,* Lexington, KY, 2002, Myers Printing.
11. Krupa D: *Flight nursing core curriculum,* Park Ridge, IL 1997, National Flight Nurses Association.
12. Ready R: Clinical competency testing for emergency nursing, *J Emerg Nurs* 20:24-31, 1994.
13. Proehl J: Assessing emergency nursing competence, *Nurs Clin North Am* 37(1):97-110, 2002.
14. Johnson R, Childress S, Herron H: Regulation of prehospital nursing practice: a national survey, *J Emerg Nurs* 19:437-440, 1993.
15. Duffy M, Snyder K: Can ED patients read your patient education materials? *J Emerg Nurs* 25:294-297, 1999.
16. Hepp H: *Flight nursing standards of practice,* St Louis, 1995, Mosby.
17. McCafferty M: Teaching tools for heart failure, *J Emerg Nurs* 22:451-453, 1996.

Additional Readings

Alspach JG: *Core curriculum for critical care nursing,* ed 5, Philadelphia, 1998, WB Saunders.

McQuillan KA, Von Rueden KT, Hartsock RL et al, editors: *Trauma nursing: from resuscitation through rehabilitation,* Philadelphia, 2002, WB Saunders.

Kelley S: *Pediatric emergency nursing,* Norwalk, CT, 1994, Appleton & Lange.

Kim MJ, McFarland G, McClane A: *Pocket guide to nursing diagnoses,* St Louis, 1993, Mosby.

Kitt S, Selfridge-Thomas J, Proehl J et al, editors: *Emergency nursing: a physiologic and clinical perspective,* Philadelphia, 1995, WB Saunders.

Semonin Holleran R, editor: *Air and surface patient transport: principles and practice,* St Louis, 2003, Mosby.

Neff J, Kidd P: *Trauma nursing: art and science,* St Louis, 1993, Mosby.

Semonin Holleran R: *Prehospital nursing: a collaborative approach,* St Louis, 1994, Mosby.

Frazier E: *Standards for accreditation for medical transport systems,* ed 5, Anderson, SC, 2002, Commission on Accreditation of Medical Transport Systems. It is important to note that these standards undergo continuous revision. The next revision is already in progress.

CHAPTER 2

Patient Assessment and Priority Setting: Triage

REVIEW OUTLINE

I. Definition of triage
   A. History of triage
      1. Military
      2. Civilian
   B. Types of triage
      1. Nursing
      2. Physician
      3. Paramedic, emergency medical technician (EMT)
      4. Disaster, multiple-casualty incident (MCI)
      5. Telephone triage
         a. Protocol-based
         b. Nursing judgment–based
         c. Levels of expertise

II. Components of triage
   A. ABCs
      1. Airway
      2. Breathing
      3. Circulation
   B. Chief complaint
   C. History
   D. Classification
   E. Documentation
   F. Pediatric triage[1-3]
      1. Based on growth and development
      2. Need to collect history from both caregiver and child
      3. Based on assessment of the ABCs, recognizing the differences between the pediatric patient and the adult patient
      4. Use of tables that provide normal pediatric values, such as blood pressure, pulse, respirations, and weight
      5. Pediatric assessment triangle
         a. Appearance
         b. Breathing
         c. Circulation to skin
      6. General inspection of the child, looking for things such as rashes or signs of abuse or neglect
      7. CIAMPEDS[2]

III. Rapid patient assessment
   A. Basic Cardiac Life Support (BCLS)
   B. Advanced Cardiac Life Support (ACLS)
   C. Pediatric Advanced Life Support (PALS)
   D. Emergency Nursing Pediatric Course (ENPC)
   E. Trauma Nursing Core Curriculum (TNCC)
   F. Basic Trauma Life Support (BTLS)
   G. Advanced Trauma Life Support (ATLS)
   H. Pediatric Education for Prehospital Professionals (PEEP)
   I. Advanced Trauma Course for Nursing (ATCN)
   J. Course in Advanced Trauma Nursing-II: a Conceptual Approach to Injury and Illness (CATN-II)

IV. Chief complaint
   A. PQRST
      1. Provocation
      2. Quality
      3. Region and radiation
      4. Severity of the problem
      5. Time

V. History
   A. History related to the chief complaint
   B. Medical history
   C. Allergies
   D. Cultural beliefs
   E. Family interactions

VI. Diversity assessment model[4]
   A. Assumptions: taking for granted the ethnic background of the patient or family
   B. Beliefs and behaviors of the patient, families, and caregivers

C. Communication: how does the patient communicate?
D. Diversity: the way in which people differ (i.e., age, race, ethnicity, gender, sexual orientation, spirituality, and so on)
E. Education: learning about the patient's differences

VII. Vital signs
A. Blood pressure
B. Pulse
C. Respirations
1. Pulse oximetry
D. Temperature

VIII. Physical assessment
A. Subjective data (see previous outline of History, and so on)
B. Objective data
1. Inspection
2. Palpation
3. Auscultation
4. Percussion
5. Olfaction (odors)
C. Secondary assessment (review of the systems)
1. Head
2. Ear, nose, and throat
3. Chest
4. Abdomen
5. Pelvis and perineum
6. Extremities
7. Integument (skin)
D. Age-specific assessment
1. Pediatric
2. Geriatric

IX. Classification
A. Emergent, urgent, nonurgent
B. Immediate, expected, delayed care
C. Acute, nonacute
D. Comprehensive triage
1. Immediate: life threatening
2. Stable: as soon as possible
3. Stable: no distress, should be reassessed every 30 minutes
4. Stable: no distress, should be reassessed every 60 minutes
E. Emergency severity index[5,6]
1. Scores range from 1 (resuscitation) to 5 (nonurgent), used along with an algorithm that includes chief complaint, vital signs, and narrative
F. Australian Triage Scale
1. Levels
a. Level 1: resuscitation
b. Level 2: emergency
c. Level 3: urgent
d. Level 4: semiurgent
e. Level 5: nonurgent
2. Time to be seen by a provider
a. Level 1: immediately
b. Level 2: seen within 10 minutes
c. Level 3: seen within 30 minutes
d. Level 4: seen within 60 minutes
e. Level 5: seen within 120 minutes

X. Documentation
A. SOAP charting
1. Subjective
2. Objective
3. Assessment
4. Plan
B. Chief complaint
C. History
D. Brief physical assessment
E. Family
F. Allergies
G. Tetanus status
H. Patients at risk for becoming violent
1. Young males
2. Gang members
3. Intoxicated patients
4. Patients with altered mental status
5. Patients with psychiatric history
6. Patients with history of violence
7. Patients and family under stress

XI. Prehospital triage[7]
A. Primary information survey[8]
1. Description of event
2. Location and environment
B. Scene survey
C. Kinematics of injury
D. Levels of trauma care from the American College of Surgeons
1. Level I trauma center
2. Level II trauma center
3. Level III trauma center
4. Level IV trauma center
E. Factors in patient assessment in prehospital triage
1. Clinical status of the patient
2. Nature and probable severity of the injury
3. Scoring systems
a. Glasgow Coma Scale (GCS)
b. Revised Trauma Score
c. Baxt Trauma Triage Rule
4. Type and availability of transportation

5. Level of availability and accessibility of hospital care

XII. Nursing diagnoses
- A. Airway clearance, ineffective
- B. Breathing pattern, ineffective
- C. Fluid volume deficit, high risk for
- D. Injury, high risk for
- E. Knowledge deficit
- F. Pain (acute, chronic)
- G. Rape-trauma syndrome
- H. Spiritual distress (distress of the human spirit)
- I. Tissue perfusion, altered

The word *triage* has its origin from the French, meaning "to pick, sort, select, or choose." The current use of triage in the emergency department is "to sort out" those in need of emergency services first.

The concept of medical triage evolved during battle, when Napoleon's surgeon developed a system that "sorted out" the wounded on the battlefield. The most critically injured were transported first. Florence Nightingale, using her now-famous lamp, went out during the night after battles during the Crimean War to "sort out" the remaining soldiers and offer them care.[3]

At the end of the nineteenth century, the English introduced casualty and clearing stations where injuries were identified and first aid initiated. Based on their injuries, patients were then sent to an appropriate place for further treatment.[2,5,6]

During World War II and the Korean War, primary triage of the injured occurred on the battlefield, with secondary triage occurring at the battalion station, and the final destination being a Mobile Army Surgical Hospital (MASH) unit.[2,8]

The introduction of helicopter transport of the injured from the battlefield during the Korean War helped to increase the speed that victims were triaged and transported for care. Many casualties could be removed at the same time. Triage was done before and after air evacuation.[9,10]

Civilian triage within hospitals formally began in the 1960s. Physicians initially did triage, but nurses quickly assumed primary triage responsibilities.[3,5,7]

The goals of triage include early patient assessment, brief overall assessment, determination of urgency need, documentation of findings during patient assessment, control of patient flow through the emergency department, assignment of patients to the appropriate care area, initiation of diagnostic measures, initiation of therapeutic interventions, infection control, promotion of good public relations, and health education for patients and families.[1] The goals and their implementation vary from emergency department to emergency department.

In the prehospital or field environment, the goals of triage are not much different. The nurse needs to be able to rapidly assess, identify, and intervene as indicated by the patient's condition. When multiple patients are involved, the transport nurse and other team members need to be able to recognize who is the emergent patient or patients and provide or assign the appropriate resources so that the patient is stabilized and transported quickly.

Of primary concern is safety, in both the prehospital and emergency department environments, before triage can occur. Surveying the scene and determining safety, whether it is at the site of the accident or at a referring facility, are the first steps in the triage process. Identifying a potentially unsafe situation or potentially violent patient is imperative to the safety of the nurse as well as emergency department staff and visitors.

Triage in the emergency department and in the prehospital care environment is based on both art and science. Experience, as well as the science of nursing and medicine, helps the emergency and flight nurse make assessment decisions. The *Journal of Emergency Nursing* contains a section entitled "Triage Decisions," which provides case studies about specific patient problems that may be seen in the emergency department. These can provide an excellent review for the nurse studying for the Certification in Emergency Nursing (CEN®) examination and the Certification in Flight Nursing (CFRN) examination. *Prehospital and Disaster Medicine* and *Air Medical Journal* offer case studies that help sharpen one's triage skills by learning from others' experiences.[10]

REVIEW QUESTIONS

Three patients come to the triage nurse at one time. The first patient is a 48-year-old man complaining of left-sided chest pain radiating down his left arm. He is awake, diaphoretic, and pale. The second patient is a 3-year-old boy who is drooling and pale and can breathe only while sitting straight up on his mother's lap. The third patient has sustained a laceration on his right hand. He currently has a dressing in place, and bright red blood is noted on the dressing. His vital signs are B/P 100/70 and P 100.

1. Which patient should be taken into the emergency department first?
   A. The patient with the chest pain
   B. The child who is drooling
   C. The patient with the laceration
   D. Any patient who is bleeding

2. The triage nurse suspects that the child may have an illness that can cause airway obstruction. What care should be provided in the triage area?
   A. Immediately remove the child from his mother and take him back to the treatment areas to prevent an airway emergency
   B. Take an oral temperature to determine if he has a fever and may require a dose of acetaminophen in the triage area
   C. Leave the child in his most comfortable position and take him as quickly as possible back to the patient care area
   D. Immediately start an intraosseous infusion to administer methylprednisolone and a normal saline bolus

3. The triage nurse should base the initial care of this child on which of the following nursing diagnoses?
   A. Self-care deficit, feeding, related to the patient not being able to swallow any liquids for several days
   B. Infection, high risk for, related to his exposure to the influenza virus and possibility of having epiglottitis
   C. Airway clearance, ineffective, related to the patient's inability to keep his airway clear
   D. Family processes, altered, related to the patient's inability to interact with his mother because he is ill

4. Focused triage documentation for a patient with potential airway problems (as in this case) should include documentation of:
   A. Insurance coverage and family physician
   B. The intravenous site and catheter size used
   C. Chest and lateral neck radiography results
   D. The patient's respiratory rate and effort

An 18-year-old man comes to the triage area complaining of upper body weakness, as well as numbness and tingling in both hands. The patient states that he was involved in a fight the previous night and that his head was shoved between his legs. The patient is alert and oriented. Vital signs are B/P 110/70, P 64, R 18, and Temp 99° F. His pupils are equal and reactive. He is unable to keep his arms extended for longer than 5 seconds, and he cannot make a fist.

5. The triage classification for this patient would be:
   A. Delayed care
   B. Emergent
   C. Urgent
   D. Nonurgent

6. The initial care provided by the triage nurse should include application of:
   A. Heat to the patient's neck
   B. Ice to the patient's neck
   C. A cervical collar for immobilization
   D. Elastic bandage wraps to the patient's hands

7. Of the following, which nursing diagnosis would be most appropriate for the care of this patient?
   A. Injury, high risk for, related to his spinal cord injury
   B. Fluid volume deficit, high risk for, related to his spinal cord injury
   C. Hyperthermia, related to his spinal cord injury
   D. Infection, high risk for, related to his spinal cord injury

8. Focused triage documentation for this patient (or any patient complaining of neurological trauma) should include documentation of:
   A. Adventitious breath sounds
   B. Peripheral and central pulses
   C. Paradoxical pulses
   D. Level of consciousness per GCS

A granddaughter brings her 83-year-old grandfather to the triage nurse. She states that he has said that he wants to kill himself. His wife died recently, and he is suffering from prostate cancer. The patient states that he has a living will and has the right to die. He is refusing to allow the triage nurse to assess him.

9. Which of the following would be an appropriate action for the triage nurse to take?
   A. Allow the patient to leave
   B. Ask the granddaughter to leave
   C. Explain to the patient why he must stay
   D. Have the patient arrested

10. All of the following would be emergent conditions except:
A. Obvious fractures without vascular compromise
B. Hemorrhage from a wound
C. Cardiopulmonary arrest
D. Respiratory distress

11. An infant with a heart rate of over 260 beats per minute with no peripheral pulses should be placed in which triage category?
A. Stable
B. Nonurgent
C. Urgent
D. Emergent

12. The goals of triage include all of the following except:
A. Control of patient flow through the emergency department
B. Assignment of patients to appropriate care areas within the emergency department
C. Performing and documenting a secondary survey on all patients who come for triage
D. Determination of the urgency of the patient's condition

The transport team has been called to the scene of a head-on motor vehicle crash. There are four victims involved. Victim 1 is a 2-year-old boy who has suffered a moderate head injury. His GCS is 12, but he is maintaining his airway. Victim 2 is an 18-year-old woman (probably the mother of the child). She has a GCS of 15, multiple orthopedic injuries, and severe abdominal pain. Her B/P is 90/40, P is 140, and R 32. Victim 3 is a 72-year-old man who is under full cardiopulmonary resuscitation. Finally, Victim 4 is a 70-year-old woman who has a GCS of 15. She is complaining of severe chest pain and shortness of breath. Her vital signs are B/P 80/50, P 120, and R 10. All victims were unrestrained. The helicopter can only transport one patient at a time. The closest facility is 40 miles from the scene of the accident.

13. Which victim should be transported first?
A. Victim 3
B. Victim 1
C. Victim 2
D. Victim 4

14. Which victim should be transported second?
A. Victim 3
B. Victim 1
C. Victim 2
D. Victim 4

15. Which patient should not be transported by helicopter?
A. Victim 3
B. Victim 1
C. Victim 2
D. Victim 4

16. Respirations that are becoming faster and deeper, followed by a period of apnea, is described as:
A. Kussmaul's breathing
B. Eupnea
C. Apneustic
D. Cheyne-Stokes respirations

17. Which of the following mnemonics may be used to determine and describe a patient's level of consciousness?
A. PQRST
B. AVPU
C. TIPPS
D. AEIOU

18. An example of objective patient data is:
A. History of diabetes mellitus
B. Complaint of pain in the left foot
C. Brief neurological examination
D. Precipitating event or onset of symptoms

19. Telephone triage:
A. Involves decision making under conditions of certainty of what is wrong with the patient based upon information gathered by talking with the patient
B. Provides unlimited sensory input from the patient's verbal descriptions of their signs and symptoms
C. Is an effective patient management tool and patients appear to be satisfied with it
D. Can be performed by any nurse who has practiced in an emergency department for a year

20. Components of an effective telephone triage protocol include all of the following except:
A. Clearly described and defined protocols addressing specific patient populations and the areas served

B. A policy that states that nurses may never use their judgment in decision making about a patient's condition
C. Experienced, educated nurses with education in telephone assessment and communication skills
D. A continuous quality improvement program that evaluates telephone triage decisions and patient outcomes

The following four patients are in the triage area at the same time. Patient 1 is a 2-week-old neonate carried in by his mother who states that the baby has a fever. The baby's skin is pink and he is sucking a bottle of formula. Patient 2 is a 25-year-old construction worker who has amputated the distal third of his left fifth finger. He has no other injuries but states it is very painful (7/10). Patient 3 is a 60-year-old man with chronic obstructive pulmonary disease (COPD) and increasing shortness of breath "since the weather became hot last week." He can speak in complete sentences but can take only 5 to 6 steps before stopping to rest. Patient 4 is an 80-year-old man complaining that he hasn't had a bowel movement for 3 days.

21. Which patient should the triage nurse assess first?
A. The 2-week-old infant with history of a fever
B. The 25-year-old construction worker with the fingertip amputation
C. The 60-year-old patient with COPD who is experiencing increasing dyspnea
D. The 80-year-old man with constipation

22. What additional information is the *most important* to obtain regarding the infant?
A. Temperature, blood pressure, weight, last bowel movement
B. Temperature, fluid intake and output, respiratory status
C. Complete vital signs, weight, pulse oximetry
D. Current medications, allergies, immunizations

23. The infant's axillary temperature is 39° C (102.2° F). You should:
A. Give him a weight-based dose of acetaminophen and recheck him in 30 minutes
B. Give him a weight-based dose of ibuprofen and recheck him in 30 minutes
C. Take him to the treatment area for further nursing and medical evaluation
D. Take him to the treatment area and insert an intraosseous needle

24. The patient with COPD probably can wait in the waiting room if he states which of the following?
A. "I'm feeling a little lightheaded."
B. "My oxygen tank ran out last night."
C. "The hot weather bothers me; air conditioning helps me breathe."
D. "I have to stop and rest when I get chest pain."

25. In the triage area, what should you do with the construction worker's amputated fingertip?
A. Pack it in ice and label the container with his name and put in the refrigerator
B. Nothing, it probably will not be replanted anyway because it is a construction accident
C. Wrap the piece in moist gauze, place in a plastic bag, and place the bag on ice
D. Wrap the fingertip in dry gauze, place it in a plastic bag, and place on dry ice

26. Which mnemonic is helpful in assessing a patient's pain?
A. PQRST
B. AVPU
C. TIPPS
D. AEIOU

27. Which of the following nursing diagnoses is the highest priority?
A. Ineffective airway clearance
B. Ineffective breathing pattern
C. Impaired gas exchange
D. High risk for infection

28. A man runs into the triage area and yells "my wife is having a baby." The triage nurse should:
A. Take gloves, the precipitous delivery kit, call for help, and evaluate the patient while she is in the car
B. Ask the husband to bring the wife to the triage area by wheelchair, because the triage nurse is not allowed to leave the designated area
C. Send an attendant to bring the patient to the triage area by wheelchair, because the triage

nurse is not allowed to leave the designated area

D. Call a labor and delivery room nurse to come down to the emergency department to evaluate the patient while she is still in the car

29. Which of the following would indicate that the baby should be delivered in the emergency department?

A. This is her first delivery and her water had just broken
B. The patient yells, "I have to push."
C. The baby's head is visible at the introitus between contractions
D. You can see the infant's hand protruding from the introitus

30. In a mass casualty situation with 100 patients, a patient in cardiac arrest is categorized as:

A. Immediate
B. Delayed
C. Urgent
D. Expectant

31. When answering telephone advice calls, the emergency nurse should always:

A. Offer the patient the option of coming to the emergency department
B. Provide recommendations for over-the-counter medications
C. Ask the patient what treatments have already been tried
D. Use institutional telephone protocols with modifications as necessary

32. Subjective data include all the following except:

A. "I'm having chest pain."
B. Skin warm, pink, and dry
C. States pain started last night
D. Denies nausea, vomiting, or dyspnea

33. The triage nurse plays an important role in:

A. Customer service for the emergency department
B. Ensuring that the sickest patients are seen first
C. Performing patient assessment in the triage area
D. All of the above

34. Which of the following patients should be taken to the treatment area first?

A. A 2-year-old child with croupy cough; her skin is pink, warm, and dry; she is alert, with moist mucosa
B. A 2-year-old child with vomiting and diarrhea; skin pink, warm, and dry; she is lethargic, with dry mucosa
C. A 2-year-old child with active bleeding from a 4-centimeter scalp laceration; she is alert and afraid of the triage nurse
D. A 2-year-old child with a right forearm deformity after falling off of a swing; there are no other injuries and she is alert and complaining of arm pain

35. When triaging a patient with chest pain, it is important to remember that some patients do not complain of the classic signs and symptoms of a myocardial infarction. Which of these patients is likely to have atypical symptoms?

A. A 41-year-old female
B. A 55-year-old male with diabetes
C. An 81-year-old man
D. All of the above patients

36. A patient with lung cancer comes to the emergency department with a fever of 38.5° C (101° F) and no specific complaints. The triage nurse should:

A. Administer acetaminophen per protocol and notify the patient's oncologist
B. Take a complete set of vital signs and have the patient wait in the waiting room if no other abnormalities are found
C. Notify the charge nurse that the patient is urgent and needs to be placed in the treatment area for further assessment and care as soon as possible
D. Instruct the patient that he should go to his physician's office as soon as possible

37. A patient with a significant psychiatric history arrives in the triage area stating that he wishes to "kill myself and anyone who tries to stop me!" Which of the following is associated with an increased risk of harm to others?

A. Previous suicide attempts by overdose
B. History of violent behaviors
C. Poor eye contact and disheveled appearance
D. Excessively neat and fastidious appearance

38. Which 41-year-old female patient whose chief complaint is a headache should be seen first?

A. "It's the worst headache of my life. It came on suddenly, like I was hit in the head with a bat."

B. "My headache has gradually gotten severe over the last day. I've had a cold for about a week."

C. "It feels like my usual migraine, but it's not responding to the medications that my doctor gave to me to take."

D. "It feels like a tight band around my head. I've been under a lot of stress at work lately and my husband was just laid off from his job."

39. Which clinical picture of back pain would be considered urgent?

A. A 26-year-old female with a history of chronic back pain, worse today with spasms and pain radiating down her left leg

B. A 76-year-old male with no known history of trauma who describes his back pain as "knife-like" and in the midsection of his back

C. A 40-year-old male with severe right-sided back pain radiating down his groin; he also complains of nausea and urinary frequency

D. A 50-year-old female who complains of low back pain after having moved furniture all weekend with her friends

40. A 19-year-old college student is brought by his friends to the emergency department. His friends state that he has not been "feeling well" and today developed a fever. They also noticed that he has a red rash all over his body. Which of the following rashes are indicative of a potentially life-threatening infection?

A. Vesicles on his trunk, arms, and legs

B. Pruritic maculopapular rash all over his body

C. Petechiae on his trunk and arms and legs

D. Target lesions on his legs and groin

ANSWERS

1. **B. Assessment.** Based on rapid patient assessment using both basic and advanced life support principles (airway, breathing, circulation, neurological deficit, exposure [ABCDE], and history), the patient having airway difficulties should be taken into the emergency department first. A child who is drooling and is able to breathe comfortably only while sitting straight up may have epiglottitis and is at great risk of complete obstruction of his airway.[1-3]
2. **C. Intervention.** Because the child is currently able to comfortably maintain his airway, the triage nurse should leave the child in the position in which he is most comfortable. By removing him from his mother or performing any unnecessary procedures, the nurse may cause the child to become agitated and his airway to become obstructed.[1-3]
3. **C. Analysis.** Because the patient is having airway difficulties, airway clearance, ineffective, should be the initial nursing diagnosis on which the emergency nurse bases care. Defining characteristics of this nursing diagnosis include abnormal breath sounds, cyanosis, tachypnea, and dyspnea.
4. **D. Evaluation.** The patient's respiratory rate is an important piece of information for the patient who is having respiratory difficulties and should be documented on the triage record. One of the responsibilities of the triage nurse is to sort patients and determine the need for emergency services. The patient's vital signs provide the emergency nurse with observed information about the patient's cardiopulmonary status.[2]
5. **B. Assessment.** Based on rapid patient assessment using ABCDE, this patient's condition would be considered emergent. He has signs and symptoms of a neurological deficit that could place him at risk for additional complications related to injury of the cervical spine.[7,9]
6. **C. Intervention.** One of the goals of triage is the initiation of therapeutic interventions. Because this patient may have suffered a cervical spine injury, initial care should include immobilization of the cervical spine.[1,3]
7. **A. Analysis.** The initial assessment of the patient demonstrates that he is currently in no acute distress but, because of his mechanism of injury and symptoms, is at great risk for additional injury. Defining characteristics of this nursing diagnosis are divided into host factors such as sensory or motor deficits, tissue hypoxia, and cognitive impairment, agent factors such as chemical and mechanical energy, and environmental factors such as unsafe design, unsafe mode of transportation, and presence of pollutants.
8. **D. Evaluation.** Documentation of a neurological examination includes the level of con-

sciousness, pupillary response, motor response, sensory response, and vital signs.

9. **C. Intervention.** The triage nurse should first try to explain to the patient that a living will does not allow the patient to deliberately harm himself. Rather, the living will allows the patient to decide whether or not medical or nursing care should be given if the patient is dying from natural causes. The emergency department is obligated to treat the patient.[10,11]
10. **A. Assessment.** One method of triage classification is the use of specific patient designations: emergent, urgent, and nonurgent. Emergent patients include those with cardiopulmonary arrest, chest pain indicative of a myocardial infarction, respiratory distress, severe trauma, and attempted suicide. Urgent patients include those with obvious fractures with vascular compromise, abdominal pain of less than 36 hours' duration, sudden headaches, vomiting, and jaundice. Nonurgent patients include those with sprains, minor burns, and closed fractures.[7,9]
11. **D. Assessment.** The normal infant's heart rate will range from 120 to 160 (newborn to 1 year of age). A heart rate without peripheral perfusion would indicate compromise in the child's circulation, making the situation emergent.[1,2]
12. **C. Intervention.** Performing and documenting a secondary survey on all patients who come to triage is an unrealistic goal. The primary goal of triage is to recognize the ill or injured patient who requires treatment in a timely manner. Triage areas generally are not set up to perform an adequate secondary assessment.[7,9]
13. **D. Assessment.** Based on ABCs, the elderly patient having shortness of breath and a decreased respiratory rate should be transported first. The child has a lower GCS, but he is maintaining his airway.
14. **B. Assessment.** Even though the child is maintaining his airway, he has the potential to deteriorate because he has a moderate head injury and a GCS of 12. Based on the length of time and distance to a receiving facility, the child may be at greater risk of additional injury.[9]
15. **A. Assessment.** Patients who suffer a traumatic arrest have less than a 1% chance of survival, which would justify the transport team's decision not to transport the patient under full CPR.[10]
16. **D. Assessment.** Cheyne-Stokes respirations gradually become faster and deeper, then slower, followed by periods of apnea. Apneustic breathing is prolonged, gasping inspiration followed by short expiration. Eupnea is a description of normal respiratory rate and rhythm.[12,13] Kussmaul's breathing is characterized by abnormally deep, very rapid sighing respirations.
17. **B. Assessment.** Many mnemonics exist that may be used in patient assessment. One that can be used to determine and describe a patient's level of consciousness is AVPU.
    - A: alert
    - V: responds to voice
    - P: responds to painful stimuli
    - U: unresponsive

    PQRST is a mnemonic that can be used to obtain information about patient history, and TIPPS and AEIOU provide descriptions of causes that may alter a patient's level of consciousness.[14]
18. **C. Assessment.** Objective data includes airway, breathing, circulation, and a brief neurological examination.[14]
19. **C. Intervention.** Telephone triage can be an effective patient management tool, and patients have expressed satisfaction with the process, especially when it has kept them from unnecessary trips to the emergency department. However, patient assessment is limited, and only experienced, skilled nurses who have received specific training related to telephone triage should perform it.[15,16]
20. **B. Intervention.** Telephone triage policies, procedures, and protocols must allow for the exercise of nursing judgment when making decisions about the disposition of the patient. Protocols should serve only as guidelines and should never be inflexible.[15,16]
21. **A. Intervention.** The 2-week-old infant with a history of a fever. Infants less than 3 months old with a temperature of 38° C (101° F) or greater are at risk for sepsis. Infants are more difficult to assess than older children and adults and may decompensate more quickly.[2] The patient with COPD is pink and able to speak in full sentences.
22. **B. Assessment.** Temperature, fluid intake and output, and respiratory status. These are all essential components of any pediatric assessment. Blood pressure is not usually helpful in infants, because it generally remains within normal limits until 25% of the baby's circulating volume is lost. Weight, last bowel movement, medications, and immunizations should

all be ascertained at some point in the patient assessment but will not significantly contribute to the triage decision.[2]

23. **C. Intervention.** Take the patient to the treatment area for further medical and nursing evaluation. Generally, a physician should be consulted before medications are given to an infant.[2]
24. **C. Assessment.** The patient who is lightheaded or has chest pain and the patient who has been without oxygen for several hours may all be at risk for cardiovascular and pulmonary compromise.
25. **C. Intervention.** Wrap the part in moist gauze, place it in a plastic bag, and place the bag on ice. The amputated part must be kept moist and cool but protected from freezing.[17]
26. **A. Assessment.** PQRST. The mnemonic commonly is used to assess pain; the letters stand for provoking or palliating factors, quality, radiation, severity (0 to 10 scale), and time (onset, duration, constant). AVPU is used to assess level of consciousness. AEIOU and TIPPS are mnemonics used to discover possible causes of altered mental status.
27. **A. Analysis.** Ineffective airway clearance. Airway is always the highest priority.[2,18,19]
28. **A. Intervention.** Immediately take gloves and the precipitous delivery kit to the car and assess the patient.[20]
29. **C. Assessment.** The baby's head is at the introitus between contractions. The bag of water may have broken hours before delivery, especially in a primiparous patient. A hand presentation indicates a complicated birth that requires the immediate expertise of obstetric personnel. Visibility of the head between contractions indicates that birth is imminent.[20]
30. **D. Analysis.** Patients in this category are not expected to survive without almost immediate critical care. In a mass-casualty situation, the resources needed to attempt cardiopulmonary resuscitation are better utilized in patients with conditions more amenable to treatment.[21]
31. **A. Intervention.** Offer the patient the option of coming to the emergency department. Telephone triage can be very risky. Any treatment recommendations offered over the telephone should be guided by institutional protocols.[22]
32. **B. Assessment.** *S*ubjective data is something that is *s*aid and *o*bjective data is what you *o*bserve or can measure.
33. **D. Intervention.** All are important functions of the triage nurse.[23]
34. **B. Assessment and Intervention.** A 2-year-old child with vomiting, diarrhea, lethargy, and dry mucous membranes has indications of serious dehydration.[2] None of the other children displays any evidence of a life-threatening problem. Direct pressure to the child's wound should be applied to control the bleeding.
35. **D. Assessment.** Women, the elderly, and patients with diabetes or hypertension may experience and come to the emergency department with atypical symptoms of a myocardial infarction.[18]
36. **C. Intervention.** Notify the charge nurse that the patient needs to come to the treatment area as soon as possible for further assessment and care. A patient with cancer is at great risk of being immunocompromised and at risk for developing sepsis.[23]
37. **B. Assessment.** A history of violent behaviors. Violence is difficult to predict. A history of violence should alert the triage nurse that this is a high-risk patient.[24]
38. **A. Assessment.** Phrases like "worst headache of my life" and "started suddenly like I was hit in the head with a bat" often are associated with intracranial bleeding.[25]
39. **B. Assessment.** Older patients with no known history of trauma and knifelike back pain should be evaluated on an urgent basis. One of the differential diagnoses may be an aortic or thoracic aneurysm. The pain of an aneurysm is many times described as knifelike, tearing, or a ripping sensation.[26]
40. **C. Assessment.** Petechiae on the extremities and trunk often are associated with meningococcemia, which is related to life-threatening meningitis and sepsis. Young children and college students are commonly affected. A vesicular rash is more consistent with the chicken pox, a widespread pruritic maculopapular rash is often an allergic reaction, and target lesions often are associated with Lyme disease.[27]

References

1. Bracken J: Triage. In Newberry L, editor: *Sheehy's emergency nursing: principles and practice,* ed 5, St Louis, 2003, Mosby.
2. Emergency Nurses Association: *Emergency nursing pediatric core course,* Des Plaines, IL, 2004, Emergency Nurses Association.

3. Thomas DO, Bernardo LM, Herman B: *Core curriculum for pediatric emergency nursing,* Boston, 2003, Jones and Bartlett.
4. Emergency Nurses Association: *Approaching diversity: an interactive journey,* Park Ridge, IL, 1998, Emergency Nurses Association.
5. Gilboy N, Travers D, Wuerz R: Re-evaluating triage in the new millennium: a comprehensive look at the need for standardization and quality, *J Emerg Nurs* 25(6):468-473, 1999.
6. Gilboy N, Tanabe P, Travers D et al: *The emergency severity index: implementation handbook*, Des Plaines, IL, 2003, Emergency Nurses Association.
7. Champion H: Prehospital triage. In *Trauma care systems,* Rockville, MD, 1986, Aspen Publications.
8. Air and Surface Transport Nurses Association: *Transport nurse advanced trauma course,* Denver, 2002, Air and Surface Transport Nurses Association.
9. Rund DA, Rausch TS: *Triage,* St Louis, 1981, Mosby.
10. Semonin Holleran R: *Prehospital nursing: a collaborative approach,* St Louis, 1994, Mosby.
11. Ramler CL, Mohammed N: Triage. In Kitt S, Selfridge-Thomas J, Proehl J et al, editors: *Emergency nursing: a physiologic and clinical perspective,* Philadelphia, 1995, WB Saunders.
12. Southard P: Legal and legislative considerations in emergency practice. In Kitt S, Selfridge-Thomas J, Proehl J et al, editors: *Emergency nursing: a physiologic and clinical perspective,* Philadelphia, 1995, WB Saunders.
13. Sedlak K: Patient assessment. In Newberry L, editor: *Sheehy's emergency nursing: principles and practice,* ed 5, St Louis, 2003, Mosby.
14. Twedell D: Nursing process: assessment and priority setting. In Jordan K, editor: *Emergency nursing core curriculum,* ed 5, Philadelphia, 2000, WB Saunders.
15. Rutenberg CD: What do we really know about telephone triage? *J Emerg Nurs* 26(1):76-78, 2000.
16. Emergency Nurses Association: *Telephone triage advice,* Des Plaines, IL, 1998, Emergency Nurses Association.
17. Proehl JA: Wound care for amputations. In Proehl JA, editor: *Emergency nursing procedures,* ed 3, St Louis, 2004, WB Saunders.
18. American Heart Association & International Liaison Committee on Resuscitation: Guidelines 2000 for cardiopulmonary resuscitation and emergency cardiovascular care: international consensus on science, *Circulation* 102(suppl):2196-2210, 2000.
19. Emergency Nurses Association: *Trauma nursing core course provider manual,* ed 5, Des Plaines, IL, 2000, Emergency Nurses Association.
20. Rossoll LR: Emergency childbirth. In Proehl J, editor: *Emergency nursing procedures,* ed 3, St Louis, 2004, WB Saunders.
21. Connor GC, Boulais LJ, editors: *Emergency nursing secrets,* Philadelphia, 2001, Hanley & Belfus.
22. Zimmerman PG, Rhodes LS: Professionalism and leadership. In Jordan KS, editor: *Emergency nursing core curriculum,* ed 5, Philadelphia, 2000, WB Saunders.
23. Zimmerman PG: Triage. In Oman KS, Koziol-McLain J, Scheetz LJ, editors: *Emergency nursing secrets,* Philadelphia, 2001, Hanley & Belfus.
24. Shawler C: Behavioral conditions. In Kidd PS, Sturt PA, Fultz J, editors: *Emergency nursing reference,* ed 2, St Louis, 2000, Mosby.
25. Snyder JA: Neurological emergencies. In Jordan KS, editor: *Emergency nursing core curriculum,* ed 5, Philadelphia, 2000, WB Saunders.
26. Doherty KA: Cardiovascular emergencies. In Jordan KS, editor: *Emergency nursing core curriculum,* ed 5, Philadelphia, 2000, WB Saunders.
27. Kidd PS: Communicable diseases. In Kidd PS, Sturt PA, Fultz J, editors: *Mosby's emergency nursing reference,* ed 2, St Louis, 2000, Mosby.

CHAPTER 3

ABDOMINAL EMERGENCIES

REVIEW OUTLINE

I. Anatomy and physiology
   A. Right upper quadrant
      1. Liver
      2. Gallbladder
      3. Pylorus
      4. Duodenum
      5. Head of the pancreas
      6. Portion of the right kidney and adrenal gland
      7. Hepatic flexure of the colon
      8. Section of the ascending and transverse colon
   B. Left upper quadrant
      1. Left lobe of the liver
      2. Stomach
      3. Spleen
      4. Body of the pancreas
      5. Portion of the left kidney and adrenal gland
      6. Splenic flexure of the colon
      7. Sections of the transverse and descending colons
   C. Right lower quadrant
      1. Appendix
      2. Cecum
      3. Lower pole of right kidney
      4. Right ureter
      5. Right ovary
      6. Right spermatic cord
   D. Left lower quadrant
      1. Sigmoid colon
      2. Section of the descending colon
      3. Lower pole of the left kidney
      4. Left ureter
      5. Left ovary
      6. Left spermatic cord
   E. Midabdomen and upper chest
      1. Oral cavity
      2. Tongue
      3. Pharynx
      4. Epiglottis
      5. Trachea
      6. Esophagus
      7. Bladder urinary
   F. Abdominal vessels
      1. Mesentery
      2. Descending abdominal aorta
      3. Inferior vena cava
      4. Iliac artery
      5. Renal artery
   G. Physiology
      1. Digestion
      2. Absorption
      3. Elimination
      4. Bile production and excretion
      5. Liver functions
      6. Insulin production and use
      7. Red and white blood cell production and destruction

II. Abdominal assessment
   A. History
      1. Pain
         a. Location
         b. Quality
         c. Severity
         d. Radiation
         e. Temporal
         f. Provocation or relief
      2. Nausea and vomiting
         a. Onset
         b. Frequency
         c. Duration
         d. Amount
         e. Color, consistency
      3. Other associated symptoms
         a. Bleeding or bruising
         b. Change in bowel habits
         c. Change in appetite
         d. Recent weight gain or loss
         e. Fever, chills
      4. Mechanism of injury
         a. Blunt
         b. Penetrating

5. Pertinent medical history
   a. Current or chronic diseases
   b. Past surgeries
   c. Current medications
      (1) Prescribed
      (2) Over-the-counter
      (3) Illicit drug use
   d. Allergies
   e. Alcohol use
   f. Recent travel: domestic, international

B. Physical examination
   1. General
      a. Position of comfort
      b. Facial expression
   2. Vital signs: postural vital signs
   3. Inspection
      a. Skin
         (1) Color
         (2) Lesions
         (3) Edema
         (4) Superficial vascularity
         (5) Open areas
      b. Contour
         (1) Symmetry
         (2) Abdominal girth measurement
         (3) Protuberance (the six Fs [fat, flatus, fetus, feces, fluid, fatal growth])
      c. Movement
         (1) Abdominal breathing
         (2) Visible peristalsis
         (3) Visible aortic pulsations (normal)
      d. Signs of abdominal trauma or illness
         (1) Cullen's sign
         (2) Grey Turner's sign
         (3) Coopernail's sign
   4. Auscultation
      a. Bowel sounds
         (1) Location
         (2) Present
         (3) Absent
      b. Bruits
      c. Venous hum
      d. Friction rub
   5. Palpation
      a. Light
      b. Deep
      c. Tenderness
      d. Guarding
      e. Rigidity
      f. Rebound tenderness
      g. Masses
      h. McBurney's point
      i. Rovsing's sign
      j. Murphy's sign
   6. Percussion
      a. Dullness or resonance
      b. Liver size
      c. Borders of any masses
      d. Fundus of urinary bladder
      e. Costovertebral angle tenderness
      f. Ballance's sign

C. Diagnostic studies and procedures
   1. Complete blood count with differential
   2. Electrolytes, blood urea nitrogen, whole blood glucose, creatinine
   3. Amylase and lipase
   4. β-human chorionic gonadotropin: blood, urine
   5. Liver function tests: aspartate amino transaminase; alanine aminotransferase, lactate dehydrogenase (LDH), alkaline phosphatase
   6. Coagulation studies
   7. Type and screen or crossmatch
   8. Blood for *Helicobacter pylori*
   9. Sickle cell screen
   10. Urinalysis
   11. Urine culture
   12. Stool for ova, parasites, occult blood, leukocytes, mucus, and protein; enzyme-linked immunosorbent assay of stool
   13. Test (guaiac) for presence of blood in feces, emesis, gastric drainage
   14. Upright chest radiograph
   15. Upright, left lateral decubitus, flat abdominal radiographic films
   16. Contrast studies
   17. Scanning: computed tomography (CT) with contrast, magnetic resonance imaging (MRI)
   18. Ultrasonography
   19. Gastroscopy, endoscopy, sigmoidoscopy
   20. Peritoneal lavage
   21. Local wound exploration

III. Related nursing diagnoses
   A. Altered nutrition: intake less than body requirements
   B. Constipation
   C. Colonic constipation
   D. Diarrhea

E. Infection: potential for
F. Altered gastrointestinal (GI) tissue perfusion
G. Fluid volume deficit
H. Tissue perfusion: altered: GI, renal
I. High risk for fluid volume deficit
J. Impaired physical mobility
K. Altered health maintenance
L. Knowledge deficit
M. Pain
N. Chronic pain

IV. Collaborative care of the patient with an abdominal emergency
A. Ongoing abdominal assessments
B. Oxygen therapy
C. Monitoring
1. Vital signs
2. Cardiac monitoring
3. Intake and output
D. Intravenous fluids
E. Blood administration
F. Gastric decompression
G. Identification and control of bleeding
1. Saline lavage
2. Balloon tamponade
H. Autotransfusion
1. Mechanical autotransfuser
2. Pneumatic antishock garment (controversial) (PAGS)
I. FAST (focused abdominal sonography for trauma) examination
J. Peritoneal lavage
K. Urinary catheter
L. Pharmacological intervention
1. Analgesics
2. Antibiotics
3. Antiemetics
4. Antispasmodics, anticholinergics
5. Histamine receptor antagonists
6. Antacids
7. Vasopressors
M. Emotional or psychological support
N. Patient and family teaching

V. Specific abdominal emergencies
A. Diarrhea
B. Inflammatory conditions
1. Gastritis
2. Gastroenteritis
3. Appendicitis
4. Pancreatitis
5. Cholecystitis
6. Diverticulitis
7. Hepatitis
8. Irritable bowel syndrome
C. Intestinal obstruction
D. Intussusception
E. GI bleeding
1. Upper GI bleeding
2. Lower GI bleeding
F. Gastroesophageal reflux disorder
G. Abdominal aortic aneurysm
H. Mesenteric ischemia
I. Abdominal trauma
1. Penetrating
a. Gunshot wounds
b. Stab wounds
c. Shrapnel wounds
2. Blunt
a. Organ contusion
b. Organ laceration
c. Organ rupture
3. Insertion of foreign bodies

Abdominal pain or discomfort is one of the most common complaints expressed by patients who come to the emergency department for care.[1] Abdominal pain may be the manifestation of an acute process or a chronic, long-standing problem. Pain may arise from one of many systems located in the abdomen. The GI, genitourinary, and reproductive systems occupy most of the organ space in the abdominal cavity. In addition, the vascular and musculoskeletal systems may be involved, especially when bleeding or inflammation is present. Likewise, trauma to the abdomen may involve multiple systems. The abdominal cavity is large and located anteriorly, making it more susceptible to both blunt and penetrating injury. As the diaphragm rises with expiration, the abdominal cavity size increases, and injury to its contents may occur with a lower chest injury. Blunt trauma results in a force being diffused throughout the abdomen. Penetrating injury is caused by any object that penetrates the abdominal wall. Usually a bullet, knife, or some type of missile injures anything in its path.[2] When solid organs of the abdomen, such as the liver, spleen, and kidneys, are injured, significant bleeding results. When hollow organs, such as the stomach and intestines, are damaged, their contents spill, causing massive irritation and infection.

Abdominal pain may be classified according to type. These include visceral, parietal, and referred abdominal pain caused by metabolic disease, and neurogenic and psychogenic pain. Visceral pain, so named because the stretching of a hollow viscus causes it, is characterized by diffuse, crampy pain varying in intensity. Many inflammatory conditions, such as appendicitis, cholecystitis, pancreatitis, and intestinal obstruction, become apparent with the onset of visceral pain. The second type, somatic or parietal pain, is a result of bacterial or chemical irritation of nerve fibers. This type of pain is sharp and localized. The patient suffering from somatic pain characteristically assumes the fetal position, either on the side or supine with knees flexed, attempting to prevent any movement that will result in increased pain. The third type of abdominal pain, referred pain, is felt some distance from the source.[1,3] A classic example of referred pain is seen in renal colic, when the pain is located in the groin and external genitalia. Metabolic diseases, such as porphyria and lead poisoning, cause abdominal pain because they irritate the alimentary tract. Neurogenic abdominal pain results from an irritation of the nerves in the abdomen. The source of the pain can be the spinal cord or caused by diseases such as diabetes. Finally, patients may suffer from abdominal pain when there is no organic dysfunction. Life stresses can contribute to intestinal spasms and hypersecretion of stomach acids.[4] Research has demonstrated that abdominal pain related to diseases such as peptic ulcer disease may actually be caused by an infection rather than excessive acid secretion. *H. pylori* has been implicated in over 80% of peptic ulcer disease cases.[4]

Diarrhea, a common symptom associated with abdominal pain and discomfort, has emerged as a potentially serious health care problem. Diarrhea from person-to-person contact (rotavirus) and from food-borne transmission causes many patients to visit the emergency department each year. Diarrhea can result from antibiotic use, travel, sexual transmission, and contact during daycare. Depending on the age of the patient and the type of diarrhea, severe and even lethal complications can occur.[5]

Initial nursing care of the patient with an abdominal emergency is based on subjective and objective assessments. When evaluating the patient, the emergency nurse needs to keep in mind what may be the source of the patient's pain by the location (e.g., the right upper quadrant). A general overview of the patient, including the position he or she assumes, facial expression, and skin color, temperature, and moisture, may give an indication as to the type and severity of pain. Vital signs give important baseline information.

A subjective assessment or history using the PQRST mnemonic (provocation, quality, radiation, severity, and timing) is a useful tool in evaluating the patient with an abdominal complaint. It is useful to have the patient point with one finger to where the pain or discomfort is located. If the problem cannot be localized, it offers some additional assessment information about the nature of the patient's complaint. Associated signs and symptoms such as nausea, vomiting, fever, or chills will assist in determining which system or systems need further evaluation.

Abdominal trauma needs to be recognized quickly. In a patient with multiple-system injury, abdominal trauma should be assumed until ruled out.

General management of the patient with an abdominal emergency is guided by evaluation of the ABCs (airway, breathing, circulation) during the initial assessment.

Intravenous access for fluid resuscitation, laboratory studies, and medication administration may be indicated. For the multiply injured patient, a FAST examination should be performed quickly after arrival in the emergency department.

Abdominal CT with contrast and ultrasonography have become a foundation for the evaluation of abdominal trauma. Fewer patients are being treated in the operating room and are instead being managed by close observation and initiation of critical interventions, as indicated by the patient's injury and condition.[6]

Gastric decompression and bladder catheterization are frequent interventions. Pain management should be addressed early in the care of the patient with an abdominal emergency. Many abdominal illnesses and injuries cause great pain and discomfort, as well as make diagnosis difficult.

The care of the patient with an abdominal emergency requires a rapid and focused care plan. In addition, follow-up information and education are important components when caring for a patient with an abdominal emergency.

REVIEW QUESTIONS

1. The correct sequence for performing a physical assessment of the abdomen is:
   A. Inspection, palpation, auscultation, percussion
   B. Inspection, auscultation, palpation, percussion
   C. Inspection, percussion, palpation, auscultation
   D. Palpation, auscultation, inspection, percussion

2. When palpating a painful abdomen, the emergency nurse should do which of the following?
   A. Begin by palpating nonpainful areas first, then proceed to the painful areas
   B. Begin with deep palpation first, then move to lighter palpation
   C. Cover the patient's face when palpating the abdomen to decrease embarrassment
   D. Never palpate the abdomen without the physician's permission

3. When assessing the abdomen, the emergency nurse remembers that:
   A. Deep palpation should never be used by any health care provider
   B. Deep palpation should be performed if splenomegaly is present
   C. Normally, one should not be able to palpate the spleen
   D. Normally, one should not be able to palpate the liver

4. When listening for bowel sounds, the emergency nurse should remember that:
   A. Adequate assessment of bowel sounds takes 5 minutes
   B. Absent bowel sounds always indicate a bowel obstruction
   C. Audible bowel sounds automatically rule out any GI obstruction
   D. It is normal to hear bowel sounds in the thoracic cavity

5. If rebound tenderness is found when assessing the abdomen, the emergency nurse knows that:
   A. It is frequently a sign of a malignancy
   B. It is normal to have abdominal rebound tenderness
   C. Rebound tenderness is a sign of peritoneal irritation
   D. Rebound tenderness occurs only when the patient is nauseated

6. Which of the following statements is true of abdominal pain?
   A. Abdominal pain location accurately reflects the patient's illness or injury
   B. Individual and cultural variations should be considered when evaluating abdominal pain
   C. A patient with abdominal pain should never receive narcotics until a diagnosis is made
   D. Elderly patients will always have pain when they have an abdominal emergency

7. The diagnostic evaluation of a woman of childbearing age with abdominal pain must include:
   A. Postural vital signs
   B. Liver function studies
   C. Pregnancy test
   D. Pap smear

8. All abdominal pain, no matter how minor, is considered to be an emergency:
   A. In the elderly
   B. In women of childbearing age
   C. Until it is relieved
   D. Until it is diagnosed

Gastritis

9. Factors that may provoke the symptoms of gastritis include all of the following except:
   A. Smoking tobacco
   B. Taking a nonsteroidal antiinflammatory drug (NSAID)
   C. A parent with gastritis
   D. Meditation and exercise

10. The most common cause of superficial gastritis is:
    A. Occasional ingestion of alcohol
    B. Inflammation caused by *H. pylori*
    C. Response to a stressful job or life change
    D. Short-term use of an NSAID for pain

11. The primary management of superficial gastritis is:
    A. Taking an over-the-counter antacid
    B. Taking only oral antibiotics
    C. Changing one's eating habits
    D. Taking a proton pump inhibitor

Bowel Obstruction

12. The four hallmark signs of a bowel obstruction are:
    A. Absent bowel sounds, nausea, vomiting, and cramping
    B. Abdominal pain, abdominal distention, vomiting, and constipation
    C. Hyperactive bowel sounds, distention, fever, and vomiting stool
    D. Anorexia, normal bowel sounds, vomiting, and cramping

13. All of the following interventions are therapeutic for a patient with a bowel obstruction except:
A. No food or drink by mouth
B. Gastric tube to low suction
C. Enemas until bowel is clear
D. Intravenous fluids for rehydration

Gastroenteritis

14. Acute gastroenteritis is considered more serious in what patient population?
A. Athletes in training
B. Infants and young children
C. Middle-aged men and women
D. Women during the postpartum period

15. With the persistent vomiting and diarrhea that accompanies acute gastroenteritis, the patient is a candidate for which nursing diagnosis?
A. Injury, potential for
B. Ineffective airway clearance
C. Fluid volume deficit
D. Impaired skin integrity

16. Discharge teaching instructions to a patient who has been treated for gastroenteritis should include all of the following except:
A. Do not eat or drink anything for 72 hours after being diagnosed in the emergency department
B. Wash hands, dishes, and eating utensils thoroughly before eating
C. Drink an electrolyte replacement solution (e.g., Gatorade, Pedialyte) for the next 24 hours, then advance to regular diet as tolerated
D. Throw out any foods that you think may be contaminated or spoiled and may have contributed to the development of the gastroenteritis

17. The most common cause of diarrhea in young children is:
A. Salmonella
B. Cryptosporidium
C. Adenovirus
D. Rotavirus

18. A 3-year-old child is brought to the emergency department by his caregiver because of continued abdominal pain and watery diarrhea. When obtaining a history related to his present illness, an important risk factor to identify would be:
A. Current diet the child has been on
B. Recent use of antibiotics
C. Time spent at a daycare center
D. All of the above

19. A clinical sign that would indicate that the child is suffering severe dehydration is:
A. Sunken eyeballs
B. Absence of urinary output
C. Slightly increased heart rate
D. Slightly increased respiratory rate

20. The child who is mildly dehydrated should initially be treated with:
A. A fluid bolus of 20 ml/kg of D5W over 20 minutes
B. A balanced electrolyte solution by mouth
C. A fluid bolus of 20 ml/kg of crystalloid solution
D. No fluids until the source of the dehydration is identified

Intussusception

A young mother brings her 18-month-old child to the emergency department. She states that he began crying and drawing his legs up. Since then he has vomited twice, and after that he had one small stool that looked like "red jelly." She also states she "felt a lump in his stomach where he hurts."

21. Based on the above information and these symptoms, you suspect:
A. Child maltreatment
B. Foreign body aspiration
C. Intussusception
D. Mesenteric injury

22. The child is taken to radiology for a hydrostatic barium enema to attempt reduction. The emergency nurse knows that:
A. A barium enema is contraindicated in children no matter what the initial clinical findings are
B. A barium enema is diagnostic for intussusception and may even reduce it and eliminate the need for surgery
C. Soapsuds enemas until clear will be required before this test can be initiated

D. A barium enema will cause intestinal perforation and contribute to the child developing peritonitis

Appendicitis

An 18-year-old man is brought to the emergency department with a 12-hour history of abdominal pain. Initially vague and generalized, the pain is now concentrated in his right lower quadrant. Vital signs are B/P 108/60, P 112, R 24, Temp 100.8° F. Acute appendicitis is suspected.

23. All of the following would be considered a normal finding in acute appendicitis except:
A. A pulsatile abdominal mass
B. Rebound tenderness
C. Nausea and vomiting
D. Low-grade fever

24. Which of the following symptoms indicate a ruptured appendix?
A. Projectile vomiting
B. Increased fever
C. Watery, mucoid diarrhea
D. Bright red vomitus

25. Five minutes after this patient arrives in the emergency department, which initial nursing action would be inappropriate?
A. Explaining upcoming tests and procedures
B. Obtaining laboratory specimens
C. Continued ongoing assessments
D. Giving parenteral analgesics

26. The possibility for unrecognized perforation of the appendix increases:
A. In the elderly patient
B. In the adolescent patient
C. In the middle-aged patient
D. In the school-aged patient

Acute Pancreatitis

A 69-year-old male arrived in triage complaining of 10/10 abdominal pain. The patient stated he had a history of acute pancreatitis.

27. Which statement about pancreatitis is true?
A. It cannot be caused by taking thiazide diuretics
B. It generally does not cause a great deal of pain
C. It is primarily caused by a biliary disease
D. It occurs only in alcoholics and patients who abuse drugs

28. The management of acute pancreatitis should include:
A. Maintaining the patient on strict nothing by mouth (NPO) and considering inserting a gastric tube
B. Fluid resuscitation with 20 ml/kg with dextrose and water to prevent dehydration from vomiting
C. Not administering any parental pain medications until the source of the pancreatitis is identified
D. Allow the patient to drink only clear liquids while in the emergency department, to prevent dehydration and electrolyte imbalance

29. A patient with acute pancreatitis is at risk for all of the following potential nursing diagnoses except:
A. Fluid volume deficit
B. Infection, potential for
C. Gas exchange, impaired
D. Cardiac output, increased

30. Currently, the diagnosis of acute pancreatitis is confirmed by:
A. An elevated white blood cell count
B. An elevated amylase level
C. Free air on the abdominal radiographs
D. Guaiac-negative emesis and stool test results

Cholecystitis

31. The most common cause of cholecystitis is:
A. Gallstones
B. Gastritis
C. Obesity
D. Smoking

32. When caring for a patient with cholecystitis, what statement made by the patient would be the most important to communicate to the doctor?
A. "I vomited twice before coming in tonight."
B. "I ate chili dogs and French fries tonight for supper."
C. "I hurt in my right side."
D. "I've wanted to see a doctor about this for weeks."

33. Cholecystitis usually affects:
A. Thin, fair-skinned, middle-aged males
B. Middle-aged, fair-skinned, obese females
C. Premature, nonbreastfed obese infants
D. Women who have never been pregnant

Diverticulitis

34. All of the following statements about diverticulitis are true except:
A. It is thought to be caused by high-fat diets and stress
B. The symptoms of an acute attack can mimic appendicitis
C. Intravenous antibiotics are usually given for acute diverticulitis
D. Diverticulitis is common in patients under 40 years of age

Esophageal Varices

A 52-year-old man is transferred to the emergency department from the local county jail after vomiting a large amount of bright red blood. History includes a long history of alcoholism and hepatitis. He is lethargic and restless. Marked ascites is present. He denies any acute pain. B/P 100/66, P 110, R 32, Temp 100.0° F. He gags and vomits 500 ml bright red blood upon arrival in the emergency department. A diagnosis of bleeding esophageal varices is suspected.

35. Based on his clinical picture, the most urgent nursing diagnosis would be:
A. Infection, potential for
B. Nutrition, altered (potential for)
C. Airway clearance, ineffective
D. Impaired physical mobility

36. Esophageal varices:
A. May rupture spontaneously, causing rapid exsanguination and death
B. Are enlarged arterial channels dilated by portal hypertension
C. Decrease as portal hypertension increases with medical management
D. Are not caused by alcoholic cirrhosis in the United States

37. Gastric decompression and lavage for this patient would be best accomplished with the use of: a
A. Salem sump gastric tube
B. Levine gastric tube
C. Linton tube
D. Gastrostomy tube

Irritable Bowel Syndrome

38. Clinical symptoms of irritable bowel syndrome include:
A. Acute abdominal pain located around the umbilicus
B. Regular disturbance of defecation with only diarrhea
C. Nausea with projectile vomiting
D. Recurrent, episodic, cramplike abdominal pain

39. Irritable bowel syndrome is diagnosed by:
A. Laboratory values that demonstrate bowel inflammation
B. A careful history and physical examination
C. An emergent abdominal CT with contrast
D. Placing the patient on laxatives for constipation

40. One of the significant differences between Crohn's disease and ulcerative colitis is:
A. Diffuse abdominal pain
B. Frequent episodes of diarrhea
C. Considerable weight gain
D. Rectal bleeding

41. The most common cause of diarrhea is:
A. Ingestion of toxins
B. Infectious agents
C. Food intolerance
D. Psychological stress

42. A common side effect of diphenoxylate and atropine (Lomotil) is:
A. Hypothermia
B. Bradycardia
C. Dry mouth
D. Renal failure

Abdominal Trauma

43. Which of the following increases a child's risk of sustaining an abdominal injury?
A. The abdominal wall is thicker and more developed than in the adult
B. The duodenum is less vascular in the child, so blood loss is less
C. The use of lap belts prevents the chance of abdominal injury in a child
D. The chest wall is more pliable and affords less protection for abdominal organs

44. A patient sustaining liver trauma may be especially prone to developing:
A. Coagulopathies
B. Hypervolemia
C. Fatty emboli
D. Peritonitis

45. Which of the following mechanisms of injury would place a patient at risk for a splenic injury?
A. Penetrating trauma to the right upper quadrant
B. Blunt trauma to the left upper quadrant
C. Blunt trauma to the pelvis
D. Penetrating trauma to the left femur

46. Referred pain in the left shoulder area is referred to as:
A. Cullen's sign
B. Grey Turner's sign
C. Chvostek's sign
D. Kehr's sign

47. The emergency nurse knows that with a ruptured spleen:
A. The patient will always arrive in shock
B. There may be a delayed rupture and no symptoms
C. Bleeding cannot occur within the splenic capsule
D. It cannot be caused by deep abdominal palpation

48. One of the most common methods used to evaluate the stable patient with abdominal trauma is:
A. Abdominal CT with contrast
B. Diagnostic peritoneal lavage
C. Flat-plate radiography of the abdomen
D. Exploratory laparotomy

49. Patients who have undergone splenectomy are especially prone to becoming ill from and need to be vaccinated against:
A. Swine influenza
B. *Vibrio parahaemolyticus*
C. Guillain-Barré syndrome
D. Pneumococcal pneumonia

50. Which of the following is an advantage for the use of ultrasonography in the diagnosis of abdominal trauma?
A. Ultrasonography does not image the retroperitoneum or diaphragmatic defects
B. It can rapidly diagnose at the bedside whether hemoperitoneum is present
C. It can easily be used to diagnose abdominal bleeding in an uncooperative patient
D. It is more sensitive than a diagnostic peritoneal lavage in revealing a hemoperitoneum

51. In caring for a patient with penetrating abdominal trauma resulting in a partial evisceration of the small intestine, the best nursing action would be to:
A. Make a gentle attempt to force the organ back into the abdomen
B. Irrigate the organs with warmed normal saline solution
C. Cover the organs with moist normal saline dressings
D. Encourage the patient to cough and breathe deeply

52. Diaphragmatic injury should be suspected when:
A. The gastric tube is visualized in the right side of the chest on radiograph
B. Bowel sounds are auscultated in the chest cavity
C. Blood is obtained upon insertion of a left-sided chest tube
D. Hematuria is obtained with insertion of a urinary catheter

53. Normal intraabdominal pressure (IAP) is:
A. 10 to 20 mm Hg
B. 2 to 10 mm Hg
C. 20 to 40 mm Hg
D. Above 40 mm Hg

Abdominal Aortic Aneurysm Rescue

Mr. West, a 70-year-old man, arrives by squad in the emergency department, complaining of intense lower back and lower abdominal pain of 1 hour's duration. No nausea or vomiting. His wife states he fainted while sitting on the commode at home. Medical history is positive for mild hypertension. The patient is rapidly being evaluated for a dissecting abdominal aortic aneurysm. B/P 100/52, P 120, R 30, Temp 96.4° F.

54. In the diagnosis of a dissecting abdominal aortic aneurysm, which emergency diagnostic test would be of most value?
A. Diagnostic peritoneal lavage
B. CT scan of abdomen

C. Abdominal ultrasonography
D. MRI

55. The most applicable nursing diagnosis for this patient would be:
A. Tissue perfusion, altered
B. Infection, potential for
C. Airway clearance, ineffective
D. Injury, potential for

56. The pain associated with a dissecting abdominal aortic aneurysm is described frequently as:
A. Stabbing
B. Dull ache
C. Sharp, tearing
D. Crushing

57. Mr. West wants to see his wife, who is out in the waiting room. The best response would be to say:
A. "You are too sick to have any visitors."
B. "You can see her after you have surgery."
C. "Ask the doctor if you can have visitors."
D. "I'll bring her in now."

58. Which of the following statements is true about the care of the patient with a ruptured abdominal aortic aneurysm?
A. A ruptured abdominal aortic aneurysm should be the primary diagnosis in patients less than 50 years of age with abdominal or back pain
B. Only large aneurysms will rupture and cause symptoms that would bring the patient to the emergency department
C. The patient with a ruptured abdominal aortic aneurysm who arrives in the emergency department hemodynamically stable generally will remain stable
D. The patient with a ruptured abdominal aortic aneurysm should remain in the emergency department until a definitive diagnose is made

Mesenteric Ischemia

59. Major contributing factors that increase the development of mesenteric ischemia include:
A. Cardiac disease
B. Sepsis
C. Coagulation disorders
D. All of the above

60. The following are symptoms of mesenteric ischemia except:
A. Generalized, vague abdominal pain
B. Abdominal distention and no bowel sounds
C. Presence of free air on abdominal radiographic films
D. No formed bowel movements and foul-smelling diarrhea

ANSWERS

1. **B. Assessment.** The correct sequence for a physical assessment of the abdomen is inspection, auscultation, palpation, and percussion. The abdomen should be auscultated prior to any hands-on assessment. Touching the abdomen may distort bowel sounds, as well as cause pain or discomfort that would impede any further attempts at an examination.[7]
2. **A. Assessment.** In palpating a painful abdomen, the nurse should do all of the following: palpate nonpainful areas first, then painful areas last; begin with light palpation, then move to deeper palpation last; and always observe the patient's face and other behaviors while palpating.[7]
3. **C. Assessment.** The spleen would have to swell to nearly 3 times its size to be palpated. In this case, deep palpation should never be used when splenomegaly is suspected because of the possibility of rupturing the organ. However, deep palpation is a routine part of the physical assessment of the abdomen.[7]
4. **A. Assessment.** The presence or absence of bowel sounds does not necessarily rule in or rule out a GI disorder. Although they are still an important part of the physical assessment of the abdomen, their diagnostic value is questionable.[7]
5. **C. Assessment.** Rebound tenderness, pain that occurs when pressure is applied to the area and then released, develops when irritated tissues and peritoneal fluid surround an inflamed appendix. It is commonly seen in patients who have peritonitis or appendicitis.[3]
6. **B. Assessment.** Abdominal pain is a symptom of an illness or injury, not a diagnosis. Research continues to demonstrate that narcotics used as a part of pain management should be provided for the patient with abdominal pain. A patient's response to pain is individual and influenced by culture.[2]
7. **C. Assessment.** In the emergency department, all women of childbearing age are assumed to

be pregnant until proven otherwise by a documented negative serum β-human chorionic gonadotropin result. Many expert clinicians have been "burned" when they forget this basic emergency care rule.[2]

8. **D. Assessment.** All abdominal pain is an emergency until it is diagnosed. It is easy for experienced emergency nurses to be unimpressed with symptoms of abdominal pain. Do not get caught in this trap. Abdominal pain has many potentially life-threatening origins and it should always be evaluated thoroughly.[1]
9. **D. Assessment.** Meditation and exercise are methods that are used to decrease patient stress and decrease the risk of developing gastritis.[4]
10. **B. Assessment.** The most common cause of peptic ulcer disease is *H. pylori.*[4]
11. **D. Intervention.** The management of superficial gastritis is based upon a combination of treatments. If it has been determined that *H. pylori* is the primary cause of the disease process, antimicrobial therapy is initiated, along with an H_2-receptor antagonist such as ranitidine. An effectiveness of about 90% was found with a combination of ranitidine, metronidazole, and amoxicillin.[4]
12. **B. Assessment.** The four hallmark signs of a bowel obstruction are (1) abdominal pain, (2) abdominal distention, (3) vomiting, and (4) marked constipation. Again, bowel sounds assessment is not completely reliable.[3,8-10]
13. **C. Intervention.** Generally enemas are contraindicated for a patient who has a bowel obstruction. They may cause more harm than good. Remember, the constipation is not necessarily the cause of the obstruction. Keeping the patient NPO, inserting a gastric tube to low suction, and administering intravenous fluids for rehydration are the basic necessities for a patient with distress caused by bowel obstruction.[8-10]
14. **B. Assessment.** Infants are less able to tolerate any change in their body fluid status than any other patient population. Closely following infants are the elderly. Infants and small children will become dehydrated rapidly, in a matter of hours.[11]
15. **C. Analysis.** Fluid volume deficit is the applicable nursing diagnosis because of the potential for dehydration that accompanies acute gastroenteritis. Potential for injury, ineffective airway clearance, and impaired skin integrity would not apply.
16. **A. Intervention.** A patient with gastroenteritis should drink plenty of fluids, especially an electrolyte replacement solution, then advance to a regular diet. Good handwashing and washing of dishes are crucial, as is disposing of any foods thought to be contaminated.
17. **D. Assessment.** The most common cause of diarrhea in young children is rotavirus, which accounts for 80% of diarrheal infections.[11]
18. **D. Assessment.** Potential causes of diarrhea in children include raw foods; recent use of antibiotics, which may cause problems from *Clostridium difficile;* and time spent at a day-care center, which can contribute to exposure to rotavirus, *Giardia,* and *Shigella.*[11]
19. **B. Assessment.** A clinical sign of severe diarrhea is the absence of urinary output. It is true that the child's heart rate will increase, but that is a significant sign of moderate dehydration, as well. It is important to find out from the child's caregivers when the child last had a wet diaper or urinated.[11]
20. **B. Intervention.** The initial management of mild dehydration should be accomplished through oral hydration with a balanced electrolyte solution, as long as the child can tolerate oral fluids.[11]
21. **C. Assessment.** This child has virtually every symptom of intussusception, a telescoping of the lumen of the bowel that occurs mainly in infants and children. It most commonly develops at or near the ileocecal valve or at the point of attachment of a colon tumor, polyp, or Meckel's diverticulum. Death can occur within 2 to 4 days because of the compromised blood supply to the bowel and mesentery and the resulting sepsis and gangrene.[12]
22. **B. Intervention.** A barium enema is diagnostic of intussusception and may even reduce it, thus eliminating the need for surgery. A soapsuds enema would not be helpful at this point.[12]
23. **A. Assessment.** A pulsatile mass is suggestive of an abdominal aortic aneurysm, not appendicitis. Symptoms of appendicitis commonly occur in children and young adults and include anorexia, nausea, vomiting, right lower quadrant pain, rebound tenderness, low-grade fever, and an elevated white blood cell count with shift.[8]
24. **B. Assessment.** A temperature spike may be seen a few hours after the appendix has ruptured. Surprisingly, there may also be an initial relief of pain after an appendix ruptures; then a

few hours later, fever occurs and abdominal pain returns and worsens.[8,9]

25. **D. Intervention.** There still is controversy related to managing pain in abdominal emergencies. Some clinicians disagree with this rule and, instead, recommend medicating the patient early, and then giving a narcotic antagonist if pain assessment is required. Explaining upcoming tests and procedures, obtaining laboratory specimens, and continuing to assess the abdomen are all appropriate actions.[9-13]
26. **A. Analysis.** Pain perception and pain patterns change with age. It is not uncommon to have a completely different clinical picture of appendicitis in the elderly or for them not to seek treatment until the appendix has perforated and they are suffering from peritonitis.[8]
27. **C. Assessment.** The most common cause of pancreatitis is alcoholism and it can occur years after the patient is sober. Other causes of pancreatitis include abdominal surgery or trauma, local infections, drugs at normal or toxic levels (especially glucocorticoids, thiazide diuretics, sulfonamides, antihypertensive agents, opiates, estrogens, antibiotics, and acetaminophen), mechanical obstruction of the biliary tract, hyperlipidemia, and hypercalcemia. Patients with a positive family history, previous bacterial infection (especially scarlet fever), a viral infection such as mumps, or a connective tissue disease such as Crohn's disease are at increased risk for pancreatitis.[13]
28. **A. Intervention.** Treatment of the patient with pancreatitis includes: fluid resuscitation and hydration with normal saline, pain management with narcotics which may include morphine, avoidance of substances such as food and alcohol that may aggravate the disease, and monitoring for complications such as respiratory failure and hyperglycemia.[13]
29. **D. Analysis.** Increased cardiac output generally does not occur with pancreatitis. Fluid volume deficit and potential for infection are problems associated with pancreatitis. The patient also has a great potential for impaired gas exchange from several factors. Because pancreatitis is an extremely painful condition, the patients tend to hypoventilate steadily, thereby affecting their oxygen saturation levels. The concurrent loss of fluids and electrolytes may also alter the delicate acid-base balance.[13]
30. **B. Assessment.** Currently, an amylase level remains the primary test to assist in the diagnosis of pancreatitis, indicated by an elevation. New tests are being developed that more specifically predict the severity of pancreatitis. The white blood cell count can rise from numerous other factors, not just pancreatitis. Air-fluid levels are indicative of abdominal perforation, and emergency surgery is required for that. Pancreatitis may or may not cause blood in the vomitus or stool, so negative guaiac test results are not indicative.[9,13]
31. **A. Assessment.** The number one cause of cholecystitis is cholelithiasis (gallstones). Other factors that can lead to the development of cholecystitis include typhoid fever, tumors, systemic staphylococcus or streptococcus infections, obesity or heavy fatty food diet, pregnancy, oral contraceptives, diabetes, celiac disease, cirrhosis of the liver, and pancreatitis.[9]
32. **B. Assessment.** An attack of cholecystitis typically is preceded by consumption of a large, fatty, spicy meal, especially before going to bed. It is not uncommon for vomiting to accompany pain in the right upper quadrant or epigastric area.[9]
33. **B. Analysis.** Obese, fair-skinned females are at greatest risk for developing cholecystitis. Pregnancy and obesity may also contribute to the development of cholecystitis.[9]
34. **D. Assessment.** Diverticulitis is not common in people under the age of 40. The symptoms can mimic appendicitis and are thought to be caused by high-fat diets and stress. Antibiotics are recommended for acute management.[14]
35. **C. Analysis.** Because of the high volume of blood in the esophagus and oropharynx, the patient is prone to ineffective airway clearance. Although the other nursing diagnoses apply, the airway involvement receives the highest priority.
36. **A. Assessment.** Esophageal varices are very serious and may rupture spontaneously, causing rapid exsanguination and death. When portal hypertension develops, small veins at the gastroesophageal junction are forced to receive large amounts of shunted blood, which causes distention and hypertrophy of these vessels. The abrupt bleeding may be caused by acid pepsin erosion, mechanical trauma (gastric tube placement), increased abdominal pressure, or coughing, retching, or vomiting. The bleeding is made worse by the fragility of the vessels and the compromised blood clotting mechanisms that accompany liver disorders.[9,15,16]

37. **C. Intervention.** When a patient is exsanguinating from esophageal varices, balloon tamponade should be initiated. A Linton tube has been found to be better than the traditional Sengstaken-Blakemore tube.[9,15,16]
38. **D. Assessment.** Clinical symptoms of irritable bowel syndrome include chronic or recurrent abdominal pain, generally in the lower abdomen. The pain is cramplike and episodic. Other symptoms associated with irritable bowel syndrome include an irregular disturbance in bowel movements, ranging from diarrhea to constipation, and nausea without vomiting.[17]
39. **B. Analysis.** A careful history and a good physical examination provide the data to make the diagnosis of irritable bowel syndrome. Limited testing should be directed at ruling out diseases such as ulcerative colitis or colon cancer.[17]
40. **D. Analysis.** Rectal bleeding is a clinical finding of ulcerative colitis. Both disease processes manifest diffuse abdominal pain and weight loss.[18]
41. **B. Assessment.** Acute diarrhea occurs in most adults. There are multiple causes including food intolerance, psychological stresses, ingestion of toxins, and adverse reactions to medications. Most cases, however, are thought to be caused by an infectious process, including those due to bacteria, parasites, and viruses.[19]
42. **C. Analysis.** Because of the atropine in Lomotil, a dry mouth is one of the most common symptoms. A delayed toxic response to Lomotil can involve bloating, constipation, and the development of a paralytic ileus or toxic megacolon.[20]
43. **D. Assessment.** Factors that may increase the risk of abdominal injury in the pediatric patient include:
    - Thinner, weaker abdominal muscles
    - More vascular duodenum, which increases the risk of blood loss when injured
    - Lap belts can cause more serious injury in children
    - Pliable chest wall affords less protection of the abdominal organs such as the liver and spleen.[11]
44. **A. Assessment.** Among numerous other physiological responsibilities, the liver plays a major role in synthesizing blood products and clotting factors. Any injuries to this organ may result in major coagulation problems.[1,2]
45. **B. Assessment.** The spleen is likely to be injured in acceleration-deceleration accidents, trauma associated with left rib fractures, and any blunt abdominal trauma. Sled-riding accidents and handlebar injuries frequently cause splenic trauma.[2]
46. **D. Assessment.** Kehr's sign is seen in patients who have a ruptured spleen and sometimes with other forms of intraabdominal bleeding. This referred pain is felt in the left shoulder and may worsen when the patient is laid flat or placed in Trendelenburg position.[3]
47. **B. Assessment.** A ruptured spleen is not always obvious in the early phases of management, and up to 20% of patients with splenic injuries may have a delayed rupture or delayed onset of symptoms.[2]
48. **A. Assessment.** Abdominal CT with contrast has become one of the most common methods of evaluating the patient with abdominal injury, particularly blunt trauma. However, if the patient is unstable, diagnostic peritoneal lavage should be performed to rule out abdominal hemorrhage.[6,21]
49. **D. Intervention.** Patients who have had their spleens removed have a tendency to develop pneumococcal infections. Because of this tendency, every effort is made to salvage the spleen whenever possible. If the spleen must be removed, the patient should receive pneumococcal polysaccharide vaccine (Pneumovax). This procedure is especially important in children, who are particularly susceptible to the pneumococcal infection. They should receive revaccination every 5 years.[1,2]
50. **B. Assessment.** Advantages of using ultrasonography to diagnose abdominal injury include: it can be used at the bedside, its sensitivity ranges from 60% to 95%, and it can be used serially to evaluate the patient. Diagnostic peritoneal lavage is still more sensitive, and with ultrasonography one cannot distinguish between blood and ascites.[21]
51. **C. Intervention.** Eviscerated organs should always be covered with dressings soaked with normal saline. This keeps the tissue viable until surgery can be performed. The organs should never be forced back into the abdominal cavity. The patient should be encouraged to lie still and not cough or vomit, because this may lead to further evisceration.[2]
52. **B. Assessment.** The presence of bowel sounds in the chest cavity is an indication of a ruptured

diaphragm. If a gastric tube has been inserted and a chest radiograph obtained, the gastric tube will be visualized in the chest cavity. If the bowel has entered the chest cavity, a chest tube may actually drain fecal material.[2]

53. **B. Assessment.**
    - Normal IAP: 2 to 10 mm Hg
    - Mildly elevated IAP: 10 to 20 mm Hg
    - Moderately elevated IAP: 20 to 40 mm Hg
    - Severely elevated IAP: over 40 mm Hg[22]
54. **B. Assessment.** A stat CT scan of the abdomen would be the most important diagnostic test. A complete blood count and an electrocardiogram are helpful but not crucial to the diagnosis of an abdominal aortic aneurysm. An MRI would not be practical at this point, because of the amount of time needed to perform this test and the urgent nature of the patient's condition.[9,21]
55. **A. Analysis.** The obvious hypotension and tachycardia are indicative of hypovolemic shock and subsequent altered tissue perfusion, all commonly associated with a ruptured abdominal aortic aneurysm. The potential for infection and injury and airway clearance problems are not applicable.
56. **C. Assessment.** Pain associated with a dissecting abdominal aortic aneurysm is frequently described as sharp and tearing and is commonly located in the lower back, lower abdomen, and possibly the upper thigh areas. It is constant and is not relieved with changes in position.[9]
57. **D. Intervention.** Because of the high mortality rate associated with a dissecting aortic aneurysm, it would be advisable to have this patient be with his wife as soon as possible. Despite the urgency of the situation, priority should be given to his emotional needs. Depending on the wife's response and behavior, she should be allowed to be with the patient as long as possible.[9]
58. **D. Intervention.** The patient with a ruptured abdominal aortic aneurysm needs to be taken as quickly as possible to the operating room.
59. **D. Assessment.** Cardiac disease, especially congestive heart failure and atrial fibrillation, place a patient at risk for developing mesenteric ischemia. Additional cardiac conditions include myocardial infarction and valvular heart disease. Other predisposing conditions are advanced age, hypovolemia, hypercoagulable states, rheumatoid arthritis, polyarteritis nodosa, sickle cell disease, and systemic lupus erythematosus. Certain medications, such as digitalis, oral contraceptives, and psychotropic medications, have also been associated with mesenteric ischemia.[9]
60. **C. Assessment.** The presence of free air on abdominal radiographic films is associated with an acute abdominal condition or possible organ perforation. It requires surgical exploration. The symptoms of mesenteric ischemia include colicky, intermittent abdominal pain out of proportion to the physical findings associated with generalized vague abdominal tenderness, voluntary guarding, and rebound tenderness. Bowel sounds may be hyperactive initially but then become decreased to absent as an ileus develops. The abdomen usually becomes distended late in the course of acute intestinal ischemia. Distention may be the only sign in a patient with ischemia not experiencing pain. Anorexia, nausea, absence of bowel movements, or diarrhea may accompany the pain.[9]

References

1. Noventy-Dinsdale J: Gastrointestinal emergencies. In Kitt S, Selfridge-Thomas, Proehl J et al, editors: *Emergency nursing: a physiologic and clinical perspective,* ed 2, Philadelphia, 1995, WB Saunders.
2. Herman ML: Gastrointestinal trauma. In Newberry L, editor: *Sheehy's emergency nursing: principles and practice,* ed 5, St Louis, 2003, Mosby.
3. Wright J: Seven abdominal assessment signs every emergency nurse should know, *J Emerg Nurs* 23:446-450, 1997.
4. Navuluri R, Yue S: Understanding peptic ulcer disease pharmacotherapeutics, *Nurs Pract* 21:128-132, 1999.
5. Powell D: Approach to the patient with diarrhea. In Goldman L, Bennett JC, editors: *Cecil textbook of medicine,* Philadelphia, 2000, WB Saunders.
6. Elliott D, Militello P: Pitfalls in the diagnosis of abdominal trauma. In Maull K, Rodriguez, Wiles C, editors: *Complications in trauma and critical care,* Philadelphia, 1996, WB Saunders.
7. Cauthorne-Burnette T, Estes MEZ: *Clinical companion for health assessment and physical examination,* Albany, NY, 1998, Delmar.
8. Pisarra VH: Recognizing the various presentations of appendicitis, *Nurs Pract* 24:42-53, 1999.

9. Newberry L: Gastrointestinal emergencies. In Newberry L, editor: *Sheehy's emergency nursing: principles and practice,* ed 5, St Louis, 2003, Mosby.
10. Jess LW: Acute abdominal pain: revealing the source, *Nursing* 93 23(9):34-42, 1993.
11. Emergency Nurses Association: *Emergency nursing pediatric course,* ed 3, Des Plaines, IL, 2004, Emergency Nurses Association.
12. Waisman Y: Intussusception. In Barkin R, editor: *Pediatric emergency medicine,* St Louis, 1997, Mosby.
13. Santen S, Hemphill R: Pancreas. In Marx J, editor: *Rosen's emergency medicine,* ed 5, St Louis, 2002, Mosby.
14. Bitterman R, Peterson M: Large intestine. In Marx J, editor: *Rosen's emergency medicine,* ed 5, St Louis, 2002, Mosby.
15. Henneman PL: Gastrointestinal bleeding. In Marx J, editor: *Rosen's emergency medicine,* ed 5, St Louis, 2002, Mosby.
16. Friedman S: Alcoholic liver disease, cirrhosis, and its major sequelae. In Goldman L, Bennett JC, editors: *Cecil textbook of medicine,* Philadelphia, 2000, WB Saunders.
17. Talley NJ: Functional gastrointestinal disorders; irritable bowel syndrome; non-ulcer dyspepsia; and non-cardiac pain. In Goldman L, Bennett JC, editors: *Cecil textbook of medicine,* Philadelphia, 2000, WB Saunders.
18. Rayhorn N: Inflammatory bowel disease, *Nursing 99* 29:57-61, 1999.
19. Kaplan MA, Prior MJ, Ash RS et al: Loperamide-simethicone vs. loperamide alone, simethicone alone, and placebo in the treatment of acute diarrhea with gas-related abdominal discomfort, *Arch Fam Med* 8:243-248, 1999.
20. *Mosby's Drug Consult 2005,* St Louis, 2005, Mosby.
21. Marx J: Abdominal trauma. In Marx J, editor: *Rosen's emergency medicine,* ed 5, St Louis, 2002, Mosby.
22. Proehl J: *Emergency nursing procedures,* ed 3, Philadelphia, 2004, WB Saunders.

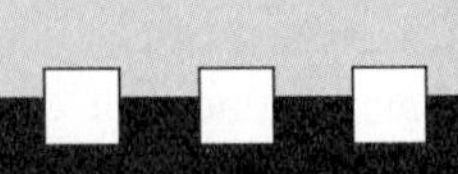

CHAPTER 4

Cardiovascular Emergencies

REVIEW OUTLINE

I. Anatomy
  A. Heart
    1. Pericardium
    2. Myocardium
    3. Endocardium
    4. Right ventricle
    5. Left ventricle
    6. Right atrium
    7. Left atrium
    8. Valves
      a. Atrioventricular (AV) valves
      b. Semilunar valves
        (1) Pulmonic
        (2) Aortic
    9. Cardiac muscle
    10. Fibrous skeleton of the heart
  B. Cardiac vasculature
    1. Superior vena cava
    2. Aortic arch
    3. Coronary arteries
    4. Inferior vena cava
    5. Pulmonary arteries
    6. Pulmonary veins
II. Physiology
  A. Cardiac cycle
    1. Diastole
    2. Systole
    3. Four phases[1]
      a. Isovolemic contraction
      b. Ventricular ejection
      c. Left ventricular relaxation
      d. Ventricular filling
  B. Preload
  C. Afterload
  D. Starling's law
III. Electrical conduction
  A. Cardiac cells
  B. Sinoatrial (SA) node
  C. Intraatrial tracts
    1. Bachmann
    2. Bundle
    3. Wenckebach
    4. Thorel
  D. AV node
  E. Right and left bundles of His
  F. Purkinje fiber
  G. P wave
  H. Q wave
  I. R wave
  J. ST segment
  K. T wave
IV. Cardiovascular assessment
  A. History
    1. Chest pain differentiation: PQRST
      a. Provocation and palliation
      b. Quality and intensity
      c. Region and radiation
      d. Severity
      e. Temporal: When did it start? How long has the pain been there? Is there any time it is not there?
    2. Medical history
    3. Risk factors for cardiac disease
      a. Hypertension
      b. Pulmonary disease
      c. Previous cardiovascular disease
      d. Smoking
      e. Family history
      f. Diabetes
      g. Renal disease
      h. Obesity: higher than average body mass
      i. Postmenopausal women
      j. Personality traits
      k. Elevated serum cholesterol level
      l. Adverse dietary pattern
      m. Lack of exercise
    4. Associated signs and symptoms
      a. Syncope
      b. Weakness
      c. Nausea and vomiting
      d. Diaphoresis

e. Dizziness
f. Orthopnea
g. Dependent edema
h. Fatigue
i. Paroxysmal nocturnal dyspnea
j. Palpitations
k. Irregular heart beat

5. Identification of possible contraindications to fibrinolytic therapy
   a. History of recent major surgery
   b. History of cerebrovascular disease or event
   c. Intracranial neoplasm
   d. Recent trauma
   e. Recent gastrointestinal or genitourinary bleeding
   f. Puncture of a noncompressible vessel such as the insertion of a central catheter
   g. Uncontrolled hypertension
   h. Pregnancy
   i. Menstruation (relative contraindication)
   j. Known bleeding diathesis
   k. Acute pericarditis

B. Physical examination
1. Obvious signs and symptoms of trauma
   a. Penetrating trauma: gunshot wound, knife wound, penetrating objects
   b. Blunt trauma: bruising and abrasions of the chest wall, anterior and posterior
   c. Obvious deformity
   d. Paradoxical movement
   e. Respiratory distress
2. Level of consciousness
3. Patient's skin color and temperature
   a. Pallor
   b. Cyanosis
   c. Diaphoresis
4. Jugular vein distention
5. Hepatomegaly
6. Clubbing of digits
7. Rate and rhythm of respirations
8. Palpation of peripheral pulses
9. Auscultation of breath sounds
   a. Comparison from side to side
   b. Presence or absence of breath sounds
   c. Rales (crackles)
   d. Rhonchi (sibilant and sonorous)
   e. Wheezes
   f. Pleural friction rub
10. Auscultation of heart sounds
   a. S_1
   b. S_2
   c. S_3
   d. S_4
   e. Friction rub
   f. Murmurs
   g. Bruits
11. Assessment of edema
   a. Location
   b. Pitting or nonpitting
12. Dysrhythmia recognition
13. Blood pressure evaluation
   a. Hypotension
   b. Hypertension
   c. Variances in pulse pressure
   d. Pulsus alternans
   e. Pulsus paradoxus
   f. Comparison of blood pressure from right to left side

C. Age-related changes[2-4]
1. Pediatric patient
   a. Infant's heart is large in relation to its size, lies horizontally, and takes up a large portion of the thoracic cavity
   b. Around age 7, the heart is closer to adult size
   c. Apical pulse more easily palpable in children
   d. S_3 is more common in children
   e. Children and young adults may have a benign systolic murmur
   f. Cardiac problems in children
      (1) Tetralogy of Fallot
      (2) Cardiac enlargement
      (3) Mitral stenosis
      (4) Aortic regurgitation
      (5) Ventricular septal defect
      (6) Patent ductus arteriosus
      (7) Truncus arteriosus
      (8) Coarctation of the aorta
      (9) Pulmonary stenosis
      (10) Myocarditis
      (11) Dilated cardiomyopathy
      (12) Endocardial fibroelastosis
   g. Blood pressure, pulse, and respirations vary depending on age of the child

2. Geriatric patient
   a. Stiffening of aorta and large arteries with age
   b. Increase in blood pressure with age
   c. Peripheral arteries lengthen and harden
   d. Some elderly develop postural hypotension
   e. Development of an aortic systolic murmur
   f. Development of a systolic murmur of mitral regurgitation
   g. Cardiac dysrhythmia common
   h. Perception of chest pain is less

D. Diagnostic studies or procedures
1. Electrocardiogram (ECG), 12 and 15 leads
2. Echocardiogram
3. Chest radiographic studies
4. Serum enzyme studies
   a. Creatine kinase
   b. Troponin complex
      (1) Troponin T
      (2) Troponin I, useful in diagnosis of an acute myocardial infarction
      (3) Troponin C
   c. Serum myoglobin
5. Cardiac angiography
6. Pericardiocentesis
7. Needle thoracostomy
8. Chest tube insertion
9. Open thoracotomy
10. Doppler ultrasonography
11. Arteriogram
12. Magnetic resonance angiography

V. Collaborative care
A. Activity intolerance
B. Airway clearance, ineffective
C. Breathing pattern, ineffective
D. Cardiac output, decreased
E. Fatigue
F. Fear
G. Fluid volume deficit, high risk for
H. Fluid volume excess
I. Gas exchange, impaired
J. Grieving, anticipatory
K. Injury, high risk for
L. Knowledge deficit
M. Pain
N. Spiritual distress (distress of the human spirit)
O. Tissue perfusion, ineffective
P. Trauma, high risk for

VI. Collaborative care of the patient with a cardiovascular emergency
A. ABCDE
1. Airway
2. Breathing
3. Circulation
4. Deficit: neurological
5. Exposure

B. Protocols
1. Basic Cardiac Life Support (BCLS)
2. Advanced Cardiac Life Support (ACLS)
3. Pediatric Advanced Life Support (PALS)
4. Emergency Nursing Pediatric Course (ENPC)
5. Trauma Nursing Core Course (TNCC)
6. Advanced Trauma Nursing Core Course (ATNC)
7. Transport Nurse Advanced Trauma Course (TNATC)
8. Basic Trauma Life Support (BTLS)
9. Advanced Trauma Life Support (ATLS)

C. Oxygen therapy
D. Cardiac monitoring
E. Pulse oximetry
F. External pacemaker
G. Transvenous pacemaker
H. Chest tube insertion
I. Open thoracotomy
J. Technological interventions
1. Biventricular pacing
2. Left ventricular assist device (LVAD)
3. Implantable cardioverter defibrillator

K. Drug therapy
1. Analgesics
2. Vasoconstrictors
   a. Epinephrine
   b. Vasopressin
   c. Norepinephrine
3. Inotropic agents
   a. Dobutamine
   b. Dopamine
   c. Milrinone
   d. Calcium sensitizers
4. Vasodilators
   a. Nitroglycerin
   b. Nitroprusside
5. Natriuretic
   a. Nesiritide

6. Antidysrhythmic agents
7. Antibiotics
8. Fibrinolytic agents
   a. Endogenous
      (1) Tissue plasminogen activator (t-PA)
      (2) Urokinase-type plasminogen activator (u-PA)
   b. Therapeutic agents
      (1) Streptokinase
      (2) Urokinase
      (3) Alteplase
      (4) Reteplase
9. Glycoprotein inhibitors: IIb/IIIa receptor antagonists
10. Digitalis antibodies
11. Antihypertensive agents
12. Calcium channel blockers
13. Anticoagulants
   a. Unfractionated heparin
   b. Low-molecular-weight heparin
14. Beta-blockers
15. Angiotensin converting enzyme inhibitors
16. Angiotensin II antagonists

L. Defibrillation and cardioversion
M. Pericardiocentesis
N. Frequent assessment
O. Arterial line insertion
P. Pulmonary artery catheter
Q. Intraaortic balloon pump
R. Cardiopulmonary bypass
S. Automatic implantable cardioverter defibrillator

VII. Specific cardiovascular emergencies
   A. Cardiac arrest
   B. Congestive heart failure, acute pulmonary edema
   C. Dysrhythmia
      1. Ventricular fibrillation
      2. Ventricular tachycardia
      3. Asystole
      4. Heart block
      5. Premature ventricular contractions (PVCs)
      6. Supraventricular tachycardia
   D. Hypertension
   E. Digitalis toxicity
   F. Thromboembolic disease
      1. Pulmonary embolus
      2. Deep vein thrombosis (DVT)
      3. Septic emboli
      4. Fat emboli
   G. Acute coronary syndrome
      1. Unstable angina
      2. Non–Q wave myocardial infarction
      3. Q wave myocardial infarction
   H. Aortic aneurysm
   I. Peripheral vascular disease
   J. Inflammation or infection
      1. Pericarditis
      2. Endocarditis
      3. Myocarditis
   K. Cardiac trauma
      1. Penetrating
         a. Gunshot wounds
         b. Stab wounds
      2. Blunt
         a. Myocardial contusion
         b. Pericardial tamponade

Cardiovascular diseases account for more deaths in the United States than the other causes of death combined.[4,5] Most of these patients seek treatment in the emergency department, which presents a particular challenge to emergency nursing practice. All of the changes that occur in the management of cardiovascular emergencies—especially chest pain and myocardial infarction—require that emergency nurses keep abreast of the current research and treatment to ensure that patients receive the best care. Diagnostic terminology has changed. What was formerly known as *rule out MI* or *unstable angina* is now called *acute coronary syndrome*. This term describes cardiac ischemia based on the patient's history, symptoms, ECG changes, and serum markers indicative of cardiac injury.[6]

A patient suffering chest pain should be treated the same as a trauma patient—rapid assessment and timely treatment. In other words, time and skill are of the essence in preventing additional injury to the patient's myocardium.[6,7] Cardiac teams, rapid treatment and diagnostic centers, and chest pain centers have reduced "door-to-treatment" times and placed patients in appropriate care areas. Management of chest pain requires knowledge about multiple medications, their effects, and what further interventions may be necessary when initial intervention fails.[6,7]

Controversy remains as to the best treatment for the patient with an acute myocardial infarction. Angioplasty appears to improve short-term outcomes after an acute myocardial infarction. However, because of limited resources (lack of a cardiac catheterization lab or interventional cardiologist), thrombolysis remains an appropriate treatment.[8]

Cardiovascular emergencies can have either a medical or a traumatic origin. Occasionally a patient may sustain a cardiovascular emergency of both a medical and a traumatic nature, such as in the case of the elderly patient who has an acute myocardial event that precipitates a motor vehicle crash.

Care of the patient who is experiencing a cardiovascular emergency begins with the assessment and stabilization of the patient's airway, breathing, and circulation (ABCs). The emergency nurse needs to possess knowledge about the anatomy and physiology of the cardiovascular system. These topics are included in the Review Outline at the beginning of the chapter. ACLS, PALS, and the ENPC offer guidelines for the care of both adult and pediatric patients experiencing cardiovascular emergencies. It is important to use the most current guidelines and revisions of any of these courses in one's practice and to be aware of any additional advisories. Most of the associations (e.g., the American Heart Association) maintain up-to-date information on their web sites.

Because the cardiovascular system affects all other body systems, inspection of the patient who is suffering from a cardiovascular emergency will encompass airway patency, breathing patterns, and perfusion. Palpation should include evaluation of both the central and the peripheral pulses. Auscultation of heart sounds, cardiac rhythm, and breath sounds should be included.

Identifying the origins of the patient's chest pain, or chest pain differentiation, presents a demanding challenge to the assessment skills of the emergency department nurse. One method that can be used to differentiate a patient's chest pain is based on four different factors: the patient's description of the pain (crushing, burning, tearing, sudden onset, location), factors that relieve the pain (stopping activity, sitting up, analgesics, relief with nitroglycerin, no relief), associated symptoms (friction rub, shortness of breath, nausea, vomiting, diaphoresis), and ECG findings (no changes, elevated ST segments, transient ST and T wave changes).[8]

Diagnostic data related to cardiovascular emergencies include an ECG, echocardiogram, chest radiograph, serum cardiac marker levels, electrolyte values (particularly potassium and calcium), and Doppler ultrasonography. The value of cardiac enzyme levels used to be limited because of the time it took to confirm their presence and significance. Bedside testing and more sophisticated laboratories with rapid turn-around times have allowed more timely diagnosis. Cardiac enzyme values are sensitive indicators of non–Q wave injury and unstable angina.[9] A recent study demonstrated that the measurement of both myoglobin and troponin during a 9-hour period was the most predictive of subsequent adverse events in patients evaluated in the emergency department for possible acute coronary syndrome.[10]

Specific collaborative procedures for the patient who is suffering from a cardiovascular emergency include the insertion of chest tubes,[3,5] pericardiocentesis, open thoracotomy, portable extracorporeal circulation,[10] and thrombolytic therapy.[4-8] The emergency nurse needs to review the indications, the nurse's role, and the nursing interventions required to provide appropriate care to patients who are undergoing these procedures.

Over the past 20 years, management of cardiovascular emergencies in the prehospital environment has expanded to include the use of automatic external defibrillators (AED). These are not only being carried by emergency services (police, fire personnel, emergency medical technicians [EMTs], and paramedics) but also are being used by flight attendants, factory workers, and many others who have received the appropriate training. The reaction to cardiovascular emergencies continues to be focused on a community response. Emergency nurses play an integral role in this response as teachers and providers of care.

Technology continues to enhance the lives of those suffering from cardiovascular disease and its complications. Witness the publicity surrounding Dick Cheney, a vice president of the United States who had an implantable defibrillator to prevent the possibility of sudden cardiac death. Other technological advances in cardiovascular management include biventricular pacing and LVADs. All of these patients and devices may arrive at some time in the emergency department for care.

Care of the patient who is suffering from a cardiovascular emergency begins with an understanding of the anatomy and physiology of the cardiovascular system. The emergency nurse needs to be able to differentiate the sources of chest pain. Recognition and management of potentially lethal dysrhythmias is a very important component of the care provided to the emergency cardiovascular patient. Finally, possessing current knowledge about the care of the patient with acute myocardial infarction, particularly fibrinolytic therapy, and recognizing and providing treatment for the patient who may have experienced blunt or penetrating cardiac trauma contribute to the emergency nurse's ability to provide optimal care to the emergency cardiovascular patient.[11,12]

REVIEW QUESTIONS

Myocardial Infarction

A 58-year-old female is transported to the emergency department by the local emergency medical services (EMS). She collapsed while working. Her co-workers applied an AED, which showed ventricular fibrillation. Three shocks were delivered before arrival of the EMS providers. The patient was intubated and an intravenous line inserted. Upon arrival in the emergency department, the patient remains in ventricular fibrillation.

1. Upon arrival in the emergency department, which of the following interventions should be performed first?
A. Check the patency of the intravenous line inserted by the EMS providers
B. Search for and treat identified reversible causes of this patient's cardiopulmonary arrest
C. Confirm endotracheal tube placement by auscultation of bilateral breath sounds
D. Prepare for administration of medication to treat the ventricular fibrillation

2. Differential diagnosis for sudden cardiopulmonary arrest include all of the following except:
A. Hypoglycemia
B. Pulmonary embolus
C. Drug induced
D. All of the above

3. The emergency department physician has ordered vasopressin. Vasopressin should be administered:
A. Only through the endotracheal tube
B. Every 5 to 10 minutes following the first dose
C. Intravenously as a single dose
D. To patients less than 50 years of age

4. Cardiopulmonary resuscitation (CPR) should not be started:
A. When a patient suffers a cardiopulmonary arrest during air or ground transport
B. When there is a valid order not to attempt resuscitation
C. When a trained professional responder arrives at the scene
D. When there are no obvious signs of death

5. After epinephrine has been administered to the patient in ventricular fibrillation, the emergency nurse should prepare to:
A. Administer amiodarone 600 mg IV over 10 minutes
B. Continue chest compressions for 5 full minutes before defibrillation
C. Resume attempts to defibrillate at 360 J within 30 to 60 seconds
D. Administer procainamide 100 mg IV over 10 minutes

A 68-year-old man comes to the emergency department complaining of midsternal chest pain. He is awake, alert, pale, and diaphoretic. His vital signs are B/P 90/62, P 64 and irregular, R 22, and Temp 98.6° F.

6. The pain pattern of myocardial infarction frequently is described as:
A. Tearing, radiating to the back
B. Sudden, sharp, increasing with a change in position
C. Sudden, crushing, radiating to the jaw and neck
D. Sudden, sharp over the lung fields, increasing with inspiration

7. All of the following risk factors correlate with the probability of cardiac disease in this patient except:
A. Male sex
B. Diabetes mellitus
C. Cigarette smoking
D. Type A personality

8. T wave inversion on a 12-lead ECG indicates:
A. Infarction
B. Dysrhythmia
C. Injury
D. Ischemia

9. A 12-lead ECG is obtained. There is ST elevation greater than 2 mm in leads II, III, and aV_F. The patient is probably having an acute:

A. Inferior wall myocardial infarction
B. Anterior wall myocardial infarction
C. Posterior wall myocardial infarction
D. Lateral wall myocardial infarction

10. Reteplase 20 units has been ordered for the patient because the closest cardiac catheterization lab is 2 hours away by air medical transport. In preparation for administration of this therapy, the emergency nurse may:
   A. Administer platelets to the patient to prevent the possibility of gastrointestinal bleeding
   B. Start an additional intravenous line of normal saline before administering the drug
   C. Draw all of the required blood studies before administering the initial 20-unit dose
   D. Initiate a lidocaine infusion at 2 mg/min in anticipation of a dysrhythmia

11. A common dysrhythmia associated with reperfusion is:
   A. Ventricular fibrillation
   B. Complete heart block
   C. Accelerated idioventricular rhythm
   D. Asystole

12. The most common complication of fibrinolytic therapy is:
   A. Dysrhythmia
   B. Bleeding
   C. Thrombosis
   D. Hypocalcemia

13. Which group of patients is at greater risk of having a stroke after treatment with fibrinolytic therapy?
   A. Elderly patients with a history of headaches
   B. Women being treated with fibrinolytic agents for myocardial infarction
   C. Men who have had previous infarctions
   D. Men who have a history of headaches

14. Because of the possibility of an intracerebral hemorrhage occurring as the result of fibrinolytic administration, the emergency nurse should evaluate the patient for:
   A. Petechiae
   B. Changes in level of consciousness
   C. Blood in the urine
   D. Fever and chills

15. The emergency nurse performs a baseline neurological assessment as part of the initial care of a patient who is to receive thrombolytic therapy for an acute anterior myocardial infarction. The patient is given reteplase (Retavase), and a weight-based heparin drip is initiated. During infusion of these drugs, the nurse notes that the patient has a sudden deterioration in mental status and weakness on his left side. What actions should the emergency nurse initiate?
   A. Notify the emergency physician and obtain an emergency computed tomography (CT) scan
   B. Discontinue the heparin drip and notify the emergency physician
   C. Continue the patient's infusions and reevaluate the patient in 15 minutes
   D. Immediately obtain blood sample for prothrombin time, partial thromboplastin time, and a platelet count from the patient

16. The most appropriate nursing diagnosis for the patient receiving fibrinolytic therapy is:
   A. Airway clearance, ineffective
   B. Fluid volume deficit, high risk for
   C. Injury, high risk for
   D. Gas exchange, impaired

17. TNK-tissue plasminogen activator:
   A. Is less likely than other fibrinolytics to cause bleeding because it is more fibrin specific
   B. Has a prolonged effect on coagulation because it depletes fibrinogen
   C. Has no effect on clotting and should not be used in fibrinolytic therapy
   D. Should not be given to patients who are allergic to streptokinase

A 53-year-old man comes to the emergency department complaining of chest pain for the past 12 hours. He states that it is crushing and goes down his left arm.

18. Which of the following statements best describes the need for pain management in the patient who is having an acute myocardial infarction?
   A. The medications used for pain management will not interfere with the patient's level of consciousness

B. Pain management will increase the fear and anxiety related to myocardial infarction
C. Pain management will decrease catecholamine release that may increase myocardial damage
D. Pain management will always cause nausea, vomiting, and increased diaphoresis

19. The patient states, "I do not know what this heart attack is going to do to my life." The most appropriate nursing diagnosis on which the emergency nurse should base care is:
A. Fear related to the implications of the patient's illness
B. Body image disturbance related to the acute myocardial infarction
C. Thought processes, altered, related to chest pain
D. Spiritual distress (distress of the human spirit) related to pain

20. After providing the patient with information about his condition, the emergency nurse should use which of the following to evaluate the effectiveness of the intervention?
A. The patient's pulse and blood pressure increases
B. The patient is able to talk about his fears
C. The patient states that he wants to be alone
D. The patient says that he does not want to see his family

A 60-year-old patient is diagnosed as having an acute inferior wall myocardial infarction and a right ventricular infarction. He is awake and alert and complaining of 10/10 chest pain. The patient develops profound hypotension while in the emergency department. His vital signs are B/P 80/50, P 60, and R 32.

21. The initial treatment of this patient should include:
A. Administration of furosemide (Lasix) to prevent the onset of congestive heart failure
B. Administration of a 200-ml normal saline fluid bolus to manage the hypotension
C. Insertion of a transvenous pacemaker to improve the patient's heart rate and hypotension
D. Administration of nitroglycerin 30 mcg/kg to decrease his chest pain and improve hypotension

22. A right ventricular infarction is diagnosed by:
A. A chest radiograph to confirm cardiomyopathy
B. Placement of right-sided precordial leads
C. Monitoring of serial cardiac markers
D. Sudden onset of pulmonary edema

23. Differentiating chest pain in the emergency setting is difficult because:
A. Most patients are able to give a clear description of their signs and symptoms
B. The severity of the pain always correlates with its life-threatening potential
C. There is little correlation between the location of the patient's pain and its cause
D. Only cardiovascular disease can cause midsternal pain that will radiate

24. Mr. J has been diagnosed with an acute anterolateral myocardial infarction. A nitroglycerin drip has been started to help manage the patient's chest pain, which he states is 8/10. When administrating nitroglycerin, the emergency nurse should:
A. Allow the patient's systolic blood pressure to drop below 90 mm Hg to increase myocardial perfusion
B. Use only nitroglycerin to manage the patient's pain instead of morphine sulfate, to prevent hypotension
C. Use the patient's description of his level of chest pain as one method of appropriately titrating the medication
D. Tell the patient that it does not matter that he took sildenafil within 24 hours of the onset of his chest pain

25. Large, inappropriate dosages of nitroglycerin may:
A. Cause reflex hypertension
B. Cause reflex tachycardia
C. Cause reflex bradycardia
D. Cause an increase in coronary perfusion pressure

26. Heparin administration is more effective when dosage is based on weight because:
A. Bleeding is less likely to occur with a smaller dosage

B. Absorption of heparin varies from patient to patient
C. Diseases such as diabetes may affect heparin
D. Bradycardia may result with inadequate dosages of heparin

27. The diagnosis of an acute myocardial infarction includes all of the following except:
A. ST segment changes or new Q waves
B. Abnormally elevated serum cardiac enzyme levels
C. No ST segment changes or new Q waves
D. Abnormally elevated serum myoglobin levels

28. When a patient has sustained a sudden cardiac arrest from ventricular fibrillation and is in the circulatory phase of resuscitation, which interventions should be initiated by the resuscitation team?
A. Immediate defibrillation at 200 J, 300 J, and 360 J with appropriately placed pads
B. Endotracheal intubation to ensure adequate oxygen delivery to the heart
C. Controlled reperfusion with apoptosis inhibitors and external cooling
D. Administration of epinephrine or vasopressin to restore electrical activity

29. Preload is measured in the right side of the heart by:
A. Pulmonary wedge pressure (PWP)
B. Central venous pressure (CVP)
C. Left atrial pressure (LAP)
D. Diastolic blood pressure (DAP)

30. Systemic vascular resistance is increased by:
A. Chronic obstructive pulmonary disease
B. Administration of nitroprusside intravenously
C. Primary pulmonary hypertension
D. Sympathetic nervous system stimulation

31. A 68-year-old female arrives in the emergency department after experiencing 4 hours of crushing chest pain, diaphoresis, and vomiting. She is diagnosed with an acute inferior myocardial infarction. She is treated with fibrinolytic therapy. Her heart rate remains at 100 without any ectopy. The emergency department physician orders metoprolol 15 mg IV to be administered over 15 minutes. The desired effect of metoprolol is:
A. To increase short-term mortality from acute myocardial infarction
B. To decrease the incidence of ventricular fibrillation and electrical storm
C. To extend the size of the patient's myocardial infarction
D. To increase cardiac metabolic demand

32. A 37-year-old obese male comes to the emergency department complaining of midsternal crushing chest pain. He has a history of diabetes controlled by diet and has been a smoker for the past 20 years. An ECG demonstrates some anterior wall ischemia. The patient is diagnosed with acute coronary syndrome. Abciximab (ReoPro) has been ordered. The physiological effect of abciximab is:
A. Lysing clots that have formed in the coronary arteries
B. Blocking fibrinogen's ability to cause platelet aggregation
C. Blocking thromboxane A_2 to stop platelet aggregation
D. Enhancing platelet aggregation in the coronary artery

33. The antiplatelet effect of glycoprotein IIb/IIIa receptor inhibitors can be reversed by:
A. Administration of platelets
B. Administration of protamine zinc
C. Administration of packed red blood cells
D. Administration of clopidogrel

34. A costly complication of myocardial infarction is:
A. Excessive medication administration in the emergency department
B. A 50% chance of suffering a cerebrovascular accident when fibrinolytic agents are administered
C. Decrease in research related to the management of myocardial infarction
D. The development of congestive heart failure after an acute myocardial infarction

35. Advantages of TNK-tissue plasminogen activator (TNKase) include:
A. The drug may cause sudden hypotension, and inline filters can remove 47% of the drug

B. The drug is more fibrin specific with less incidence of bleeding than rt-PA
C. The half-life of the drug is 18 minutes, and it has a prolonged effect on clotting
D. It can be administered in two doses, which decreases the risk of medication errors

36. Resuscitation can be withheld in which of the following circumstances?
A. In emergency departments where policies permit resuscitation to be withheld without consulting the patient or his or her family
B. In emergency departments where "slow" resuscitation is allowed until the patient or family is consulted
C. For patients who have clear advance directives directing health care providers not to begin resuscitation in the event of a cardiac arrest
D. For patients whose body temperature is less than 90° F (32° C) and who have a heart rate of 20 beats per minute

37. The immediate general treatment for a patient who comes to the emergency department and is diagnosed with acute coronary syndrome should include:
A. Administration of meperidine to manage the patient's chest pain
B. Administration of aspirin orally unless the patient has an allergy to aspirin
C. Administration of oxygen by mask to maintain oxygen saturation below 90%
D. Preparation of the patient for a chest CT scan to rule out the presence of a thoracic aneurysm

Advanced Cardiac Life Support

A family pulls up to the emergency department entrance and asks for help. They state that their 65-year-old mother would not wake up. The patient is removed from the car and brought into the resuscitation room. The patient is not breathing and does not have a pulse.

38. The patient's monitor shows a bradycardic wide-complex rhythm, but a pulse cannot be palpated. What intervention should the emergency nurse consider first?
A. Prepare the patient for defibrillation at 200 J, 300 J, and 360 J
B. Prepare the patient for insertion of a transvenous pacemaker
C. Prepare the patient for insertion of a central venous line
D. Prepare the patient for endotracheal intubation

39. A 52-year-old man comes to the emergency department complaining of a "funny feeling in his chest." When placed on the monitor, he demonstrates an irregular rhythm (see bottom of page). What rhythm is it?
A. Atrial tachycardia
B. Atrial fibrillation
C. Sinus tachycardia
D Sinus rhythm

40. His heart rate is 110 and his systolic blood pressure is 90 by palpation. The patient begins to complain of chest pain and shortness of breath. Which of the following interventions should be used to manage this patient?
A. Application of anteroposterior pad and defibrillation at 200 J
B. Insertion of a central venous line and administration of digoxin
C. Insertion of a central venous line and administration of adenosine
D. Application of anteroposterior pads and cardioversion at 360 J

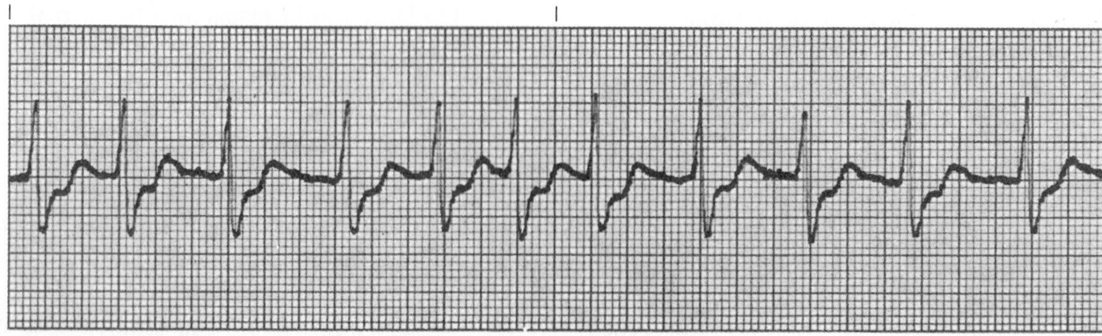

Question 39

41. A 56-year-old woman complains to the triage nurse of shortness of breath. Her heart rate is too rapid to count. A monitor is applied. What cardiac rhythm is the patient in?
A. Ventricular tachycardia
B. Ventricular fibrillation
C. Atrial fibrillation with a rapid ventricular response
D. Sinus rhythm with frequent PVCs

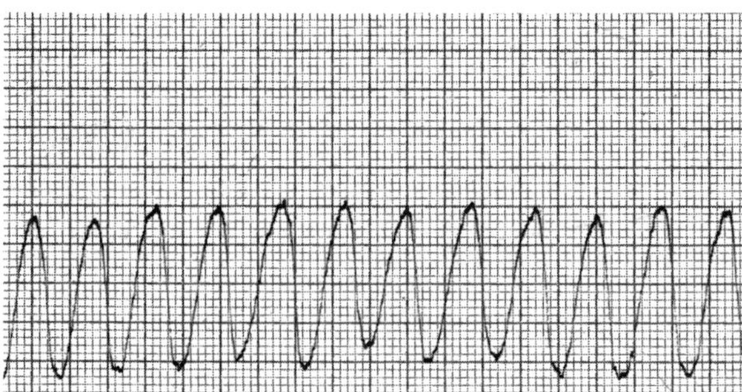

42. The emergency department physician orders a dose of amiodarone to manage this patient's dysrhythmia. How should it be administered?
A. 300 mg IV over 5 minutes
B. 150 mg IV over 10 minutes
C. 150 mg IV over 5 minutes
D. 450 mg IV over 15 minutes

43. The most common side effect of amiodarone is:
A. Hypertension
B. Tachycardia
C. Hypotension
D. Hepatic failure

44. The patient continues to respond intermittently to the amiodarone; however, a diagnosis of polymorphic ventricular tachycardia is made. What other medication may be considered to manage this patient's dysrhythmia?
A. Aminophylline 5 mg/kg infusion
B. Morphine 1 to 3 mg IV
C. Digoxin 0.25 mg IV
D. Magnesium sulfate 1 to 2 g IV

45. An 82-year-old man is brought to the emergency department after having collapsed while mowing the lawn. When his family found him, he was apneic and pulseless, and CPR was initiated. An AED had been applied and used by the local EMS provider. When the patient arrives in the emergency department, the monitor shows the following rhythm. What is it?
A. Asystole
B. Ventricular tachycardia
C. Sinus rhythm
D. Ventricular fibrillation

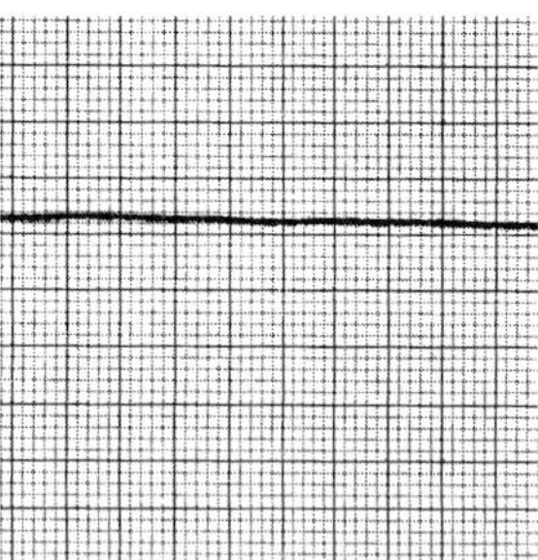

46. The patient is intubated, but an intravenous line has not yet been established. All of the following drugs can be administered via the endotracheal tube except:
A. Lidocaine
B. Atropine
C. Naloxone
D. Sodium bicarbonate

47. A 78-year-old woman is brought to the emergency department after having passed out at home. She has no history of any cardiac disease and has not seen a doctor for over 20 years. When monitoring is initiated, the following rhythm is found. What is it?
A. Asystole
B. First-degree heart block
C. Third-degree heart block
D. Sinus rhythm

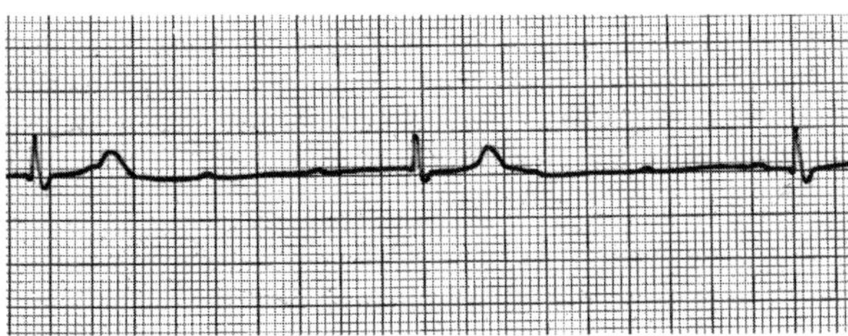

48. The patient has a blood pressure of 80/50, with P 30 and R 12. She is complaining that she feels "dizzy." An external pacemaker is placed and pacing is initiated. A common complication of external pacing in the conscious patient is:
A. Failure to capture through the patient's skin because of decreased elasticity

B. Failure of pacing pads to stick to the patient's chest wall because of age
C. Pain from muscle spasms induced by the external pacemaker
D. Shortness of breath because the patient has to lie flat during pacing

49. External pacemaker mechanical capture is demonstrated by:
A. A palpable femoral pulse
B. A decreased level of consciousness
C. A decreased blood pressure
D. Pacemaker spikes on the monitor

50. Interventions to improve external pacemaker mechanical capture include:
A. Decreasing the milliamperage until a pulse can be palpated
B. Increasing the rate setting of the external pacemaker
C. Checking the battery power of the external pacemaker
D. Adding an additional set of pads in a different position on the chest

51. An 82-year-old woman comes to the emergency department complaining of a "funny" feeling in her chest and shortness of breath. The patient's B/P is 80/60, P is 200. Her monitor shows a narrow-complex tachycardia. Which of the following drugs may be ordered to treat this dysrhythmia?
A. Epinephrine 1 mg/kg IV push
B. Atropine 1 mg IV push
C. Adenosine 6 mg IV push
D. Lidocaine 1 mg/kg IV push

52. After 2 minutes, the patient's rhythm has not changed and her blood pressure remains the same. The next treatment she would be given is:
A. Verapamil 10 mg IV push
B. Digitalis 0.5 mg slow IV push
C. Lidocaine 50 mg IV push
D. Adenosine 12 mg IV push

53. Emergency nursing care of the patient receiving adenosine, based on a common side effect of this drug, would include which of the following nursing diagnoses?
A. Injury, high risk for, related to the generalized seizures adenosine may cause
B. Hyperthermia related to the thermoregulatory side effects of adenosine
C. Self-care deficit related to the dizziness that is a side effect of adenosine
D. Fear related to the sudden change in cardiac rhythm that precedes conversion

54. A 55-year-old woman is brought to the emergency department after complaining of "weakness." The basic life support squad reported that her heart rate was around 75 and very irregular. Upon arrival in the emergency department, monitoring is initiated and the patient is in this rhythm. What is the rhythm?
A. Atrial fibrillation
B. Atrial flutter
C. Normal sinus rhythm
D. Nodal tachycardia

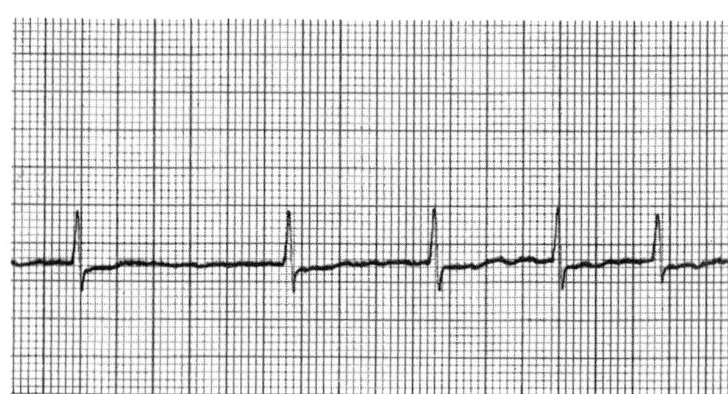

55. The patient has no history of any medical problems, and her ECG shows no evidence of previous injury. She states she exercises every day and thought that her irregular heart rate may have been related to physical exertion. During her evaluation, her heart rate increases to 120 beats per minute, and she complains of chest pain. This rhythm leaves the patient at risk for:
A. Developing complete heart block
B. Developing congestive heart failure
C. Having a transient ischemic attack
D. Developing ventricular fibrillation

56. The patient refuses cardioversion and would prefer to try pharmacologic cardioversion. Which of the following medications is the emergency physician most likely to order to manage this patient's dysrhythmia?
A. Disopyramide
B. Quinidine
C. Amiodarone
D. Digoxin

57. A 3-month-old infant is brought to the emergency department because of respiratory distress. The infant's pulse is over 260 beats per minute. The mother states that the child has not been ill and that this incident started suddenly. The infant is lethargic and cyanotic. The emergency physician has decided to perform cardioversion. The emergency nurse would calculate the joules to be used to cardiovent the child using the following:

A. 2 J/kg
B. 0.5 J/kg
C. 3 J/kg
D. 25 J/kg

58. A 10-year-old boy collapses while playing baseball. The basic life support team finds that he is apneic and pulseless. Which of the following statements is true related to the use of an AED in the pediatric patient?

A. The AED should never be used in a pediatric patient less than 18 years of age
B. When using an AED in a child with an implantable cardioverter defibrillator, the pad should be placed over the device
C. An AED can be programmed to deliver a specific amount of energy, so it can be used in infants
D. An AED may be used in children 8 years of age or older and who weigh more than 25 kg

59. The mother of a 4-week-old infant brings the child to the emergency department. She states that the baby has been "turning blue" when she cries. Today, she "turned blue" when she was sucking on her bottle. The baby is tachypneic, with R 60 and P 150, diaphoretic, and becomes cyanotic when she cries. The mother has not had any follow-up care since she was discharged home 24 hours after her daughter's birth. A loud heart murmur is auscultated. The initial treatment of this infant should include:

A. Obtain an anteroposterior and lateral chest radiograph to rule out pulmonary edema
B. Place the child in position of comfort and administer supplemental oxygen therapy
C. Obtain venous access to draw appropriate specimens for analysis and administer medications
D. Weigh the infant or ask the mother what the baby's last weight was

60. How should the paddles be placed for the patient who has an implanted cardioverter defibrillator and who needs to be defibrillated?

A. The patient should not be defibrillated
B. The paddles should be placed on the apex and sternum
C. The paddles should be placed anteriorly and posteriorly
D. The patient's chest should be opened for internal defibrillation

61. A 50-year-old man with a history of a heart transplant arrives in the emergency department in complete heart block. His B/P is 78/52, P 42, R 16. He is lethargic but can be aroused. An external pacemaker has been placed but is not effectively pacing the heart. Which medication would provide chronotropic support and increase his heart rate until a transvenous pacemaker can be inserted?

A. Isoproterenol 2 mcg/min
B. Dobutamine 10 mcg/min
C. Diltiazem 2 mg/min
D. Dopamine 1 mg/kg/min

62. A 63-year-old man has an LVAD in place and is brought to the emergency department by his wife because he is not "feeling well." As soon as monitoring is begun, the patient becomes unresponsive and the monitor shows a wide-complex rhythm. There is no palpable pulse. The emergency nurse should:

A. Initiate chest compressions in order to provide the patient with a heart rate between 80 and 100 beats per minute
B. Pump the device by hand but first feel the patient's abdomen to make sure the pump is functioning
C. Disconnect both of the cables that connect the controller of the LVAD to its power source at the same time
D. Prepare the patient for defibrillation with the LVAD batteries still connected

Hypertension

The family of a 47-year-old African American male brings him to the emergency department. He is complaining of a headache, blurred vision, and chest pain. He has no known medical problems and is not taking any medication. He states his brother has been treated for high blood pressure and a myocardial infarction. His vital signs are B/P 220/142 (right arm), P 100, and R 22. The emergency nurse takes his blood pressure in his left arm and finds it to be 218/138.

63. An adult patient is considered to have severe hypertension when:
A. The diastolic blood pressure is less than 90 mm Hg and there are no end-organ effects
B. The systolic blood pressure is 140 to 159 mm Hg and there are no end-organ effects
C. The diastolic blood pressure is greater than 110 mm Hg with end-organ effects
D. The systolic blood pressure is 140 to 159 with end-organ effects

64. Which of the following statements is true for the patient with chronic mild-to-moderate hypertension?
A. Acute elevations in diastolic blood pressure will decrease cardiac afterload and myocardial workload
B. Aggressive management of the patient's blood pressure may impair his cerebral blood flow
C. The kidneys are subject to arteriolar vasodilation, which will decrease renal function
D. Excessive elevation of the patient's blood pressure produces cerebral hyperperfusion

65. The emergency physician orders labetalol 20 mg IV push for the patient. A possible side effect of this drug is:
A. Orthostatic hypotension
B. Tachycardia
C. Excessive salivation
D. Headache

66. The labetalol has not effectively lowered the patient's blood pressure. His chest pain continues, but a 12-lead ECG shows no acute changes with evidence of left ventricular hypertrophy. A nitroprusside drip is initiated at 0.2 mcg/kg/min. The most accurate blood pressure readings would be obtained by:
A. Placing a noninvasive blood pressure cuff on the patient's left arm
B. Placing a noninvasive blood pressure cuff on the patient's right arm
C. Inserting an arterial line for continuous blood pressure monitoring
D. Connecting the patient to a continuous 12-lead ECG monitor

67. A toxic effect of the long-term use of intravenous nitroprusside is:
A. Hypocalcemia leading to muscle weakness
B. Hyperkalemia leading to peaked T waves
C. Thiocyanate and cyanide toxicity
D. Bradycardia leading to asystole

68. The emergency physician prescribes hydrochlorothiazide (HydroDIURIL) 50 mg bid for a patient with newly diagnosed hypertension. The patient states, "I have never taken any medication for my blood pressure before." The emergency nurse should base discharge instructions on which of the following nursing diagnoses?
A. Knowledge deficit related to the use of a new drug for a newly diagnosed disease process
B. Body image disturbance related to physical changes that occur with hypertension
C. Thought processes, altered, related to the cerebral changes brought about by chronic hypertension
D. Family processes, altered, related to the need for a family member to take a new medication

69. The emergency nurse provides information to the patient about his disease process and refers him for follow-up care. Which of the following actions could the emergency nurse use to evaluate the effectiveness of this intervention?
A. The patient returns to the emergency department for follow-up care
B. The patient keeps his appointment at the hypertension clinic
C. The patient does not take his medicine and returns in a hypertensive crisis
D. The patient leaves his referral information at the emergency department

70. A 72-year-old male is brought to the emergency department by the local EMS. He was found unresponsive, and a CT scan demonstrates an acute ischemic cerebrovascular accident. His blood pressure is 180/110.

Which of the following statements is true related to the management of this patient's blood pressure?

A. Blood pressure management should be undertaken with medications with a long half-life to prevent the need for medication titration

B. Reducing the patient's blood pressure will ensure that he maintains adequate cerebral perfusion, thus decreasing the size of the stroke

C. Current recommendations from the American Heart Association state that blood pressure should be decreased only when the mean arterial pressure is greater than 130 mm Hg or systolic blood pressure (SBP) is greater than 220 mm Hg

D. Hypertension in acute ischemic stroke is a serious problem and may actually increase the size of the stroke, leading to further ischemic damage

Congestive Heart Failure

A family brings their 77-year-old mother to the emergency department. She was awakened by shortness of breath. On arrival in the emergency department she is alert, pale, diaphoretic, and extremely short of breath. Her B/P is 170/112, P 110, sinus tachycardia with an occasional PVC, R 30, and oxygen saturation 88% on room air. She has bilateral basilar crackles and is complaining of 8/10 chest pain. Her family states she was diagnosed 2 weeks ago with an acute myocardial infarction.

71. Which of the following disease processes most often contributes to congestive heart failure in the adult patient?

A. Cardiomyopathy
B. Congenital cardiac disease
C. Myocardial infarction
D. Atrial fibrillation

72. Morphine 4 mg is administered by IV push by the emergency nurse. Morphine is an effective drug for the patient with congestive heart failure because it:

A. Produces respiratory arrest
B. Produces myocardial depression
C. Increases the patient's heart rate
D. Reduces venous return

73. The emergency department physician prescribes a nesiritide infusion. One of the effects of this drug is that:

A. It will increase the patient's heart rate and oxygen consumption
B. It causes vasodilation of venous, arterial, and coronary vessels
C. It can cause lethal cardiac dysrhythmias such as ventricular fibrillation
D. It can be administered only by the oral route (not IV or IM) in the emergency department

74. The patient's blood gas results are as follows: pH 7.37, PCO_2 25, PO_2 60, and HCO_3- 18. Using the data collected from these blood gas results, which of the following nursing diagnoses would the emergency nurse use to base the initial care of this patient?

A. Fluid volume deficit related to diuresis with furosemide and fluid intake restrictions
B. Gas exchange, impaired, related to the patient's acute congestive heart failure
C. Activity tolerance related to the patient's normal oxygen tension and saturation
D. Tissue integrity, impaired, related to the patient's acute congestive heart failure

75. The patient's oxygen is changed from a nasal cannula to a 100% nonrebreather mask. In addition to arterial blood gases (ABGs), what other data could the emergency nurse use to evaluate improvement in the patient's condition?

A. Level of consciousness
B. Hemoglobin and hematocrit values
C. Urinary output
D. Palpation of peripheral pulses

76. Recent research has demonstrated that the emergency management of acute or decompensated heart failure in the emergency department should include the administration of:

A. Loop diuretic, nesiritide, and nitroglycerin
B. Beta-blockers, calcium channel blockers, and aldosterone receptor blockers
C. Ethacrynic acid, loop diuretics, and digitalis
D. Digitalis, beta-blockers, and loop diuretics

77. The best marker for identifying heart failure as the cause of a patient's shortness of breath is:
A. C-type natriuretic peptide
B. Atrial natriuretic peptide
C. N-terminal atrial natriuretic peptide
D. B-natriuretic peptide

Thrombophlebitis and Arteriovascular Disease

78. Risk factors that would contribute to the development of thrombosis include all of the following except:
A. Blood clots from cancer
B. Taking oral contraceptives
C. Chronic urinary tract infections
D. Prolonged bedrest

79. Signs and symptoms of venous thrombosis include:
A. No palpable peripheral pulses
B. Lack of pain in the affected extremity
C. Absence of Homans' sign
D. An extremity that is red, hot, and swollen

80. A 25-year-old patient with a history of DVT once again has an abnormal duplex ultrasonographic result. The patient is to be treated at home with enoxaparin (Lovenox) subcutaneously and warfarin orally. The advantages of low-molecular-weight heparin (enoxaparin) over unfractionated heparin include:
A. Enoxaparin has a shorter half-life than heparin
B. Enoxaparin has a predictable anticoagulant response
C. Enoxaparin has lower bioavailability than heparin
D. Enoxaparin can only be administered orally

81. The patient is taught how to administer the enoxaparin subcutaneously. She performs the return demonstration well. What other instructions should the patient be able to demonstrate with full understanding before discharge from the emergency department?
A. Because the patient is on anticoagulant therapy, she may resume her normal physical activities without concern of additional injury
B. If excessive bruising develops around the injection site, she should ignore it because that is a common side effect of anticoagulation medications
C. Complete blood counts, platelet count, and stool for occult blood test should be performed periodically to monitor her treatment course
D. If she has any blood in her stool, this should not be reported until it has occurred for several days or turns from black to bright red

82. The advantage of using the international normalized ratio (INR) to monitor warfarin therapy instead of a prothrombin time includes:
A. It can only be used to monitor anticoagulant therapy for patients taking warfarin for the management of pulmonary embolus
B. It is reliable anywhere the patient may require treatment, allowing the patient more flexibility during the course of treatment
C. It is governed by the sensitivity of the reagents used to measure the effectiveness of the amount of warfarin the patient is taking
D. There is no advantage to using INR over prothrombin time to monitor the effectiveness of anticoagulant therapy

83. An 82-year-old man is brought to the emergency department because of severe pain in his left leg from his groin downward. He has a history of atrial fibrillation and hypertension. He states that the pain began suddenly when he got out of bed prior to arrival in the emergency department. The physical examination of a patient with an acute arterial occlusion would reveal:
A. Palpable peripheral pulses
B. A red, warm extremity
C. A pale, cold extremity
D. Intermittent claudication

84. The patient's leg is pale and cold. No pulses are palpated and the patient is in severe pain. The emergency nurse should prepare the patient with an acute arterial occlusion for:
A. An invasive procedure to relieve the occlusion, such as percutaneous transluminal angioplasty or a thromboendarterectomy

B. Anticoagulant therapy using low-molecular-weight heparin as an outpatient, with an appointment with a surgeon within 24 hours
C. Application of a posterior splint to immobilize the extremity until he can be seen in the surgical clinic within 24 hours
D. Application of antiembolic hose to decrease the risk of pulmonary embolus and pressure ulcers on the effected extremity

85. The appropriate nursing diagnosis on which the emergency nurse should base the care of this patient is:
A. Gas exchange, impaired, related to an acute arterial occlusion
B. Tissue perfusion, altered (peripheral), related to an acute arterial occlusion
C. Fluid volume deficit related to an acute arterial occlusion
D. Disuse syndrome, potential for, related to an acute arterial occlusion of a lower extremity

Digitalis Toxicity

A 4-year-old child has ingested an unknown amount of his grandmother's digitalis. The family is unsure when the child took the pills. He is currently awake, nauseated, and vomiting.

86. The most common dysrhythmia seen in patients with digitalis toxicity that do not have cardiac disease is:
A. Ventricular bigeminy
B. Ventricular tachycardia
C. Sinus bradycardia
D. AV junctional tachycardia

87. The child's monitor shows a sinus bradycardia. He progresses to a third-degree block with a blood pressure of 70/40. Which drug should the emergency team administer?
A. Lidocaine 1 mg/kg IV push
B. Isoproterenol drip of 4 mg in 250 D_5W IV
C. Atropine 0.5 mg IV push
D. Epinephrine 0.1 mg/kg IV push

88. Digibind is to be administered to this child. All of the following are indications for the use of digoxin-specific antibody fragments except:
A. Cardiac arrest from digitalis toxicity
B. Bradydysrhythmia unresponsive to atropine
C. Severe hyperkalemia
D. Conversion to sinus rhythm after atropine administration

89. Plants that contain cardiac glycosides include all of the following except:
A. Foxglove plant
B. Lily of the valley
C. Ramp
D. Hellebore

Cardiac Trauma

A 24-year-old man is brought to the emergency department following an accident in which he was struck by a car while riding his bicycle. The patient was thrown from the bike, landing on his chest. He was wearing a helmet. On arrival in the emergency department the patient is awake, moving all his extremities and complaining of midsternal chest pain. His vital signs are B/P 100/79, P 132, R 28.

90. One of the most common signs associated with myocardial contusion is:
A. Chest wall contusion
B. Pericardial effusion
C. Multiple lower rib fractures
D. Abdominal wall contusion

91. Laboratory studies that may assist in the identification of a myocardial contusion include:
A. Troponin I level
B. Clotting studies
C. Liver function tests
D. Serial hematocrit values

92. Beck's triad includes:
A. Increased blood pressure, distended neck veins, and muffled heart sounds
B. Decreased blood pressure, distended neck veins, and muffled heart sounds
C. Decreased blood pressure, flat neck veins, and audible heart sounds
D. Increased blood pressure, flat neck veins, and muffled heart sounds

93. A 52-year-old mother was stabbed in the upper left chest by her son, who believed she was a vampire. Upon arrival in the emergency department, she is alert and oriented but deteriorates quickly. The patient is hypotensive, has distended neck veins, and is still breathing. Bilateral breath sounds are auscultated.

The emergency nurse should prepare the patient for:
A. Needle decompression
B. Pericardiocentesis
C. Chest radiograph
D. Insertion of a CVP line

94. A 7-year-old boy was brought to the emergency department in full arrest. He was playing baseball and was struck in the chest with a baseball. He immediately collapsed, and bystander CPR was initiated. He was transported in a private car to the emergency department. Monitoring showed him to be in ventricular fibrillation. Despite aggressive resuscitation, including an open thoracotomy, the child expired. The most likely cause of his arrest is:
A. Pulmonary contusion from the ball that struck him in the chest
B. Cardiac concussion from a blunt blow to the chest
C. Cerebral embolus from being struck with the ball
D. Congenital cardiac problem brought on by playing baseball

95. A 24-year-old man has been brought to the emergency department with a stab wound in his midsternum. Initially awake, he has become unresponsive. He has a palpable pulse. The emergency nurse should prepare the patient for:
A. Insertion of a trauma catheter
B. Insertion of bilateral chest tubes
C. Emergency thoracotomy
D. Insertion of a CVP line

96. A 19-year-old woman is brought to the emergency department after having been involved in a head-on collision with a truck. She was entrapped for over an hour and has obvious signs of severe chest trauma. All of the following would indicate an aortic injury except:
A. Chest wall bruising
B. A first rib fracture
C. The trachea in the midline
D. Paraplegia

97. An 85-year-old woman comes to the emergency department with a complaint of severe abdominal pain. Her vital signs are B/P 110/40, P 100, R 24. Upon physical examination, a palpable pulsating mass is felt in her lower abdomen. The patient will need to be transferred to another facility for further treatment. What medications may be used to manage the patient's pain?
A. Esmolol to decrease the patient's blood pressure, which will decrease the pressure on the arterial wall and relieve her pain
B. Morphine sulfate for analgesia and a benzodiazepine to manage her anxiety related to being transferred
C. Norepinephrine to increase her blood pressure and decrease the risk of shock, which may cause further vasoconstriction and pain
D. No pain medication should ever be given to a patient with an aortic aneurysm

98. Cardiac arrest due to electrolyte abnormalities results from:
A. Hypercalcemia
B. Hypernatremia
C. Hyperkalemia
D. Hyperphosphatemia

99. A 20-year-old man was working on some electrical connections in his house. His friends found him unresponsive and called 911. Initial treatment of this patient would include:
A. Securing the patient's airway through endotracheal intubation
B. Starting chest compressions after checking for a pulse
C. Defibrillating the patient before connecting him to the monitor
D. Turning off the electrical power before rescue attempts are started

100. Which of the following is the most effective method of managing hyperkalemia in the emergency department?
A. Peritoneal dialysis
B. Administration of sodium polystyrene sulfonate (Kayexalate)
C. Administration of insulin and glucose
D. Administration of calcium chloride

ANSWERS

1. **C. Intervention.** The patency of the endotracheal tube should be evaluated before performing any of the other stated interventions. Hypoxia must be avoided in order to provide

the patient the greatest chance of survival and prevention of hypoxic injuries.[11]

2. **D. Assessment and Analysis.** The causes of sudden cardiac arrest are many and complex. Causes include hypoglycemia, pulmonary embolus, electrolyte imbalance such as hyperkalemia and hypocalcemia, drug induced from tricyclic agent toxicity, narcotic overdose, tension pneumothorax, structural heart disease, hypertrophic cardiomyopathy, and congenital anomalies. These are only a small number of causes.[5,12]
3. **C. Intervention.** Vasopressin should be administered at a dose of 40 units IV as a single dose.[10]
4. **B. Intervention.** CPR should not be started if there is a valid order not to attempt resuscitation; if there are obvious signs of death such as rigor mortis, dependent livedo, or injuries incompatible with life; or if the rescuer's life may be put at risk. That would not negate starting CPR in transport, as long as the provider could be safe during at-risk periods, for example in air medical transport on take-off and landings, when restraints are required.[10]
5. **C. Intervention.** After administration of epinephrine, defibrillation should be attempted at 360 J within 30 to 60 seconds.[10]
6. **C. Assessment.** The pain pattern described by the patient having a myocardial infarction is usually sudden in onset, crushing, and substernal; the pain may radiate to the patient's neck, jaw, and back.[5]
7. **D. Assessment.** Personality type is no longer considered a risk factor.[10]
8. **D. Assessment.** ST segment elevation indicates injury, T wave inversion indicates ischemia, and pathological Q waves indicate infarction.[5]
9. **A. Assessment.** ST elevation in leads V_2, V_3, and V_4 is indicative of an anterior infarction.[2,5] ST elevation in II, III, and AVF is indicative of an inferior infarction. ST elevation in leads I, aV_F, V_5, and V_6 is indicative of a lateral infarction. Leads showing wave changes in V_1 and V_2, a tall, broad initial R wave, ST segment depression, and a tall upright T wave would indicate a posterior infarction.[5,10]
10. **B. Intervention.** All blood should be drawn before administration of fibrinolytic agents; however, reteplase is given in two 10-unit doses. When administering reteplase, normal saline should be administered before and after the drug is given.[5]
11. **C. Evaluation.** Accelerated idioventricular rhythm is frequently associated with reperfusion. The usual rate is 60 to 100 beats per minute.[10]
12. **B. Assessment.** The most common complication of thrombolytic therapy is bleeding. Intracranial hemorrhage is the most dangerous complication of thrombolytic therapy.[5]
13. **B. Assessment.** Women who have had a myocardial infarction and are treated with fibrinolytic agents have a greater incidence of having a stroke.[13]
14. **B. Evaluation.** Because intracranial hemorrhage is one of the most serious complications of thrombolytic therapy, it is important that the emergency nurse assess the patient for changes in level of consciousness, nausea and vomiting, headache, and confusion.[12]
15. **B. Intervention.** If during the course of infusion of fibrinolytic agents the patient should exhibit signs and symptoms of intracerebral hemorrhage, the emergency nurse should immediately stop the infusions and notify the emergency physician.[12]
16. **C. Analysis.** Because the patient is receiving a drug that has several serious potential side effects, the emergency nurse's care needs to be directed at preventing any injury that could result. Examples of this prevention are drawing blood from the intravenous site, minimizing the number of intravenous sites, minimizing the number of punctures, and performing invasive procedures such as a urinary catheter insertion before the administration of the drug.[14]
17. **A. Assessment.** TNK-tissue plasminogen activator has more fibrin specificity. It is a direct activator of plasminogen, converting it to plasmin.[5]
18. **C. Intervention.** Pain stimulates the release of catecholamines, which can lead to additional oxygen demands on an already compromised myocardium.[1,5]
19. **A. Analysis.** The defining characteristics of this nursing diagnosis include increased tension, verbalization of fear, decreased self-assurance, and sympathetic stimulation. A related factor that would contribute to the use of this nursing diagnosis is that the patient is separated from his support system in a potentially life-threatening situation.[14]

20. **B. Evaluation.** One of the expected outcomes for emergency nursing interventions related to this diagnosis would be that the patient is able to verbalize his feelings about the source of his fear and how he is able to deal with it.[14]
21. **B. Intervention.** Right ventricular infarction occurs in about 40% of patients who suffer inferior wall myocardial infarctions. Management of the hypotension that occurs with right ventricular infarction is the administration of fluids.[5]
22. **B. Assessment.** Right ventricular infarcts are diagnosed by the changes seen in the right-sided precordial lead recordings of an ECG.[5]
23. **C. Assessment.** The diagnosis of an acute myocardial infarction is based on three factors: history, clinical examination, and a 12-lead ECG. The history and clinical evaluation help the emergency nurse identify risk factors for heart disease, such as smoking and hypertension. A 12-lead ECG recording may show ischemia, injury, or infarction.[5]
24. **C. Intervention.** The benefits of nitroglycerin in the management of myocardial infarction include a reduction in myocardial oxygen consumption, an increase in flow to ischemic myocardium, and a decrease in coronary artery spasm.[15]
25. **B. Intervention.** Nitroglycerin administered in large, inappropriate doses may cause reflex tachycardia, which will increase myocardial oxygen consumption.[15]
26. **B. Intervention.** The absorption of heparin varies from patient to patient. Weight-based heparin helps to ensure that the patient is receiving an effective dosage.[15,16]
27. **D. Analysis.** The World Health Organization definition of the diagnosis of an acute myocardial infarction includes (1) ST segment changes and new Q waves, (2) chest pain characteristics, and (3) abnormally elevated serum cardiac enzyme levels. However, some patients experience acute myocardial infarctions with no ECG changes or chest pain. Myoglobin may also be elevated by strenuous exercise, renal failure, IM injections, or heavy use of alcohol. The patient's age and sex also may influence myoglobin levels.[9]
28. **B. Intervention.** Research continues to demonstrate that in order to improve cerebral and cardiovascular perfusion, a new approach must be taken toward resuscitation. This includes the use of a three-phase time-sensitive model of resuscitation. The electrical phase of arrest occurs within 4 minutes of the onset of ventricular fibrillation, for which defibrillation will work best. In the circulatory phase (4 to 10 minutes post arrest), oxygen delivery should precede attempts to normalize the cardiac rhythm. After 10 minutes of arrest, interventions should be directed at controlling reperfusion in order to decrease the additional damage that can occur from resuscitation.[11]
29. **B. Assessment.** Preload is measured in the right side of the heart by the right atrial pressure or the central venous pressure. This reflects the blood being returned from the systemic circulation.[1]
30. **D. Assessment.** Systemic vascular resistance is increased by compensatory constriction of peripheral blood vessels caused by epinephrine.[5]
31. **B. Intervention.** Metoprolol is a beta-blocker, and its effects provide a protective mechanism for an injured myocardium by decreasing the heart rate, oxygen consumption, and metabolic demand.[15]
32. **B. Intervention.** Abciximab (ReoPro) is a glycoprotein IIb/IIIa receptor inhibitor. This drug inhibits platelet aggregation by binding with the site where fibrinogen binds when platelets are activated. This stops platelet aggregation and thrombus formation. Research has demonstrated that glycoprotein IIb/IIIa receptor inhibitors, along with aspirin and weight-based heparin, are effective in preventing thrombosis.[17,18]
33. **A. Intervention.** Administration of platelets will inhibit the antiplatelet effect of glycoprotein IIb/IIIa receptor inhibitors. Protamine zinc is the antidote for heparin, and clopidogrel is an oral antiplatelet drug.[18]
34. **D. Evaluation.** Congestive heart failure after acute myocardial infarction is becoming a growing and costly epidemic in the United States. Approximately 20% of patients who suffer a myocardial infarction will develop congestive heart failure within 6 years of the event. The annual cost of caring for patients with congestive heart failure is estimated to be more than $35 billion. This points to the important role emergency nurses can play in

early recognition of potential myocardial injury and the need to teach preventive strategies such as diet, exercise, and blood pressure management to at-risk patients who come to the emergency department for care.[19]

35. **B. Intervention.** Bolus administration of fibrinolytic agents offers some advantages over continuous infusion, including ease of administration and less risk of a medication error because the dosage does not have to be adjusted for patient weight. However, the longer half-life of these other fibrinolytics make it more difficult to reverse the effects of bleeding complications.[20]
36. **C. Intervention.** Resuscitation may be withheld in the following circumstances: patients who have a clear advance directive asking health care workers not to begin resuscitation in the event of a cardiac arrest, and patients with signs of irreversible death such as rigor mortis or decapitation.[10]
37. **B. Assessment.** Aspirin targets the platelet, and fibrinolytic therapy targets the fibrin component of the clot.[20]
38. **D. Intervention.** When electrical activity is detected but no pulse is palpated, the patient is in pulseless electrical activity (PEA). When the patient is in PEA, the emergency nurse needs to consider the possibility of hypovolemia, cardiac tamponade, tension pneumothorax, acidosis, pulmonary embolism, and hypoxemia, as well as what interventions could be used to correct any of these possible causes of PEA.[10]
39. **B. Assessment.** The patient is in atrial fibrillation with a rapid ventricular response.
40. **D. Intervention.** Electrical cardioversion has been recommended as one of the safest ways to restore normal rhythm. The paddles should be placed anteroposteriorly. The timing of the cardioversion may improve its effectiveness. Application of the energy when the patient has exhaled reduces pulmonary resistance to the current. The current guidelines also recommend the use of biphasic energy, because it transfers more efficiently to the atrial tissues, leading to use of lower cumulative energy discharge.[21]
41. **A. Assessment.** Ventricular tachycardia.
42. **B. Intervention.** Amiodarone is administered in three phases: rapid infusion of 150 mg over 10 minutes, early maintenance infusion 1 mg/min for 6 hours, and late maintenance infusion 0.5 mg/min for 18 hours.[10]
43. **C. Evaluation.** Hypotension is the most common side effect of amiodarone. It is not dose related.[15]
44. **D. Intervention.** Torsades de pointes should be considered when patients display ventricular tachycardia refractory to management with lidocaine and amiodarone. Magnesium sulfate may abolish torsades. It is administered IV for 1 to 2 minutes at a dosage of 1 to 2 g. Up to 4 to 6 g may be administered to treat torsades.[10]
45. **A. Assessment.** Asystole.
46. **D. Intervention.** Lidocaine, atropine, naloxone, and epinephrine can be administered via the endotracheal tube.[10]
47. **C. Assessment.** Third-degree heart block.
48. **C. Evaluation.** A common problem with an external pacemaker in the conscious patient is pain from the muscle spasms caused by the pacemaker. Patients may need to be sedated until a transvenous pacemaker can be placed.[22,23]
49. **A. Evaluation.** A palpable pulse demonstrates that there has been mechanical capture. Pacemaker spikes on the monitor demonstrate electrical capture but not mechanical capture or functional myocardial contraction.[10,23]
50. **C. Intervention.** The battery may be low and not generating enough power to effectively pace the heart. Adding a set of pacemaker pads would not be helpful, but changing the current pads and repositioning them may increase the chance of capture.[23]
51. **C. Intervention.** Adenosine slows conduction through the AV node. It is indicated for the management of paroxysmal supraventricular tachycardia because it can interrupt the reentry pathway and restore sinus rhythm.[10]
52. **D. Intervention.** If there is no change in the patient's rhythm 1 to 2 minutes after administration of the adenosine, the next step is to double the dose to 12 mg.[10]
53. **D. Analysis.** Adenosine causes conversion dysrhythmia, including sinus bradycardia, heart block, and a brief period of asystole. If the patient is not warned about this side effect, it can be very frightening. In addition, many patients complain of feeling warm and experience flushing, another common side effect.[10]
54. **A. Assessment.** Atrial fibrillation.

55. **C. Assessment.** Atrial fibrillation leaves the patient at risk for developing clots and emboli. If they enter the circulation, these may result in a transient ischemic attack or stroke.[5]
56. **C. Intervention.** Amiodarone is recommended for pharmacological management of atrial fibrillation when the situation is acute.[20]
57. **B. Intervention.** Synchronized cardioversion is the treatment of choice for a child with unstable tachydysrhythmia. The recommended dose is 0.5 to 1 J/kg.[24]
58. **D. Intervention.**
59. **B. Intervention.** The child should receive oxygen and measures to keep her calm to decrease her oxygen consumption.[2,24]
60. **C. Intervention.** The paddle position for the patient who has an implanted cardioverter defibrillator is the anteroposterior position. The batteries of the LVAD should be disconnected before defibrillation.[25,26]
61. **A. Intervention.** Isoproterenol is recommended for the management of bradycardia in the denervated transplanted heart. It has both inotropic and chronotropic properties. The dosage needed for chronotropic support in complete heart block begins at 2 mcg/min and should not exceed 10 mcg/min. Because isoproterenol markedly increases myocardial oxygen demand, it should be used only temporarily.[4,27,28] It is also important to note here that in the 1999 International Liaison Committee on Resuscitation Advisory Statements: Special Resuscitation Situations,[23] the treatment for brady asystolic rhythms in a denervated heart is administration of an adenosine-blocking agent such as aminophylline 250 mg IV bolus if pacing, atropine, and epinephrine fail.
62. **B. Intervention.** When a patient with an LVAD loses his pulse, the emergency nurse should not initiate cardiac compressions because it may disconnect the device. The family should have a hand pump available and the device should be pumped by hand, but the patient's abdomen should be felt to determine whether the device is working. The pump mechanism of the device is surgically implanted in the left upper abdomen with the inflow cannula attached to the left ventricle and the outflow cannula to the ascending aorta. If the patient requires defibrillation, the LVAD batteries should be disconnected.[29]
63. **C. Assessment.** From the National High Blood Pressure Education Program, hypertension is classified in stages:
    - Stage 1 (mild) SBP 140 to 159 or DBP 90 to 99
    - Stage 2 (moderate) SBP 160 to 179 or DBP 100 to 109
    - Stage 3 (severe) SBP ≥180 or DBP ≥110[27]
64. **B. Assessment.** Complications of hypertension include papilledema, left ventricular hypertrophy, congestive heart failure, impaired renal function, and intracranial or subarachnoid hemorrhage.[30,31]
65. **A. Evaluation.** Side effects of labetalol include orthostatic hypotension at the beginning of therapy, facial flushing, dry mouth, bradycardia, and fatigue.[15]
66. **C. Intervention.** When a nitroprusside infusion is initiated, an arterial line should be inserted to provide the most accurate assessment of the patient's blood pressure.[5]
67. **C. Analysis.** Toxic side effects of long-term infusions of nitroprusside are thiocyanate and cyanide toxicity.[15]
68. **A. Analysis.** The defining characteristics of this nursing diagnosis include verbalization of inadequate information about one's illness and the patient's requesting information about the disease process. Related factors include lack of exposure to accurate information, lack of motivation to learn, and cultural and language barriers.[14]
69. **B. Evaluation.** The expected outcome for nursing interventions related to this diagnosis would be the patient following through as instructed.[16]
70. **C. Intervention.** Research has demonstrated that hypertension may actually be a protective mechanism in acute ischemic stroke and should not be treated unless the mean arterial pressure is greater than 130 mm Hg or SBP is greater than 220 mm Hg. Decreasing the blood pressure may actually lead to further ischemic damage.[21]
71. **C. Assessment.** Congestive heart failure is a common consequence of acute myocardial infarction. As many as 20% of patients who suffer a myocardial infarction will develop congestive heart failure. Because of the increased incidence of congestive heart failure, it is being viewed as a serious epidemic in this country and costs billions of dollars each year in patient care.[5,27]

72. **D. Intervention.** Morphine produces peripheral vasodilation that decreases preload and helps in decreasing myocardial oxygen consumption.[15]
73. **B. Intervention.**
74. **B. Analysis.** Based on the data provided by the blood gas analysis, the patient is hypoxic, probably as a result of impairment of gas exchange. Related factors contributing to this nursing diagnosis include alveolar capillary membrane changes and altered capacity of the blood to carry oxygen.[14]
75. **A. Evaluation.** Defining characteristics of gas exchange, impaired, include confusion, restlessness, hypoxia, and irritability. Evaluation of the patient's level of consciousness would provide information about the effect of 100% oxygen delivery by mask.[15]
76. **A. Intervention.** Based on the recommendations of the Stat Heart Failure Consensus Panel, the care of the patient with acute or compensated heart failure in the emergency department should include oxygen, loop diuretic, nesiritide, and nitroglycerin or nitroprusside.[28,31]
77. **D. Assessment.** The natriuretic peptides are promising markers that can help discover the cause of a patient's shortness of breath when the cause is not clear. Because not every emergency department has the equipment, such as a cardiac catheterization lab, to make a rapid diagnosis of heart failure, emergency department diagnosis generally is based on history, physical examination, chest radiograph, and ECG. Natriuretic peptides are secreted by the heart in response to hemodynamic stress, such as the stretching that occurs with heart failure. B-type natriuretic peptide is the marker currently used to differentiate the diagnosis of heart failure in dyspnea.[28,31]
78. **C. Assessment.** Risk factors or common causes for blood clots are prolonged immobility, an inherited tendency for blood clots, pregnancy, and use of contraceptives.[5]
79. **D. Assessment.** Signs and symptoms of venous thrombosis include swelling; a red, warm extremity; Homans' sign; and pain that may be aggravated by walking.[5]
80. **B. Analysis.** The advantages of low-molecular-weight heparin over unfractionated heparin include its predictable anticoagulant response, high bioavailability, and longer half-life, which require fewer daily doses. Absorption of heparin varies from patient to patient.[15,32,33]
81. **C. Evaluation.** The patient who is being treated for DVT at home must demonstrate a thorough understanding of how the medications work, their potential side effects, allowed physical activities, and how the medication should be monitored. Any excessive bruising or bleeding must be reported immediately. Periodic complete blood count, platelet level, and stool guaiac test should be performed.[15]
82. **B. Analysis.** The INR is reliable anywhere. Prothrombin time results vary from place to place and even sometimes within the same lab, depending on the reagents used. The INR can be used to monitor the effectiveness of warfarin and low-molecular-weight heparin in the management of DVT or pulmonary emboli and for prevention of systemic emboli from myocardial infarction, atrial fibrillation, or mechanical valves.[33]
83. **C. Assessment.** The physical examination of an extremity that has an acute arterial occlusion would show a cool, pale limb; pain; changes in motor and sensory function; lack of pulses distal to the occlusion; and slow capillary filling.[34,35]
84. **A. Intervention.** Management of acute arterial occlusion is surgical removal of the clot, or embolectomy. The quicker the occlusion is relieved, the better the patient will do. However, if surgery is delayed, the patient may be started on a regimen of heparin.[35]
85. **B. Analysis.** The defining characteristics of this nursing diagnosis include decreased or absent arterial pulses, pale extremities, cold extremities, loss of motor or sensory function, and pain.[14]
86. **C. Assessment.** Digitalis toxicity can cause numerous types of cardiac dysrhythmia even in the patient who does not have preexisting cardiac disease (such as the pediatric patient), especially AV conduction disturbances. The patient with cardiovascular disease is more likely to have a lethal dysrhythmia.[36,37]
87. **C. Intervention.** Atropine is the drug of choice. The recommended dose is 0.5 mg to 2 mg IV.[36,37]
88. **D. Intervention.** Digibind, or digoxin-specific antibody fragments, is indicated for the management of life-threatening digitalis

overdose. Digibind works by increasing the speed of excretion and reversing tissue affinity for digitalis.[37]

89. **C. Assessment.** Plant toxicity can be a source of many types of problems. Some plants contain toxins that affect the heart in the same manner as cardiac glycosides do. These include the foxglove plant, lily of the valley, and hellebore.[26]
90. **A. Assessment.** The most common sign or symptom of myocardial contusion is sinus tachycardia. Other signs and symptoms of myocardial contusion include severe chest pain, chest wall contusion, hypotension, and dyspnea.[26]
91. **A. Evaluation.**
92. **B. Assessment.** Beck's triad includes decreased blood pressure, distended jugular veins, and muffled heart sounds. These signs may be indicative of cardiac tamponade.[26,38,39]
93. **B. Intervention.**
94. **B. Assessment.** Cardiac concussion is a rare occurrence. It results from a blunt blow to the chest, such as being struck by a baseball. The dysrhythmia caused by cardiac concussion is very hard to convert, and the mortality rate is high.[38]
95. **C. Intervention.** Thoracotomy is indicated for penetrating cardiac trauma, tension pneumothorax, and crush injuries to the chest.[37]
96. **C. Assessment.** Indications of aortic injury include first and second rib fractures, signs of hypovolemic shock, tracheal deviation to the right, chest wall bruising, paraplegia, and sternal fracture.[26]
97. **B. Intervention.** The patient with an aortic aneurysm should receive both pain management and blood pressure management, when indicated. The patient's blood pressure should be maintained between 100 and 120 mm Hg. Because her vital signs are adequate, her pain should be managed with an analgesic and a sedative to prevent any further detrimental side effects from pain.[5,26]
98. **C. Assessment.** Cardiac arrests from electrolyte abnormalities are not very common except for hyperkalemia. Hyperkalemia can be identified by ECG changes (peaked T waves, bradycardia) and by history (presence of renal failure).[10]
99. **D. Intervention.** The electrical power or the energy source must be stopped before rescue is attempted.[5]
100. **D. Intervention.** Administration of calcium chloride 5 to 10 ml of 10% solution, which is a potassium antagonist, will work in 1 to 3 minutes and last 30 to 60 minutes.[10]

References

1. McCance KL, Huether SE: *Pathophysiology: the biological basis for disease in adults and children,* St Louis, 2002, Mosby.
2. Thomas DO, Bernardo LM, Herman B: *Core curriculum for pediatric emergency nursing,* Boston, 2003, Jones and Bartlett.
3. Bickley LS: *Bates: a guide to physical examination and history taking,* Philadelphia, 2002, Lippincott.
4. Newman P: Trauma in the elderly. In Neff J, Kidd P, editors: *Trauma nursing: the art and science,* St Louis, 1993, Mosby.
5. Barnason S: Cardiovascular emergencies. In Newberry L, editor: *Sheehy's emergency nursing: principles and practice,* St Louis, 2003, Mosby.
6. Smith DD: Acute coronary syndromes in the emergency department: new millennium, new mentality, *J Emerg Nurs* 26:535-538, 2000.
7. Howland-Gradman J, Kitt S: Cardiac emergencies. In Kitt S, Selfridge-Thomas J, Proehl J et al, editors: *Emergency nursing: a physiologic and clinical perspective,* Philadelphia, 1995, WB Saunders.
8. Gallagher EJ: Angioplasty versus intravenous thrombolysis for acute myocardial infarction, *Ann Emerg Med* 39:299-301, 2002.
9. McCord J, Nowak RM, Hudson MP et al: The prognostic significance of serial myoglobin, troponin 1, and creatine kinase-MB measurements in patients evaluated in the ED for acute coronary syndrome, *Ann Emerg Med* 42:343-350, 2003.
10. American Heart Association: *ACLS provider manual,* Dallas, 2002, American Heart Association.
11. Callans DJ: Management of the patient who has been resuscitated from sudden cardiac death, *Circulation* 105:2704-2707, 2002.
12. Kosnik L: Treatment protocols and pathways: improving the process of care, *Crit Care Nurse* 19(5 suppl):3-7, 1999.
13. Pickett S: Women, thrombolytic therapy, and the gender gap: recommendations for practice, *J Emerg Nurs* 19:491-497, 1993.
14. Kim M, McFarland G, McLane A: *Pocket guide to nursing diagnoses,* St Louis, 1993, Mosby.

15. *Mosby's drug consult 2005,* St Louis, 2005, Mosby.
16. Horvanessian H: New-generation anticoagulants: the low molecular weight heparins, *Ann Emerg Med* 34(6):768-779, 1999.
17. MacCallum E, Hanlon S, Byrne K: How glycoprotein inhibitors ease coronary syndromes, *Nursing 99* 29(12):34-40, 1999.
18. Gibler BW, Wilcox RG, Bodie C et al: Prospective use of glycoprotein IIb/IIIa receptor blockers in the emergency department setting, *Ann Emerg Med* 32(6):712-722, 1998.
19. Moser DK, Frazier SK, Worster PL et al: The role of the critical care nurse in preventing heart failure after acute myocardial infarction, *Crit Care Nurse* 19(5 suppl):11-15, 1999.
20. Dracup K, Cannon C: Combination treatment strategies for management of acute myocardial infarction: new directions with current therapies, *Crit Care Nurse* (suppl):3-17, 1999.
21. Aizer A, Fuster V: Atrial fibrillation, WebMD Scientific American Medicine 2004, WebMed.
22. Kloeck W, editor: *ILCOR advisory statements: special resuscitation situations,* Dallas, 1999, American Heart Association.
23. Gamarth B, Del Monte L, Richards K: Noninvasive pacing: what you should know, *J Emerg Nurs* 24(3):223-233, 1998.
24. Hazinski M: *PALS provider manual, Dallas,* 2002, American Heart Association.
25. Schuster DM: Patients with an implanted cardioverter: a new challenge, *J Emerg Nurs* 16:219-225, 1990.
26. Sherwood SF, Hartsock RL: Thoracic injuries. In McQuillan K, Von Rueden KT, Hartsock RL, Flynn MB, Whalen E, editors: *Trauma nursing: from resuscitation through rehabilitation,* ed 3, Philadelphia, 2002, WB Saunders.
27. Wellens JJ, Anton PG, deMunter H: Cardiac arrest outside of the hospital: can we improve results of resuscitation? *Circulation* 107:1948-1950, 2003.
28. Collins SP, Ronan-Bentle S, Storrow A: Diagnostic and prognostic usefulness of natriuretic peptides in the emergency department patients with dyspnea, *Ann Emerg Med* 41(4):532-545, 2003.
29. Bond EA, Nelson K, Germany CL et al: The left ventricular assist device, *Am J Nurs* 103(1):32-41, 2003.
30. Shayne PH, Pitts SR: Severely increased blood pressure in the emergency department, *Ann Emerg Med* 41(4):513-529, 2003.
31. Peacock WF: *Management of acute decompensated heart failure in the emergency department,* Cleveland, OH, 2003, UNITECH.
32. Zed PJ, Tisdale JE, Borzak S: Low-molecular-weight heparins in the management of acute coronary syndromes, *Arch Intern Med* 159:1849-1857, 1999.
33. Ortel L: Monitoring warfarin therapy: how the INR keeps your patient safe, *Nursing 99* 29:41-44, 1999.
34. Colucciello S: Protocols for deep vein thrombosis (DVT): a state-of-the-art review. Part II: patient management, anticoagulation, and special considerations, *Emerg Med Rep* 20(3):25-32, 1999.
35. Go S: Extremity pain. In Davis M, Votey S, Greenough P, editors: *Signs and symptoms in emergency medicine,* St Louis, 1999, Mosby.
36. Goodman LS: Digitalis. In Haddad L, Shannon M, Winchester J, editors: *Poisoning and drug overdose,* ed 3, Philadelphia, 1998, WB Saunders.
37. Edgerton PH: Symptoms of digitalis-like toxicity in a family after accidental ingestion of lily of the valley plant, *J Emerg Nurs* 15:220-223, 1989.
38. Flynn MB, Bonni S: Blunt chest trauma: case report, *Crit Care Nurse* 19:68-77, 1999.
39. Snyder O: A 17-year-old man with history of trauma and dizziness, *J Emerg Nurs* 24(4):371-373, 1998.

CHAPTER 5

DENTAL, EAR, NOSE, AND THROAT EMERGENCIES

REVIEW OUTLINE

I. Anatomy and physiology
   A. Anatomical structures
      1. Oral cavity and contents
      2. Deciduous and permanent teeth
      3. Pharynx
      4. Larynx
      5. Salivary glands
      6. Thyroid cartilage and gland
      7. Cricoid cartilage and membrane
      8. Trachea
      9. Mastoid process
      10. Nose, nasal cavity, and contents
      11. Four paranasal sinuses
      12. Temporomandibular joint
      13. External, middle, and inner ear
      14. Cranial nerves
   B. Physiology
      1. Process of taste
      2. Process of hearing
      3. Process of smell
      4. Process of mastication
      5. Process of swallowing

II. Assessment
   A. Primary survey
      1. ABCD
         a. Airway
         b. Breathing
         c. Circulation
         d. Deficit: neurological
      2. Stabilization
   B. Secondary survey
      1. History of illness or injury
         a. Mechanism and time
         b. AMPLE history
      2. Chief complaint
         a. Pain: PQRST
            (1) Provocation
            (2) Quality
            (3) Region and radiation
            (4) Severity
            (5) Temporal
         b. Bleeding
         c. Shortness of breath
         d. Edema or ecchymosis
         e. Foreign body
         f. Asymmetry
         g. Fever, chills
         h. Nausea, vomiting
         i. Dysphasia, dysphagia
         j. Paresthesia
         k. Foul odor or taste in mouth
         l. Loss of hearing
         m. Tinnitus or vertigo
         n. Trismus
         o. Loss of smell
         p. Deformity or dislocation
      3. Physical examination
         a. General appearance
         b. Teeth
            (1) Number and condition
            (2) Dental prosthesis
            (3) Gaps between existing teeth
         c. Gingiva
         d. Oral mucosa
         e. Lips
         f. Tongue
         g. Floor of mouth
         h. Hard palate
         i. Soft palate
         j. Salivary glands
         k. External ear
            (1) Position
            (2) Drainage
         l. Tympanic membrane
            (1) Intact
            (2) Abnormalities
         m. External nose
            (1) Position, size, symmetry
            (2) Drainage

n. Internal nose
   (1) Septum, turbinates, mucosa
   (2) Abnormalities
o. Neck
   (1) Symmetry of structures
   (2) Abnormalities
p. Palpation
   (1) Symmetry
   (2) Localized point tenderness
   (3) Abnormal mobility
   (4) Crepitus
   (5) Mobility of teeth
   (6) Temporomandibular joint mobility

III. Diagnostic methods for dental, ear, nose, and throat emergencies
   A. Radiology
   B. Laboratory
   C. Visualization
      1. Pharyngeal mirror
      2. Tongue blades
      3. Otoscope
      4. Nasal speculum
      5. Laryngeal mirror
      6. Suction

IV. Related nursing diagnoses
   A. Alteration in comfort, pain
   B. Anxiety
   C. Airway clearance, ineffective
   D. Fluid volume deficit, high risk for
   E. Infection, high risk for
   F. Nutrition, alteration in
   G. Sensory deficit

V. Age-related changes
   A. Pediatric patient
      1. Foreign bodies are common and should be considered in children under 3 years during ear, nose, and throat examinations[1]
   B. Geriatric patient
      1. Decrease in hearing due to aging process needs to be considered during assessment
      2. Most dental and ear, nose, and throat injuries are related to falls, motor vehicle accidents, and assaults[1]

VI. Dental, ear, nose, and throat emergencies
   A. Odontalgia
   B. Gingivitis
   C. Dental trauma
   D. Ludwig's angina
   E. Acute otitis media
   F. Ruptured tympanic membrane
   G. Ménière's disease
   H. Rhinitis
   I. Epistaxis
   J. Nasal fracture
   K. Pharyngitis
   L. Tonsillitis
   M. Fractured larynx
   N. Peritonsillar abscess

VII. Foreign bodies

Dental, ear, nose, and throat emergencies are not generally life-threatening emergencies unless there is a risk of airway obstruction from swelling, blood, or fluids. However, to the patient arriving in the emergency department with a chief complaint involving one of these structures, an emergent situation exists, because the patient or family (especially of a crying infant) believes the condition must be alleviated immediately. It is important for the emergency nurse to realize the patient's perception of an emergent situation and to intervene rapidly. By doing so, the nurse will meet the patient's and the family's needs and expectations and engender trust. Patients with dental, ear, nose, and throat emergencies frequently need education and referral to a specialist as part of their emergency care.

Dental, ear, nose, and throat conditions are emergent when they obstruct the airway, cause hypovolemia, or have the potential to cause permanent sensory loss.

REVIEW QUESTIONS

Odontalgia

Mr. Brown, a 19-year-old man, comes to the emergency department at 3:00 AM complaining of a severe toothache (odontalgia) for 1 week. His vital signs are as follows: B/P 130/80, P 90, and R 18. His skin is warm, pink, and dry.

1. Which is a serious complication of odontalgia?
   A. Pain when drinking a cold beverage
   B. Loss of the tooth from decay and damage
   C. Pain when drinking a hot beverage
   D. An abscess and facial cellulitis

2. The appropriate nursing diagnosis applicable to Mr. Brown is:
   A. Swallowing, impaired
   B. Fluid volume deficit, high risk for
   C. Alteration in comfort, pain
   D. Alteration in thought processes

3. The most appropriate nursing action would be to:
   A. Administer an analgesic agent
   B. Administer an antibiotic
   C. Administer an antiemetic drug
   D. Administer an antiinflammatory agent

4. A patient suffered a fractured tooth that exposed the dentin. Which of the following statements is true?
   A. The fractured tooth will appear chalky white
   B. This type of fracture is more serious in a child
   C. Cosmetic restoration is possible in 24 to 48 hours
   D. Bacteria cannot pass easily through this type of fracture

5. Baby Brown, 1 year old, is brought to the emergency department by his parents for a "cold." The parents report that the baby has a clear nasal discharge and is drooling, is irritable, and has trouble sleeping, a normal temperature, and reddened, swollen gums. You suspect:
   A. Epiglottitis
   B. Odontalgia
   C. Tooth eruption
   D. Nasal foreign body

A 43-year-old female is triaged to the Fast Track Area with the complaint of painful, swollen, and bleeding gums. She states that her teeth are "coming loose."

6. Systemic risk factors for periodontal disease include:
   A. Adequately fitting upper and lower dentures
   B. Good daily fluid and nutrient intake
   C. Untreated cardiovascular disease
   D. Pregnancy and hormone changes

7. No evidence of acute infection is identified after evaluation in the emergency department, and she is sent home and instructed to rinse her mouth with an over-the-counter mouthwash. She returns 48 hours later with extensive facial swelling and cellulitis over the lower part of her jaw. Her tongue is swollen, and she is complaining of difficulty swallowing and shortness of breath. The most probable cause of her symptoms is:
   A. Pericoronitis
   B. Vincent's disease
   C. Ludwig's angina
   D. Multiple dental abscesses

8. The emergency nurse should prepare for a potential:
   A. Circulatory compromise
   B. Airway compromise
   C. Neurological compromise
   D. Febrile seizure

Acute Otitis Media

An 18-month-old infant is brought to the emergency department by her parents for complaints of fever, irritability, vomiting, and diarrhea. The parents relate that the child has a history of frequent ear infections.

9. Risk factors that contribute to the development of recurrent otitis media in children include:
   A. Age older than 4 years
   B. Consistent care provided in the home
   C. Recent use of antimicrobial agents
   D. No previous antimicrobial treatment

Further assessment reveals a child who is awake with hot, moist skin and a purulent nasal discharge. Her vital signs are as follows: P 150, R 32, Temp 103.2° F (rectal).

10. Your priority nursing diagnosis for this child would be:
    A. Anxiety
    B. Hyperthermia
    C. Swallowing, impaired
    D. Airway clearance, ineffective

11. Which of the following statements is true about managing a foreign body that has lodged in a patient's ear?
    A. If the foreign body is of vegetable material, the ear should be irrigated with water to assist in removal of the material
    B. If there is an insect in the ear, it can be irrigated with mineral oil even if the tympanic membrane is not intact
    C. Patients who have had objects removed from the ear may be at risk for otitis externa and should be treated with combined antibiotic-cortisone ear drops
    D. Irrigation is one of the first things that should be tried to remove a foreign body, even if the tympanic membrane is ruptured

12. Symptomatic management of acute otitis media for a child who is clinically stable and not toxic may include:
A. Liquid aspirin 3 times a day
B. Steroid ear drops bought in the pharmacy
C. Warm ear drops to the affected ear
D. Ear cleaning with cotton-tipped applicators 3 times a day

Nosebleed (Fracture)

Ms. Lee, a 27-year-old woman, is admitted per Life Squad with severe epistaxis. She was the unrestrained passenger in the front seat of a car that was struck from behind. Ms. Lee's face reportedly struck the dashboard. She is awake and oriented. Her vital signs are as follows: B/P 110/70, P 92, and R 24. She is appropriately immobilized on a backboard with a cervical collar in place. Ms. Lee has an obvious nasal deformity and moderate nasal bleeding.

13. Your initial nursing assessment should be directed toward:
A. Patency of the patient's airway
B. Effectiveness of her breathing
C. Any changes in mental status
D. Obtaining a manual blood pressure

14. Ms. Lee's cervical spine is cleared, and her cervical collar and backboard are removed. Her nose continues to bleed. Your initial nursing intervention to stop the epistaxis should be:
A. Apply direct pressure
B. Prepare for cauterization
C. Provide a suction device
D. Prepare for nasal packing

15. Once the bleeding stops, Ms. Lee's nose should be inspected internally for:
A. Blood clots
B. Bone chips
C. A septal hematoma
D. Purulent discharge

16. Ms. Lee requests a mirror so she can look at her nose. Upon observation, Ms. Lee becomes very upset. An appropriate nursing diagnosis would be:
A. Knowledge deficit related to her injury
B. Pain related to a potential nasal fracture
C. Anxiety related to possible permanent alteration in facial appearance
D. High risk for injury related to the patient's behavior

17. Ms. Lee is referred to an ear, nose, and throat specialist for treatment after 48 hours, when the edema has subsided. To prevent further epistaxis during this 48-hour period, Ms. Lee should be instructed to:
A. Avoid cold food to prevent further bleeding
B. Take aspirin for the pain from her injury
C. Open her mouth when sneezing to relieve pressure
D. Blow her nose forcefully to remove all clots on a routine basis

Pharyngitis

Mr. Blue, age 31, comes to the triage desk with complaints of a sore throat for 5 days. Mr. Blue reports he has tried throat lozenges and aspirin for pain, but nothing has helped.

18. To assist in differentiating an urgent versus nonurgent condition, the triage nurse should ask Mr. Blue if he has had:
A. A sinus headache
B. Posterior neck tenderness
C. To lie flat in bed
D. Difficulty swallowing

Mr. Blue states he is having increasing difficulty swallowing. He is taken immediately into the emergency department for care. His vital signs are as follows: B/P 110/70, P 104, R 28, Temp 102° F. While assessing his vital signs you note that Mr. Blue is drooling.

19. Your initial nursing diagnosis for Mr. Blue would be:
A. Violence, high risk for
B. Infection, high risk for
C. Body image disturbance
D. Airway clearance, ineffective, high risk for

20. Mr. Blue is diagnosed as having a peritonsillar abscess. Your initial nursing intervention for Mr. Blue should be:
A. Have Mr. Blue lie flat on his side
B. Have Mr. Blue lie on his stomach
C. Elevate the head of the bed 60 to 90 degrees
D. Place Mr. Blue in Trendelenburg position

Mr. Blue is given oxygen, antibiotics, an analgesic, and an antipyretic agent. You realize the importance of monitoring Mr. Blue's respiratory status.

21. To evaluate the effectiveness of your nursing interventions, you would want to see:
A. Pale, diaphoretic skin
B. A decrease in pulse rate
C. A decrease in blood pressure
D. An increase in respiratory rate

22. The most effective tool in the prevention of epiglottitis is:
A. Administration of prophylactic antibiotics when other children become sick
B. Receiving recommended childhood immunizations in a timely manner
C. Taking large amounts of vitamin C during the cold and flu season each year
D. Providing a cool mist when the child sleeps at night

23. When antibiotic, antipyretic, and analgesic therapies are administered to manage epiglottitis, which of the following would indicate patient improvement?
A. An increase in drooling
B. An increase in capillary refill time
C. A decrease in blood pressure
D. A decrease in respiratory rate

Trauma

24. Mrs. Bush brings her 5-year-old son to the emergency department. He has a history of falling in the hospital parking lot and knocking his tooth out. She hands you the tooth. In order to "save" the tooth, you immerse it in:
A. Cold milk
B. Iced tap water
C. Normal saline
D. Lactated Ringer's solution

25. For successful reimplantation, the avulsed tooth should be reinserted into the socket within:
A. 15 minutes
B. 30 minutes
C. 60 minutes
D. 120 minutes

26. The most common cause of tympanic membrane rupture is:
A. Trauma
B. Infection
C. Self-induced
D. Exposure to a loud sound

27. A 15-year-old boy is brought to the triage desk by his parents. He is complaining of difficulty swallowing and a hoarse voice. He states that earlier in the day he was struck in the throat by a baseball bat during a game. You suspect:
A. Fractured larynx
B. Peritonsillar abscess
C. Cervical spine injury
D. Upper respiratory tract infection

28. Your triage classification of this adolescent is:
A. Urgent
B. Emergent
C. Nonurgent
D. Delayed care

29. Objective signs of a fractured larynx include:
A. Normal respiratory rate
B. Neck swelling or edema
C. Distended neck veins
D. Oxygen saturation of 100%

30. Palpation of the neck when the larynx has been injured would reveal:
A. No tenderness in the injured area
B. Subcutaneous emphysema
C. Normal tracheal position
D. Normal and equal breath sounds

ANSWERS

1. **D. Assessment.** An abscess and facial cellulitis will require more aggressive management. The patient is at risk for tooth and jaw bone loss and for developing a systemic infection.[1,2]
2. **C. Analysis.** Fluid volume deficit is a potential problem for Mr. Brown if his tooth is sensitive to hot or cold, causing him to decrease his fluid intake. However, a review of his vital signs and skin signs demonstrates that he is not dehydrated at this time.[1]
3. **A. Intervention.** Because it is 3:00 AM, the patient's most obvious need is pain relief. After this primary need is met, associated needs can be addressed.[1]
4. **B. Assessment.** This type of fracture is more serious in a child, because there is little dentin to protect the pulp. With this type of fracture, bacteria can pass easily into the pulp to cause an abscess.[1,2]

5. **C. Assessment.** Baby Brown has classic signs of tooth eruption. These patients frequently are seen in the emergency department with first-time parents.[1,2]
6. **D. Assessment.** Systemic risk factors that contribute to periodontal disease include pregnancy, diabetes mellitus, human immunodeficiency infection, advanced age, male gender, and heredity. Ill-fitting dentures and neoplasm also contribute. Periodontal disease, on the other hand, is a risk factor for diabetes mellitus and coronary artery disease.[3]
7. **C. Assessment.** Ludwig's angina is characterized by bilateral swelling of the jaw and neck, marked elevation the tongue, shortness of breath, and difficulty swallowing. Vincent's disease, or acute necrotizing ulcerative gingivitis, presents signs and symptoms that include bleeding, edematous gums, poor oral hygiene, and bad breath. Ludwig's angina results from a secondary infection involving the second and third molars.[1]
8. **B. Intervention.** Displacement of the patient's tongue because of the extensive swelling places the patient at risk of airway compromise. Emergency airway equipment, particularly for emergent cricothyrotomy, should be placed at the patient's bedside.[1]
9. **C. Assessment.** Risk factors for recurrent otitis media include recent use of microbial agents, age younger than 2 years, and daycare attendance.[4]
10. **B. Analysis.** Your initial nursing diagnosis should address the patient's priority problem. For this baby, the initial nursing concern should be her fever, because febrile children have a high potential for seizure.[1]
11. **C. Intervention.** Patients who have foreign bodies removed may suffer some degree of damage to the epithelium in the canal. The patient should be treated with antibiotic-cortisone ear drops. An ear should never be irrigated with anything if the tympanic membrane is not intact.[5]
12. **C. Intervention.** Because of the emergence of antibiotic-resistant bacteria causing acute otitis media, symptomatic management alone in a stable, nontoxic patient may prove useful for improving the condition. Measures include administering warm oil ear drops, acetaminophen or ibuprofen for pain relief, and normal saline nose drops, and applying warmth by holding a hair dryer on low setting over the affected ear.[4-7]
13. **A. Assessment.** For any trauma patient, the initial assessment should address the airway while maintaining cervical spine immobilization. Ms. Lee's mouth should be opened and observed for blood or broken teeth, because foreign bodies can obstruct the airway. Ms. Lee's airway should especially be inspected for blood from her obvious nasal fracture.[1]
14. **A. Intervention.** Nasal packing or cauterization may be required. Direct pressure, however, is the first nursing intervention. Suctioning may exacerbate the bleeding.[1]
15. **C. Assessment.** A septal hematoma is a grape-like hematoma located on the nasal septum. It is imperative that the hematoma be recognized and drained, or septal necrosis may occur.[1]
16. **C. Analysis.** Patients with facial fractures are frequently anxious due to a fear of permanent facial deformities.[1]
17. **C. Intervention.** Other measures Ms. Lee should be taught include: avoiding straining (lifting, stooping); avoiding further nasal trauma, such as could be caused by inserting a cotton-tipped applicator; and avoiding forceful nose blowing, hot liquids, and high altitudes.[1]
18. **D. Assessment.** Patients complaining of sore throats should be assessed for stridor, fever, dehydration, and difficulty swallowing or talking. These symptoms indicate serious illness, so the patient should be given an urgent status if any are present.[6]
19. **D. Assessment.** Mr. Blue exhibits muffled voice, reports difficulty swallowing, is drooling, and has a fever. These are all symptoms of an infectious process in the throat, which should alert the nurse to the potential for airway obstruction.[6,7]
20. **C. Intervention.** This is the best position to maintain an open airway.
21. **B. Evaluation.** A return of vital signs to within normal range is an indicator of successful treatment. All other choices are indicators for reevaluation and further interventions.[5,6]
22. **B. Intervention.** In many communities, epiglottitis has been eradicated because of immunization.[8-10]
23. **D. Evaluation.** A return to normal respiratory rate indicates that therapies are working.[8]
24. **A. Intervention.** Avulsed teeth should be placed in a cell preservative solution when pos-

sible. If the patient does not have access to this type of solution, cold milk can be used until the patient gets to the emergency department.[11]

25. **B. Intervention.**[1,11]
26. **B. Assessment.** [5]
27. **A. Assessment.**[5,6]
28. **B. Assessment.** The patient should be treated emergently due to his potential for airway obstruction.[12]
29. **B. Assessment.** Loss of the normal prominence of the thyroid cartilage is a classic sign of fractured larynx.[12]
30. **B. Assessment.** Subcutaneous emphysema indicates a fractured larynx and may be a precursor to tension pneumothorax.[12]

References

1. Coimbra-Emanuele DM: Dental, ear, nose and throat emergencies. In Jordan KS, editor: *Emergency nursing core curriculum,* ed 5, Philadelphia, 2000, WB Saunders.
2. Olson C: Dental, ear, nose, and throat emergencies. In Newberry L, editor: *Sheehy's emergency nursing: principles and practice,* St Louis, 2003, Mosby.
3. Cavendish R: Periodontal disease, *Am J Nurs* 99(3):36-37, 1999.
4. Parshall M: Ear, nose, throat, and facial/dental conditions. In Kidd P, Sturt P, editors: *Mosby's emergency nursing reference,* Philadelphia, 1996, WB Saunders.
5. Hamilton G, Sanders A, Strange G et al: *Emergency medicine: an approach to clinical problem-solving,* Philadelphia, 2003, WB Saunders.
6. Fitzgerald MA: Acute otitis media in an era of drug resistance: implications for NP practice, *Nurs Pract* 24(10 suppl):10-14, 1999.
7. Dowell SF, Butler JC, Giebink S et al: Acute otitis media: management and surveillance in an era of pneumococcal resistance, *Nurs Pract* 24(10 suppl):1-9, 1999.
8. Normandin P, Brown J: A 19-year-old with a cough and hemoptysis, *J Emerg Med* 24(4):306-308, 1998.
9. Greenough G: Sore throat. In Davis M, Votey SR, Greenough PG, editors: *Signs and symptoms in emergency medicine,* St Louis, 1999, Mosby.
10. Emergency Nurses Association: *Emergency nursing pediatric course,* Des Plaines, IL, 2004, Emergency Nurses Association.
11. Proehl J, editor: *Emergency nursing procedures,* ed 3, St Louis, 2004, Mosby.
12. Emergency Nurses Association: *Trauma nursing core course,* Des Plaines, IL, 2000, Emergency Nurses Association.

Additional Readings

Kitt S, Selfridge-Thomas J, Proehl J et al, editors: *Emergency nursing: a physiological and clinical perspective,* Philadelphia, 1995, WB Saunders.

Lower J: Maxillofacial trauma, *Nurs Clin North Am* 21(4):611-628, 1986.

CHAPTER 6

ENVIRONMENTAL EMERGENCIES

REVIEW OUTLINE

I. General management of the patient who is experiencing an environmental emergency
  A. Assess the safety of the environment
    1. Safety of the rescue crew
    2. Safety of the health care providers
      a. Care providers should be appropriately dressed for the particular environmental emergency
    3. Control of the environment
    4. Additional hazards that may be in the environment
    5. Contact and use of appropriate authorities and experts (e.g., zoo, Environmental Protection Agency, poison information center)
    6. Preparation of the emergency department for the victim(s)
  B. General patient management
    1. ABCDE (airway, breathing, circulation, deficit [neurological], exposure): exposure of the patient could be particularly important to identify the cause of the problem and any additional injuries
    2. Vital signs: blood pressure, pulse, respiratory rate, temperature
    3. History
      a. What happened and when did it occur?
      b. Where was the patient found?
        (1) Enclosed space
        (2) Water temperature
      c. What type of environment was the patient found in?
        (1) Outside ambient temperature
        (2) Inside ambient temperature
      d. Symptoms experienced before coming to the emergency department
        (1) Nausea and vomiting
        (2) Headache
        (3) Dizziness
        (4) Temperature
        (5) Skin lesions
        (6) Seizures
      e. Medical history
        (1) Tetanus status
        (2) Diabetes
        (3) Cardiovascular disease
        (4) Cancer
        (5) Alcoholism
        (6) Obesity
        (7) Spinal cord injury
        (8) Medications
      f. Social situation
      g. Witnesses
      h. History suggestive of abuse
    4. Physical assessment
      a. Inspection
        (1) Airway
          (a) Patent
          (b) Maintainable
          (c) Nonmaintainable
        (2) Breathing
          (a) Rate
          (b) Work of breathing
        (3) Circulation
        (4) Level of consciousness
        (5) Pupillary function
        (6) Motor function
        (7) Skin appearance
          (a) Hyperemia
          (b) Blistering
          (c) Edema
          (d) Ulceration
          (e) Rash
          (f) Hives
          (g) Ticks
          (h) Fang or bite marks
          (i) Stingers
        (8) Wounds
          (a) Size
          (b) Shape

(c) Depth
(d) Visible skin structures
(e) Debris: fangs, teeth
b. Palpation
(1) Heart rate and rhythm
(2) Pulses, central and peripheral
(3) Blood pressure
(4) Motor and sensory response
(5) Skin temperature
(6) Crepitus
(7) Deformities
(8) Sensation to injured area
c. Percussion
(1) Chest
(2) Abdomen
d. Auscultation
(1) Breath sounds
(2) Blood pressure
(3) Bowel sounds

C. Age-related characteristics
1. Pediatric
a. Skin is thinner and temperature control immature
b. Drowning is a leading cause of death in the pediatric population
c. Alcohol abuse is related to disability and death in the adolescent
d. Weight places children at greater risk of suffering complications from envenomation
e. Size leaves children at greater risk for complications from bite injuries
2. Geriatric
a. Changes in senses such as vision and peripheral sensation leave older patient at risk for injury
b. Thermoregulatory changes leave elderly at risk
c. Changes in peripheral sensation from aging leave elderly at risk for burn injury
d. Age changes leave patient at greater risk for complications from envenomation
e. Age changes leave patient at risk for complications from bite injuries

D. Diagnostic procedures
1. Complete blood count, prothrombin time, partial thromboplastin time
2. Platelet, fibrin, fibrin split products
3. Electrolytes
4. Whole blood glucose
5. Toxicology screen
6. Arterial blood gas analysis
7. Chest radiograph
8. Cervical spine radiograph
9. Computed tomography
10. Electrocardiography

II. Related nursing diagnoses
A. Airway clearance, ineffective
B. Breathing pattern, ineffective
C. Fluid volume deficit
D. Thermoregulation, ineffective
E. Knowledge deficit related to specific environmental emergency and prevention
F. Injury, high risk for
G. Infection, high risk for
H. Poisoning, high risk for
I. Spiritual distress

III. Collaborative care for the patient experiencing an environmental emergency
A. Determine priorities of care
1. Safety of the rescuers and the health care providers
2. Control and maintain ABCs, provide cervical spine immobilization as indicated
3. Monitor vital signs, including temperature
4. Obtain a history related to the environmental emergency
5. Prepare the patient for interventions specific to the environmental emergency
a. Airway and ventilation management
b. Fluid resuscitation
c. Wound care
(1) Dressings
(2) Fasciotomy
(3) Escharotomy
d. Warming procedures
e. Cooling procedures
6. Medications
a. Antibiotics
b. Tetanus prophylaxis
c. Medications for anaphylaxis
d. Antivenin
e. Rabies prophylaxis
7. Sedation or pain management
8. Consult experts as indicated

IV. Selected environmental emergencies
A. Thermoregulatory emergencies
1. Heat cramps
2. Heat exhaustion
3. Heat stroke
4. Frostbite
5. Hypothermia

B. Near drowning
C. Diving emergencies
   1. Air embolism
   2. Nitrogen narcosis
   3. Decompression sickness
D. Lightning injuries
E. Electrical injuries
F. Thermal injuries
   1. Thermal
   2. Chemical
   3. Radiation
G. Bites and stings
   1. Human bites
   2. Animal bites
      a. Dogs
      b. Cats
      c. Exotic pets
   3. Snake bites
   4. Insect stings
   5. Tick bites
   6. Spider bites
   7. Aquatic organisms

The environment that surrounds us not only provides us with beauty but is a source of potential danger, as well. Throughout human evolution, we have learned to adjust to our surroundings; one method of doing this is by controlling our environment. However, there are still forces in the environment that cannot be controlled. In these circumstances, humankind has had to learn to live within the environment or suffer the consequences. To understand the effects of the environment on a patient, one must be familiar with how the body interacts with the environment. Body temperature, or thermoregulation, is maintained by the hypothalamus. The preoptic anterior hypothalamus receives body temperature information from the peripheral and central nervous systems. Several systems interact to help control or adjust the body temperature. These include the pituitary and adrenal glands and the sympathetic nervous system. The sympathetic nervous system manages vasodilation and vasoconstriction. In addition, convection, radiation, and evaporation contribute to the regulation of body temperature.[1]

The integumentary system provides sensation, regulation, and protection from the environment. Age, chronic illnesses, and medications can influence the integumentary, cardiovascular, neurological, and pulmonary systems, which may leave patients at risk for suffering an environmental emergency.

Other living organisms that coexist in the environment in which we live may cause illness or injury, such as snakes, spiders, and ticks. As humans venture into new environments either to live or for pleasure, they encounter animals that may inflict trauma and require specific treatments, such as rabies prophylaxis.

The initial care of the patient who has suffered an illness or injury begins with ensuring the safety of the rescuers and those who will be providing care. Next the victim should be taken to a safe care environment. The caregivers need to be appropriately dressed; additional hazards such as radiation or chemical toxins need to be contained; and the appropriate authorities need to be notified so that the victim receives the best possible care.

General treatment of the patient who has suffered an illness or injury related to the environment is based on the initial evaluation and stabilization of the ABCs. It is important to remove all clothing and expose the patient, because exposure will help the emergency nurse identify the cause of the problem, as well as any additional injuries. Vital signs, particularly the patient's temperature, should be evaluated.

Obtaining a history of what happened will help the emergency nurse recognize the type of environmental illness or injury the patient has suffered. Information should include the type of environmental surroundings in which the patient was found, any significant exposure to toxins, the length of time the patient was exposed, the patient's medical history, currently used medications, and any recent use of alcohol or drugs.

Initial emergency nursing interventions are based on the specific illness or injury suffered by the patient. Intravenous access will need to be established and medications administered as needed. A baseline neurological assessment should be made to set the foundation for further assessment and to evaluate the effects of specific treatments. Wound care is initiated in the prehospital care environment and continued in the emergency department. Finally, the appropriate authorities or experts will need to be notified or consulted to provide additional information for patient care.[1-3]

REVIEW QUESTIONS

Heat-Related Emergencies

A 14-month-old infant is found unresponsive in the back seat of a locked car with all of the windows rolled up. The outside temperature is 104° F (40° C). Upon arrival in the emergency department, the child remains unresponsive. His vital signs are a B/P of 60 by palpation, heart rate 180 beats per minute, respiratory rate of 40 breaths per minute, and a rectal temperature of 107.6° F (42° C).

1. The major difference between heat exhaustion and heat stroke is the patient's:
A. Level of consciousness
B. Blood pressure and pulse
C. Inability to dissipate heat
D. Age and skin integrity

2. One of the primary interventions in the care of the patient who is suffering from heat stroke is:
A. Removing all of the child's clothes and cooling him as quickly as possible with cold water
B. Inserting a rectal temperature probe to monitor the patient's temperature during resuscitation
C. Administering acetaminophen or ibuprofen based on the child's weight to decrease his core temperature
D. Inserting an intravenous line to administer medication to prevent shivering when warming the child

3. Based on this patient's blood pressure and pulse, the following is the most appropriate nursing diagnosis:
A. Airway clearance, ineffective related to airway obstruction from airway edema
B. Pain related to an increase in the body's temperature; interventions needed to decrease the body's temperature
C. Fluid volume deficit, related to decreased circulating blood volume from a fluid shift
D. Breathing pattern, ineffective related to hypoxia from an increase in body temperature

4. Which of the following is a common electrolyte imbalance found in heatstroke?
A. Hyperphosphatemia
B. Hypernatremia
C. Hypercalcemia
D. Hypermagnesemia

5. Which of the following drugs increase heat production?
A. Narcotics
B. Benzodiazepines
C. Amphetamines
D. Antihistamines

6. Monitoring for rhabdomyolysis during resuscitation from heat stroke would include monitoring:
A. For changes in the patient's level of consciousness
B. The color of the patient's urine and output
C. The patient's electrolytes for hypokalemia
D. The patient for rhonchi and rales

Heat Cramps

An 18-year-old man comes to the emergency department complaining of weakness and cramps in his legs. He has been out working with a paving crew. The outside temperature is 90° F, and the humidity is 80%.

7. The major cause of heat cramps is:
A. Fluid retention in the general circulation and that causes swelling in the lower extremities
B. Loss of salt in thermal sweat without adequate replacement in food and oral fluids
C. Hyperventilation tetany that occurs with trying to decrease the body's temperature
D. Drinking excessive amounts of a sports drink during outside exercise in a hot environment

8. The preferred management for the patient with heat cramps is:
A. Inserting two large-bore IV needles and giving a fluid bolus of hypertonic saline
B. Using ice packs on the extremities that are causing the patient discomfort
C. Oral rehydration with a balanced electrolyte solution
D. Insertion of a gastric tube and irrigation with cool saline solution

9. The patient is treated for heat cramps. On what nursing diagnosis should the emergency nurse base the patient's discharge planning?
A. Fear related to suddenly experiencing a heat-related emergency
B. Knowledge deficit related to the causes of heat cramps
C. Fluid volume deficit related to the hot environment

D. Self-esteem disturbance related to becoming ill on the job

10. One evaluation criterion the emergency nurse could use to assess whether this patient understood his discharge instructions would be that the patient:
A. States methods to prevent heat cramps while working
B. Returns the next day with heat cramps and continues to work
C. Quits his job because it is too hot outside
D. Returns in a hypernatremic state to the emergency department

11. Infants and young children are at greater risk than an adult for suffering a heat-related emergency because they have:
A. A slower metabolic rate while they are young
B. Less subcutaneous tissue
C. A larger body surface area in proportion to circulating volume
D. A better ability to protect themselves from the environment

12. A 45-year-old female, who has a history of severe depression that has been managed with antidepressants, is brought to the emergency department because of fever and altered mental status. Her family states that she has been getting worse. Upon arrival in the emergency department, the patient is unresponsive and rigid. Her core body temperature is 42° C (107° F). Which of the following is the most likely cause of her symptoms?
A. Heat-induced syncope
B. Neuroleptic seizure
C. Catatonic reaction
D. Exertion-induced heatstroke

Cold-Related Emergencies

13. Superficial frostbite is managed by:
A. Warming the tissue in warm water
B. Rubbing the affected area with snow
C. Covering the affected area with wool
D. Protecting the patient from infection

14. Signs and symptoms of frostbite include all of the following except:
A. Erythemic tissue
B. Blistering of the injured tissue
C. Blackened dry tissue
D. Soft and pliable tissue

15. Tissue injury occurs in frostbite because of:
A. Enhanced circulation to the injured extremity as a response to the cold
B. Indirect injury to the protoplasm of the tissue as a response to the cold
C. Disruption of the cell and tissue structures by ice formation
D. Direct thermal injury to the tissue from rewarming with hot water

Hypothermia

A 40-year-old man is brought to the emergency department after having been found lying under a bridge in a sleeping bag. The outside temperature has ranged from 20° to 35° F. No one knows how long the man was lying there. The patient is alone and no medical history is available. He is responding only to deep pain. Vital signs are B/P 100/70, P 48, R 10, Temp 86° F (30° C) rectally.

16. What is the potentially lethal cardiac dysrhythmia associated with hypothermia?
A. Ventricular fibrillation
B. Paroxysmal atrial tachycardia
C. Complete heart block
D. Multifocal premature ventricular contractions

17. Which of the following systems is affected first by a drop in body temperature?
A. Renal system
B. Neurological system
C. Pulmonary system
D. Cardiovascular system

18. During the initial rewarming of the hypothermic patient, the most appropriate nursing diagnosis is:
A. Knowledge deficit related to proper dress during the winter
B. Pain related to the increase in circulation to the extremities after rewarming
C. Injury, high risk for, related to the effects of rewarming
D. Infection, high risk for, related to being outside in the winter

19. Because of the sludging of blood that can occur in the hypothermic patient, fluid resuscitation

will be needed to prevent complications such as acute tubular necrosis. What criteria should the emergency nurse use to evaluate the effectiveness of the fluid resuscitation?
A. Decreased mental status
B. Increase in body temperature
C. Decrease in peripheral pulses
D. Increase in central venous pressure and urinary output

20. Signs and symptoms of "afterdrop" include:
A. Cardiac dysrhythmia and hypotension
B. Hypertension and hypoventilation
C. Shivering and hyperthermia
D. Sinus rhythm and normothermia

21. Active external rewarming involves:
A. Using warm humidified oxygen by mask
B. Removing the patient's wet clothing
C. Performing peritoneal lavage with warm fluids
D. Using cardiopulmonary bypass

22. Active core rewarming involves:
A. Putting on dry clothes
B. Turning on a radiant heater
C. Using "body-to-body" contact
D. Inhalation rewarming

23. When using active external rewarming devices, caution must be exercised to prevent:
A. Additional vasoconstriction in the affected extremities from the application of heat
B. Decrease in patient's core body temperature from the application of heat
C. Injury to the patient's skin from heating devices because of peripheral vasoconstriction
D. Development of hypertension from heat application

24. All of these drugs may place the patient at risk of becoming hypothermic except:
A. Phenothiazines
B. Benzodiazepines
C. Amphetamines
D. Tricyclic antidepressants

Submersion Injuries

An 18-month-old boy is brought to the emergency department after having been found at the bottom of a swimming pool. Cardiopulmonary resuscitation was initiated by his mother and continued by the basic life support (BLS) squad. On arrival in the emergency department, he is intubated and high-dose epinephrine administered. He now has a palpable peripheral pulse. His B/P is 82/50, P 150 and regular, Temp 95° F (rectal). He has no spontaneous respirations.

25. Significant predictors for survival of a near drowning include:
A. Sex and race of the victim
B. Swimming ability of the victim
C. Fresh water instead of salt water
D. No associated injuries

26. Initial critical interventions for the near-drowning victim should include:
A. Rewarming the patient immediately upon arrival of the rescue squad
B. Immobilizing the cervical spine to protect the cervical spine
C. Drawing blood gases upon arrival in the emergency department
D. Obtaining a radiograph before the child is intubated

27. This child's initial blood gases are pH 7.25, PO_2 78, PCO_2 30, and HCO_3 25. The most appropriate nursing diagnosis is:
A. Gas exchange, impaired, related to aspiration
B. Fluid volume deficit related to fluid loss
C. Cardiac output, decreased, related to fluid loss
D. Tissue perfusion, altered (cerebral), related to hypoxia

28. Which of the following is a poor prognostic indicator for a submerged victim?
A. On-scene advanced life support initiated
B. Older child or an adult
C. Submerged for longer than 5 minutes
D. Alert on admission to the emergency department

29. The most effective intervention to manage near-drowning incidents among pediatric patients is:
A. Teaching BLS to babysitters of children under 5 years of age so that appropriate resuscitation can be performed
B. Placing the patient on extracorporeal membrane oxygenation (ECMO) to manage the

pulmonary injury after aspiration of water or toxic substances in the water
C. Developing and implementing community prevention programs, including education about pool barriers
D. Administering surfactant upon arrival in the emergency department for management of the pulmonary complications that may occur

30. Favorable prognostic factors in near-drowning incidents include:
A. Conscious on arrival in the emergency department
B. Submersion longer than 10 minutes
C. Preexisting medical problems
D. Arterial blood gas pH 7.10 or less

31. Pulmonary dysfunction may be exacerbated when a patient suffers a submersion injury in:
A. Salt water in a fish tank
B. Fresh water in a lake
C. Bath water with bubble bath
D. Fresh water in a toilet bowel

Thermal Injuries

A 17-year-old boy is brought to the emergency department after having been pulled out of a burning car. He is unconscious and has sustained second-degree and third-degree burns to his face, chest, and arms. The BLS squad has wrapped him in wet sheets and is maintaining his ventilation with a bag-valve-mask and an oral airway.

32. Signs and symptoms of a potential inhalation injury include:
A. First-degree burns to the neck
B. Second-degree burns to the chest
C. Normal respiratory effort
D. Carbonaceous sputum

33. Based on this patient's history, what additional laboratory test should be obtained during his initial evaluation?
A. Hepatic profile
B. Carboxyhemoglobin level
C. Toxicology screen
D. Cardiac enzyme values

34. Full-thickness burns:
A. Involve the epidermis and upper layers of the dermis
B. Involve damage only to the dermis
C. Involve damage to the epidermis and most of the dermis
D. Destroy all layers of the skin

35. A partial-thickness burn causes injury to:
A. Muscles and tendons
B. Subcutaneous tissues
C. Regenerative epithelial cells
D. The upper portion of the dermis

36. The patient has suffered circumferential burns to his chest. For this type of injury, the most appropriate nursing diagnosis on which to base this patient's emergency care is:
A. Breathing pattern, ineffective
B. Fluid volume deficit
C. Cardiac output, decreased
D. Family processes, altered

37. Using the fluid resuscitation formula (Parkland formula) of 4 ml of Ringer's lactate solution times total body surface area burned times patient's weight in kilograms: how much fluid should this patient receive in the first 8 hours (rounded to the nearest 10 ml)? His body weight is 150 pounds. The amount of body surface burned is 35%.
A. 10,500 ml
B. 4760 ml
C. 8000 ml
D. 5000 ml

38. Because of the potential pulmonary injury this patient has suffered, what would be the best evaluative criterion the emergency nurse could use to monitor this patient?
A. A capillary refill time longer than 2 seconds
B. The patient's ability to cough
C. The patient's ventilatory pattern
D. The patient's tidal volume

39. The patient has received 3000 ml of fluid while awaiting transfer to the burn center. In order to determine if the fluid resuscitation is adequate, the patient's urinary output should be:
A. 25 ml per hour
B. 20 ml per hour

C. 30 ml per hour
D. 10 ml per hour

40. Wound care of a minor burn (partial thickness less than 15% in the adult and less than 10% in the child) would consist of:
A. Putting crushed ice directly on the wound
B. Pouring povidone-iodine solution directly on the wound
C. Washing with a mild soapy solution
D. Rinsing the wound with turpentine and distilled water

41. A patient has suffered a chemical burn from an unknown wet chemical. The initial management of this patient should include:
A. Inserting an intravenous line for antidote administration
B. Applying lidocaine jelly to decrease the pain caused by the burns
C. Flushing the affected area with copious amounts of water
D. Calling the local poison information center before beginning treatment

42. The most common type of thermal burn in children under age 3 is:
A. Scald burn
B. Chemical burn
C. Flame burn
D. Petroleum burn

43. Factors that may alert the emergency nurse that a burn injury in a child may be intentional include:
A. Lower socioeconomic background
B. Burn injuries match the history given
C. Up-to-date immunizations
D. Symmetrical burn injury

44. In infants, the head and neck represent what percentage of the body surface area?
A. 14%
B. 36%
C. 9%
D. 18%

45. What type of ultraviolet radiation causes sunburn?
A. Ultraviolet C radiation
B. Ultraviolet B radiation
C. Ultraviolet E radiation
D. Ultraviolet D radiation

46. Which of the following burns should be managed at a burn center?
A. Inhalation injury with a burn injury
B. Second-degree and third-degree burns less than 10%
C. Third-degree burns less than 3%
D. No circumferential burns of the chest

47. An 18-month-old girl is brought to the emergency department by her parents after having bitten into an electrical cord. The child has a large blister and a charred wound on the right side of her lip. A delayed consequence of this type of burn would be:
A. Cardiac dysrhythmia
B. Hypovolemic shock
C. Bleeding
D. Cataracts

Electrical Injuries

A 30-year-old construction worker is brought to the emergency department by the rescue squad after having sustained an electrical shock of 10,000 volts. On arrival, he is alert and oriented, complaining of tingling in his left foot. His vital signs are B/P 120/70, P 100, R 18.

48. All of the following factors determine the nature and severity of electrical injuries except the:
A. Age of the patient
B. Amperage of the current
C. Type of current
D. Duration of contact with the current

49. Initial management of a patient who has suffered an electrical injury should include:
A. Preparation for escharotomy due to the severity of the burn wounds found in victims who have been electrocuted
B. Immobilization of the cervical spine because many victims of electrical injuries have fallen
C. Electrocardiogram upon admission in the emergency department to rule out any cardiac injury
D. Removal of all of the patient's clothes to identify the path of the electricity that passed through the patient

50. The tissue in the body with the least resistance to current flow is:
A. Bone tissue
B. Muscle tissue

C. Nerve tissue
D. Cardiac tissue

51. Because of the effects of electricity on the cardiovascular system, the most appropriate nursing diagnosis that the emergency nurse could use in planning the care of this patient is:
A. Injury, high risk for
B. Infection, high risk for
C. Fear
D. Cardiac output, decreased

Lightning Injuries

Every day there are approximately 8,000,000 lightning flashes throughout the world. About 100 people are killed each year by lightning in the United States. However, 70% to 80% of people struck by lightning survive.[4]

Even though this is not a common environmental emergency seen by the emergency nurse, it is important to be aware of the possibility of a lightning strike occurring no matter where one works. People at risk include campers, golfers, farmers, forest rangers, and construction workers.[4]

52. All of the following are early indications that a person may have been struck by lightning except:
A. Vaporized rain water
B. Feathery skin burns
C. Ruptured tympanic membrane
D. Bilateral cataracts

53. Initial treatment of the patient who is suspected of having been struck by lightning includes:
A. Applying antibiotic ointment and loose dressings to the burns
B. Managing the airway after effecting cervical spine immobilization
C. Inserting two large-bore IV needles for aggressive fluid resuscitation
D. Connecting the patient to a cardiac monitor and managing any life-threatening dysrhythmia

Bites and Stings

54. Most bites managed in the emergency department result from:
A. Human bites to the metacarpophalangeal joint
B. Cat bites to the fingers and hands
C. Snake bites to the feet and ankles
D. Dog bites to the face, hands, and legs

55. Which of the following is the *least* likely to be a complication of a bite?
A. Transmission of hepatitis B
B. Transmission of HIV
C. Exposure to rabies
D. Exposure to tetanus

56. For the patient who has suffered a dog bite wound to the hand, the most appropriate nursing diagnosis would be:
A. Ineffective airway clearance
B. Fluid volume deficit
C. Risk for infection
D. Ineffective thermal regulation

57. Injury prevention strategies that the emergency nurse may use to teach patients how to avert a dog bite would include:
A. Always run from a dog and scream when it chases you
B. If knocked over by a dog, roll into a ball and lie still
C. Always approach an unfamiliar dog to ascertain its intentions
D. Always look an unfamiliar dog directly in the eyes

58. The most common source of exposure to rabies virus in humans in the United States is from:
A. Dogs
B. Skunks
C. Raccoons
D. Bats

59. The human diploid cell vaccine (HDCV) should always be administered in adults and older children:
A. In the deltoid area
B. In the outer aspect of the thigh
C. Directly into the wound
D. In the gluteal area

60. A simple method that may be used to remove the stinger from an insect bite is:
A. Anesthetizing the affected area and using a scalpel
B. Scraping it off with a hard-edged object like a credit card

C. Applying an over-the-counter salve to loosen the stinger
D. Pulling it with a set of eyebrow tweezers

61. A 15-year-old boy who was stacking wood 2 days ago comes to the emergency department complaining of painful ulceration on the dorsal surface of the second digit of his right hand. He has no other complaints. Based on this history, the most likely thing to have bitten him is a:
A. Black widow spider
B. Blue scorpion
C. Brown recluse spider
D. Wolf spider

62. A 30-year-old female arrives in the emergency department with complaints of fatigue, headache, and fever and chills. She also states that she has a "ringlike" reddened area on her right arm. A tick bite is suspected. Important pieces of history related to tick bite that should be obtained from this patient would include all of the following except:
A. Season of onset of her symptoms
B. Description of her outdoor activities
C. Travel in known tick area
D. Type of stinger removed from any wounds

63. A simple method to remove a tick in the emergency department is:
A. Pull out the tick with a pair of tweezers
B. Coat the tick with fingernail polish
C. Suffocate the tick with gasoline or kerosene
D. Apply a hot match head to the tick

64. The primary management of Lyme disease is:
A. Methylprednisolone IV for 3 days
B. Amoxicillin PO for 14 to 28 days
C. Tetracycline PO for the patient who is pregnant
D. Topical antibiotics to the lesions for 2 weeks

65. A 5-year-old child is brought to the emergency department by his parents. They state that he has been unable to walk for the last few days and has had a low-grade fever and lack of appetite. They state that they went camping recently and noticed the symptoms after they returned. Tick paralysis is suspected. The primary management of tick paralysis is:
A. Admission to the ICU and methylprednisolone IV for 1 month
B. Admission to the ICU and IV antibiotics for 3 weeks
C. Removal of the tick and provision of supportive care
D. Removal of the tick and oral antibiotics for 2 months

66. A 16-year-old male was snorkeling in the ocean and was stung by a jellyfish. Wound care of this patient would include:
A. Rinsing the wound immediately with fresh water and administering epinephrine subcutaneously
B. Rubbing the affected area to remove all the remaining nematocysts
C. Removing all the remaining nematocysts with ungloved hands to decrease the risk of skin irritation
D. Applying acetic acid 5% (vinegar) to deactivate the toxin from the nematocysts

67. The initial management of decompression sickness includes:
A. Administration of a large dose of morphine sulfate for pain management
B. Administration of 100% oxygen via nonrebreather mask
C. Transport of the patient by air in an unpressurized cabin for recompression
D. Administration of acetaminophen prophylactically to prevent platelet aggregation

68. Which of the following is not a characteristic of a pit viper native to the United States?
A. Round pupils
B. Elliptical pupils
C. Heat-sensing pit
D. Fang sheath

ANSWERS

1. **C. Assessment.** Patients with heat exhaustion and heat stroke may have similar symptoms, which include changes in mental status, hypotension, and tachycardia. The patient suffering from heat exhaustion, however, sweats freely and may even complain of chilling.[1,2]
2. **A. Intervention.** In addition to initial management of the ABCs, primary care of the patient with heat stroke includes rapid cooling. Several methods are available for cooling the patient: wetting the patient down with cool water, using large fans, ice water immersion, and rectal and

gastric lavage with cold water. However, despite great controversy, research has demonstrated that ice water immersion works quickly. It must be used with great care in special populations such as the elderly.[4]

3. **C. Analysis.** Because of the large volume of fluid that has been lost through sweating, the patient with heat stroke will develop hypotension. Defining characteristics of fluid volume deficit include hypotension, tachycardia, dry skin, dry mucous membranes, and decreased skin turgor.[4]
4. **B. Evaluation.** Because of the dehydration that occurs in heat stroke, hypernatremia is the most common electrolyte imbalance of the ones presented. However, not all patients with heat stoke will be hypernatremic.[4]
5. **C. Assessment.** Amphetamines increase heat production, as do thyroid hormone replacement medications, tricyclic antidepressants, and lysergic acid diethylamide (LSD).[4]
6. **B. Evaluation.** Monitoring the patient for rhabdomyolysis would include monitoring the patient's urinary output, color changes in the urine (dark yellow, brown, red), complaints of muscle cramps, and hyperkalemia.[1]
7. **B. Assessment.** Heat cramps are related to the loss of salt in thermal sweat from working in a hot environment. Heat cramps differ from exercise cramps in that they tend to occur while the person is resting and do not resolve spontaneously.[1,2]
8. **C. Intervention.** Heat cramps usually are managed with oral ingestion of a salt solution. The emergency nurse must keep in mind that the patient with heat cramps may be hypochloremic. Careful evaluation of all the patient's electrolytes is important.[1-4]
9. **B. Analysis.** The most appropriate nursing diagnosis on which to base this patient's discharge planning is knowledge deficit related to the causes of heat cramps.[5]
10. **A. Evaluation.** The best criterion to use in evaluating discharge instructions is to have the patient explain the instructions to the emergency nurse.
11. **C. Assessment.** Pediatric patients are at greater risk than adults for developing heat-related emergencies because they have a smaller relative amount of subcutaneous fat, a higher metabolic rate, less ability to protect themselves from environmental changes, a larger TBSA-to-volume ratio. Children with chronic illnesses such as cystic fibrosis are also at risk for developing heat-related illnesses.[6]
12. **B. Assessment.** Neuroleptic seizure is an uncommon, but potentially fatal, complication related to antidepressant use. It is important for the emergency nurse to be aware of this syndrome, particularly in departments that treat a lot of patients with psychiatric problems. Signs and symptoms include altered mental status, skeletal muscle rigidity, dyspnea, extrapyramidal syndrome, and severe metabolic acidosis.[4]
13. **A. Intervention.** The affected part should be rewarmed in water at a temperature of 104° to 108° F (40° to 42° C). In addition, the patient's core temperature should be monitored.[4]
14. **D. Assessment.** Signs and symptoms of frostbite include firm to hard tissue, pale to erythemic tissue, and blistering and blackening of the injured tissues.[4]
15. **C. Assessment.** The mechanism of injury in frostbite involves three processes. These include:
    - Disruption of the cell and tissue structures from the formation of ice crystals
    - Direct injury to tissue protoplasm from the cold, probably from dehydration
    - Injury from impaired circulation[4,7]
16. **A. Assessment.** A patient whose core body temperature is below 86° F is at risk of developing ventricular fibrillation. This dysrhythmia can be stimulated easily by procedures, such as the insertion of monitoring lines. At temperatures between 82.4° and 86° F, ventricular fibrillation may not respond to drugs or countershock.[1,8]
17. **B. Assessment.** When the body temperature drops and a patient becomes hypothermic, initial changes in the level of consciousness are seen. The patient will become apathetic, weak, and fatigued, and may become confused and actually remove clothing instead of putting it on to get warmer.[1,4,8,9]
18. **C. Analysis.** During the rewarming process the patient is at great risk of being injured. Rewarming mechanics can cause injury, seizures can occur, and the patient can aspirate.[4]
19. **D. Evaluation.** Fluid resuscitation is best monitored by changes in the patient's central venous pressure and urinary output. These parameters help prevent fluid overload.
20. **A. Assessment.** Afterdrop may occur while rewarming a patient with moderate to severe hypothermia. It occurs when the periphery is

rewarmed and acidotic blood is dumped into the central circulation. Signs of afterdrop include hypotension and cardiac dysrhythmia.[5,8]

21. **B. Intervention.** Active external rewarming includes "buddy warming," using heated blankets and heating pads, immersion in hot water, and exposure to forced circulated hot air.[1,4]
22. **D. Intervention.** Active core rewarming includes airway rewarming with warm humidified oxygen by mask or into the endotracheal tube, peritoneal lavage with warm fluids, and cardiopulmonary bypass.[4]
23. **C. Intervention.** Because of the peripheral vasoconstriction that occurs with hypothermia, heating devices may cause burns.[1]
24. **C. Assessment.** Amphetamine ingestion contributes to the development of hyperthermia.[4]
25. **D. Assessment.** Factors that predict survival from a near drowning include time to resuscitation, water temperature, contaminants in the water, length of time immersed, less struggle, and no associated injuries.[1,2,9-12]
26. **B. Intervention.** The cervical spine should be immobilized in the unconscious near-drowning victim until possible injury to the cervical spine can be evaluated. The child was found unconscious at the bottom of the pool. He could have fallen into the pool or struck his head on the bottom of the pool.[1]
27. **A. Analysis.** The defining characteristics of impaired gas exchange include hypercapnia and hypoxia. Because of the aspiration of water, the child's lungs have sustained an alteration in alveolar capillary membrane function.[5]
28. **C. Evaluation.** Poor prognostic indicators for submerged victims include:
    - Age under 3 years
    - Coma upon admission to the emergency department
    - Submersion longer than 5 minutes
    - No resuscitation attempts for longer than 10 minutes.[4]
29. **C. Intervention.** The most appropriate intervention is to develop and implement community programs to teach prevention. Many pediatric drowning incidents occur because of lack of adult supervision, lack of fences around swimming pools, and lack of swimming instruction for young children.[1,9-11]
30. **A. Analysis.** Favorable prognostic factors include:
    - Age under 3 years
    - Submersion shorter than 3 minutes
    - Colder water
    - Conscious on arrival in the emergency department
    - Presence of pulse in the emergency department.[10,11]
31. **C. Assessment.** Even though many articles point out that hypertonic or hypotonic solutions, in and of themselves, cause additional injury in drowning, research in animals has shown that it would take a large amount of aspirated fluid to cause additional injury. Most near-drowning victims aspirate only a small amount of fluid. However, water containing chemicals, such as caustic cleaning fluids or soapsuds, may cause chemical pneumonitis and surfactant destruction.[4,11]
32. **D. Assessment.** Signs of injury to the respiratory tract from thermal exposure include facial burns, singed nasal hairs, carbonaceous sputum, hypoxemia, intercostal retractions, rales, rhonchi, and a hoarse voice.[1,4,13]
33. **B. Intervention.** Because the injury occurred in an enclosed space and because the patient is unconscious, a carboxyhemoglobin level should be obtained so that he can be evaluated for carbon monoxide poisoning. Carbon monoxide will bind with hemoglobin 240 times faster than will oxygen, causing the patient to become hypoxic.[13,14]
34. **D. Assessment.** See 35 for explanation.
35. **D. Assessment.** Partial-thickness, or second-degree, burns cause injury to the upper portion of the dermis. First-degree burns cause injury to the epidermal layer of the skin. Full-thickness burns cause injury through the epidermis, dermis, subcutaneous tissues, and into the muscles. These burns will damage the regenerative epithelial cells, destroy nerve endings, and cause vessel thrombosis.[13-15]
36. **A. Analysis.** Circumferential burns of the body, particularly of the chest and neck, can impair respiratory function. A defining characteristic of this nursing diagnosis is altered chest excursion. The constriction caused by the burn injury prevents the patient from ventilating properly.[13-16]
37. **B. Intervention.** This calculation would be:

    4 ml × 68 kg × 35 (percentage of TBSA burned)

    One half of this should be given during the first 8 hours. The volume would be 4760 ml.[13]

38. **C. Evaluation.** The most useful evaluative criterion for this patient would be his ventilatory pattern. Because he is at risk for ventilation problems from circumferential burns and for hypoxia from inhalation injury and carbon monoxide poisoning, the pattern of his ventilatory efforts must be monitored closely.
39. **C. Evaluation.** Urinary output is one of the best methods available to monitor fluid resuscitation. Adult urinary output should be 30 to 50 ml per hour.[13]
40. **C. Intervention.** Ice or povidone-iodine (Betadine) directly on the wound would only cause additional damage to the skin. The skin is the largest organ system, and when it is intact, it prevents toxins from entering the body and helps regulate body temperature. When it has been damaged, as in a burn injury, these functions are compromised. Washing with mild soap will help remove any debris from the burn and help prevent infection.[13]
41. **C. Intervention.** Wet chemical burns should be flushed with copious amounts of water to remove the chemical as quickly as possible. Caregivers need to be covered to prevent exposure and the water should be appropriately contained.[9]
42. **A. Assessment.** The most common type of thermal injury seen in children under age 3 is scald injuries. Children over age 3 are more often injured by a flame.[14]
43. **D. Assessment.** A symmetrical burn injury should alert the emergency nurse to the possibility that the burn injury was intentional. For example, symmetrical burns to the lower extremities are generally an indication that the child may have been held in hot water. Unintentional splash or scald burns are rarely symmetrical.[6]
44. **D. Assessment.** In infants, the head and neck represent 18% of the body surface area. In the adult, this is only 9% of the body surface area.[6,13]
45. **B. Assessment.** Ultraviolet B waves are the main cause of sunburn and skin cancer.[13]
46. **A. Assessment.** According to the American Burn Association, the following burns should be managed at a burn center:
    - Second-degree and third-degree burns over 20% or more
    - Third-degree burns over 5% or more
    - Electrical burns, including lightning injuries
    - Inhalation burns with burn injury
    - Circumferential burns of the extremities and chest[14]
47. **C. Assessment.** A delayed complication of this type of burn would be bleeding. The labile arteries can begin bleeding 3 to 5 days after the injury. The emergency nurse will need to teach the parents to use direct pressure to control the bleeding and bring the child for further evaluation if it does not stop.[13,14]
48. **A. Assessment.** Six major factors determine the nature and severity of an electrical injury: voltage, amperage, type of current, duration of contact, current path through the victim, and skin resistance.[13]
49. **B. Assessment.** Many victims of an electrical shock may have fallen or been thrown against something, so the cervical spine should be immobilized until injuries can be ruled out.[4]
50. **C. Assessment.** Bone is the tissue with the greatest resistance to current flow. Nerve tissue has the least resistance to current flow.[13]
51. **D. Analysis.** Because of the effects of electricity on the cardiovascular system, close monitoring is important. Defining characteristics of this nursing diagnosis include dysrhythmia, electrocardiographic changes, hypotension, cold, clammy skin, and variations in hemodynamic parameters.[5,15]
52. **D. Assessment.** A late sign of injury caused by lightning strike is cataract formation. Four types of injuries occur initially after a lightning strike: cardiac injuries, neurological injuries, burns, and blunt trauma.[4,17]
53. **B. Intervention.** Many times when patients are struck by lightning, they become apneic. Because of the possibility of trauma to the cervical spine, immobilization must precede airway management. [4,17]
54. **D. Assessment.** Most animal bites managed in the emergency department are from dogs. In 1994, approximately 4.7 million people in the United States were bitten by dogs.[18,19]
55. **B. Assessment.** Bites and stings can lead to multiple complications, including anaphylaxis, envenomation, local tissue damage, and disease transmission. Some of the organisms transmitted include hepatitis virus, rabies virus, Lyme disease spirochete, and numerous types of bacteria, such as *Staphylococcus aureus.* The risk of transmission of HIV from a bite is considered low.[1]
56. **C. Analysis.** The location of the wound increases the risk of infection.[1]

57. **B. Intervention.** The Centers for Disease Control and Prevention guidelines for safety around dogs include:
    - Never approach an unfamiliar dog
    - Never run from a dog and scream
    - Stay still when an unfamiliar dog comes up to you
    - If knocked over by a dog, roll into a ball and lie still; do not look a dog in the eye[19]
58. **D. Assessment.** Between 1990 and 2000 there was a total of 3 cases of human rabies in the United States. Most deaths were caused by exposure to bats.[20]
59. **A. Intervention.** HDCV and rabies vaccine absorbed (RVA) must be given in the deltoid area in adults and older children. In younger children, they may be given in the outer aspect of the thigh.[18]
60. **B. Intervention.** Many stingers will continue to secrete venom until removed. It is important to remove a stinger without causing it to break apart. Using a hard edge, such as that of a credit card, to scrape it out is one of the simplest methods.[1]
61. **C. Assessment.** Black widow spiders live in secluded, dark areas such as garages, barns, and outhouses. The brown recluse spider resides in woodpiles and storage areas. The bite of a black widow spider generally produces systemic symptoms such as abdominal pain, hypertension, nausea, vomiting, and tachycardia. A brown recluse bite will produce a distinct type of wound that begins with painful purpura and develops into a necrotic ulcerating wound.[1,21]
62. **D. Assessment.** History that should be obtained from a patient when a tick bite or tick-related disease is suspected should include:
    - Season of onset, usually from May through September
    - Outdoor activities, such as hiking in woods or fields
    - Geography of outside activities, such as known tick areas
    - Symptoms related to the tick bite
    - Fatigue
    - Weakness
    - Headache
    - Photophobia
    - Fever or chills
    - Muscle or joint pain
    - Rash[4]
63. **A. Intervention.** Over the years, people have used a variety of methods to remove ticks, including gasoline, kerosene, and matches (hopefully without the gasoline and kerosene). The tick-removal method recommended in *Wilderness Medicine* is to grasp the tick as close as possible to the skin surface with blunt curved forceps, tweezers, or protected fingers. It should be pulled out with a steady pressure so as not to crush it and release any fluids that may transmit disease. Devices that can be used for removal are commercially available.[4]
64. **B. Intervention.** Lyme disease is managed with oral amoxicillin for 14 to 28 days. Tetracycline is not recommended for the pregnant patient.[4]
65. **C. Intervention.** Management of tick paralysis is immediate removal of the tick. As long as the tick is attached to the patient, it is secreting toxin, which blocks the release of acetylcholine. Symptoms of tick paralysis include ascending symmetrical weakness of the lower extremities and ataxia. Death can occur from respiratory arrest. Once the tick is removed, management is supportive.[4]
66. **D. Intervention.** Stings from jellyfish should be managed by:
    - Washing the wound immediately with sea water, because rubbing and fresh water will activate remaining nematocysts
    - Cleansing with vinegar 5% to inactivate the toxin
    - Applying shaving cream or a paste of baking soda, flour, or talc and shaving off the remaining nematocysts

    Rescuers and health care providers should always wear gloves to protect themselves[22]
67. **B. Intervention.** Initial management of decompression sickness is 100% oxygen by nonrebreather mask. Recompression is the definitive management. If air transport is required, the patient should be carried in a pressurized cabin. Narcotics should be avoided to prevent respiratory depression. Aspirin may be given for its antiplatelet action.[9]
68. **A. Assessment.** Round pupils are not a characteristic of pit vipers native to the United States.[9]

References

1. Semonin Holleran R: Environmental emergencies. In Jordan KS, editor: *Emergency nursing core curriculum,* ed 5, Philadelphia, 2000, WB Saunders.
2. Proehl JA: Environmental emergencies. In Kitt S, Selfridge-Thomas J, Proehl J et al, editors:

Emergency nursing: a physiologic and clinical perspective, Philadelphia, 1995, WB Saunders.

3. Stewart C: *Environmental emergencies,* Baltimore, 1990, Williams & Wilkins.
4. Auerbach PS, Geehr EC: *Management of wilderness and environmental emergencies,* ed 4, St Louis, 2001, Mosby.
5. Kim MJ, McFarland GK, McLane AM: *Pocket guide to nursing diagnoses,* St Louis, 1993, Mosby.
6. Emergency Nurses Association: *Emergency nursing pediatric course,* Des Plaines, IL, 2004, Emergency Nurses Association.
7. Mills W, Whaley R: Frostbite with rapid rewarming and ultrasonic therapy, *Wilderness Environ Med* 9(4):226-247, 1998.
8. Weissenberger EV: A 17-year-old with severe hypothermia and cardiac arrest from exposure, *J Emerg Nurs* 18:380-382, 1992.
9. Morris J: Environmental emergencies. In Newberry L, editor, *Sheehy's emergency nursing: principles and practice,* ed 5, St Louis, 2003, Mosby.
10. Young L: A 22-month-old victim of near-drowning, *J Emerg Nurs* 18:197-198, 1992.
11. Dickison AE: Near-drowning, predictors of survival, *Wilderness Med Let* 16(2):1, 6-9, 1999.
12. Beyda DH: Childhood submersion injuries, *J Emerg Nurs* 24(2):140-144, 1998.
13. Wraa C: Burns. In Newberry L, editor: *Sheehy's emergency nursing: principles and practice,* ed 5, St Louis, 2003, Mosby.
14. American Burn Association: *Prehospital burn life support,* Lincoln, NE, 1996, American Burn Association.
15. Bryant KK: Burn injuries. In Kitt S, Selfridge Thomas J, Proehl J et al, editors: *Emergency nursing: a physiologic and clinical perspective,* Philadelphia, 1995, WB Saunders.
16. Dries DJ, Holleran R: Burn care pearls, *Air Med J* 16(3):68, 1997.
17. Lewis AM: Understanding the principles of lightning injuries, *J Emerg Nurs* 23(6):535-541, 1997.
18. Dog-bite related fatalities in the United States, 1995-1996, *MMWR* 46:463-467, 1997.
19. National Center for Injury Prevention and Control: Unintentional injury prevention fact sheet on dogs, www.cdc.gov/ncipc/diup/dogbite2.htm, 1999.
20. Gibbons RV: Cryptogenic rabies, bats and the question of aerosol transmission, *Ann Emerg Med* 39(5):528-536, 2002.
21. Clowes TD: Wound assessment of the *Loxosceles reclusa* spider bite, *J Emerg Nurs* 22(4):283-287, 1996.
22. Auerbach P: Envenomations from jellyfish and related species, *J Emerg Nurs* 23:555-568, 1997.

CHAPTER 7

Facial Emergencies

REVIEW OUTLINE

I. Anatomy and physiology
  A. Anatomical structures
    1. Mandible
    2. Maxilla
    3. Zygoma
    4. Zygomatic arch
    5. Nasal bones and structures
    6. Orbit
    7. Orbital rim
    8. Sinuses
      a. Frontal
      b. Maxillary
      c. Ethmoid
      d. Sphenoid
    9. Ethmoid
    10. Cranial nerves
    11. Cranial bones
    12. Oral cavity and contents
    13. Auditory bones and structures
    14. Major blood vessels
  B. Physiology
    1. Central nervous system
      a. Cranial nerves
      b. Functions of brain stem, cerebrum, and cerebellum
    2. Process of sight
    3. Process of speech

II. Assessment
  A. Primary survey
    1. ABCD
      a. Airway
      b. Breathing
      c. Circulation
      d. Deficit, neurological
    2. Critical interventions
  B. Secondary survey
    1. History of illness or injury
      a. Mechanism and time
      b. AMPLE history
    2. Chief complaint
      a. Pain: PQRST
        (1) Provocation
        (2) Quality
        (3) Radiation
        (4) Severity
        (5) Timing
      b. Bleeding
      c. Edema or ecchymosis
      d. Asymmetry
      e. Fever or chills
      f. Paresthesia
      g. Diplopia
      h. Malocclusion
      i. Trismus
      j. Deformity
    3. Physical examination
      a. General appearance
      b. Mental status and level of consciousness
      c. Glasgow Coma Scale
      d. Vital signs
      e. Inspection
        (1) Symmetry of facial features
        (2) Ecchymosis
        (3) Edema
        (4) Eyes: subconjunctival hemorrhage, pupillary height, pupillary reaction, extraocular eye movements
        (5) Nose
        (6) Mouth malocclusion (visualize gross dental occlusion)
        (7) Ears
        (8) Cranial nerves
        (9) Neck
        (10) Head
      f. Palpation
        (1) Symmetry
        (2) Localized point tenderness

(3) Abnormal mobility
(4) Crepitus
(5) Temporomandibular joint
(6) Foreign bodies
(7) Lacerations or hematomas

III. Diagnostic methods for facial emergencies
  A. Radiology
    1. Facial radiographs
      a. Panorex
      b. Waters' view
    2. Computed tomography
    3. Magnetic resonance imaging
  B. Laboratory
    1. Complete blood count with differential
    2. Electrolytes
    3. Toxicology screen
    4. Blood alcohol level
    5. Cultures

IV. Related nursing diagnoses
  A. Airway clearance, ineffective
  B. Alteration in comfort, pain
  C. Anxiety
  D. Fluid volume deficit, high risk for
  E. Infection, high risk for
  F. Knowledge deficit
  G. Sensory-perceptual alteration
  H. Skin integrity, impairment of

V. Age-related changes
  A. Pediatric patient
    1. Facial bones in children are softer and more pliable than in adults; therefore, facial fractures tend to be less severe[1]
  B. Geriatric patient
    1. Elderly have a decrease in pain perception
    2. Elderly tend to dismiss complaints as normal aging, so all complaints should be investigated

VI. Selected facial emergencies
  A. Sinusitis
  B. Trigeminal neuralgia
  C. Facial lacerations and soft tissue injuries
  D. Mandibular fractures
  E. Maxillary fractures
  F. Zygomatic fractures
  G. Blow-out fractures

Maxillofacial emergencies are common in any emergency department. Most injuries are not life threatening, but the potential for disfigurement and emotional despair is great. The most common cause of facial injuries is blunt trauma secondary to motor vehicle accidents. Other mechanisms of injury include those that produce both blunt and penetrating trauma, such as altercations, domestic violence, falls, and sports-related accidents.

Maxillofacial emergencies produce life-threatening situations when they obstruct the airway or cause hemorrhagic shock. Mechanical obstruction of the airway occurs due to anatomical displacement of normal structures secondary to trauma or disease. Broken teeth or a swollen epiglottis are examples. Because the head is rich in vasculature, profuse bleeding is a natural occurrence with any injury. Maxillofacial trauma can cause severe hemorrhage, which may be occult, because patients have a tendency to swallow blood rather than expectorate it.

Assessment and stabilization of clients with maxillofacial emergencies follow the same sequence, the ABCs, as for any trauma patient.

REVIEW QUESTIONS

Facial Trauma

1. Which of the following is the most common indicator of a facial fracture?
A. Edema
B. Laceration
C. Asymmetry
D. Ecchymosis

A 26-year-old woman is brought to your emergency department via Life Squad. She was the unrestrained driver of an automobile that ran into a bridge abutment. The car's windshield was reportedly cracked. The victim, Ms. Green, is awake and oriented. A large scalp laceration and facial trauma are obvious. Ms. Green's vital signs are B/P 90/60, P 100, and R 28. Ms. Green has been appropriately immobilized on a backboard, with a cervical collar in place.

2. Your first priority for this patient is:
A. Airway assessment and management
B. Breathing assessment and management
C. Circulation assessment and management
D. Neurological assessment and management

3. Which of the following is the most appropriate way to begin assessment of Ms. Green's airway?
A. Ask the patient if she is able to bite down evenly or if she has pain with jaw movement

B. Listen to the patient's lungs for indications of possible aspiration of blood or vomitus
C. Draw arterial blood gases to evaluate her oxygenation as soon as she is in the trauma room
D. Ask the patient to open her mouth and look for any foreign objects, loose debris, or blood

4. When assessing Ms. Green's airway, you discover that she has a large amount of bleeding in the oropharynx, which she is swallowing. Your immediate intervention would be:
A. Prepare for intubation to protect the airway
B. Insert a nasogastric tube to empty the stomach
C. Suction frequently and teach the patient to expectorate the blood
D. Wait until the cervical spine is cleared, and then place Ms. Green in a semi-Fowler's position

5. Based on the mechanism of injury and Ms. Green's vital signs, the most appropriate nursing diagnosis is:
A. Anticipatory grieving
B. Hyperthermia
C. Fluid volume deficit, high risk for
D. Impaired thought processes

Ms. Green is diagnosed as having a bilateral LeFort III fracture, also known as craniofacial dysjunction. *As its name implies, the facial and cranial skulls become disjoined. A LeFort I fracture produces a horizontal detachment of the maxilla at the level of the nasal floor, leaving the maxillary alveolar ridge and hard palate mobile. A LeFort II fracture, or pyramid fracture, involves fractures of the maxilla, nasal bones, the medial half of the interior orbital rim, the orbital floor, and lacrimal bones.*

6. A common emergency nursing intervention is to monitor airway patency. What criterion is the first indicator of airway compromise?
A. Change in color
B. Change in mental status
C. Change in respiratory rate
D. Change in blood pressure and pulse

Blow-out Fractures

The police bring Mr. Plant, a 32-year-old man, to your emergency department after his involvement in an altercation. He has sustained facial trauma and is diagnosed with a right-sided blow-out orbital fracture. He is awake and alert, with periorbital ecchymosis on the right side of his face. Mr. Plant's vital signs are B/P 120/80, P 84, R 18.

7. Common signs and symptoms of a blow-out orbital fracture include:
A. Permanent loss of vision of the affected eye
B. Exophthalmos of the affected eye
C. Lowered pupil position on the affected side
D. Extraocular eye movements limited bilaterally

8. The most appropriate nursing diagnosis for Mr. Plant would be:
A. Hopelessness
B. Fluid volume deficit
C. Alteration in comfort, pain
D. Impaired thought processes

9. The patient who has sustained a blow-out orbital fracture and has periorbital crepitus should have visual acuity monitored to evaluate for involvement of the:
A. Optic nerve
B. Intraorbital nerves
C. Central retinal artery
D. Extraocular eye muscles

Bell's Palsy

Mrs. Jones, a 45-year-old woman, comes in with peripheral facial paralysis, fever, chills, and flulike symptoms. She is diagnosed as having Bell's palsy. This is Mrs. Jones' first episode of any type of disorder and she is very anxious.

10. Bell's palsy affects which cranial nerve?
A. Seventh: facial
B. Fourth: trochlear
C. Fifth: trigeminal
D. Ninth: glossopharyngeal

11. Common signs and symptoms associated with Bell's palsy include:
A. Unilateral, flaccid facial paralysis
B. Gradual onset of symptoms
C. Increased lacrimation on the affected side
D. Lid lag on the opposite side, especially noted when closing the eyes

12. The most appropriate nursing diagnosis for Mrs. Jones is:
   A. Hopelessness
   B. Infection, high risk for
   C. Airway clearance, ineffective
   D. Anxiety, related to knowledge deficit

13. The most appropriate nursing intervention related to the above nursing diagnosis involves education. Mrs. Jones should be taught that:
   A. She must be admitted to the hospital to rule out a cerebrovascular accident
   B. Recovery is usually spontaneous and occurs within 3 weeks
   C. To facilitate recovery, she must enter a rehabilitation program immediately
   D. She will never recover and must learn to live with permanent Bell's phenomenon

Facial Laceration

A 10-year-old child, Tommy, is brought to the emergency department by his mother after a bicycle accident. Tommy fell head-first on a gravel road. He was not knocked unconscious and is awake and oriented. He has sustained a deep facial laceration extending from the forehead through the left eyebrow. He also has multiple facial abrasions. His vital signs are stable, and Tommy has no other obvious injuries.

14. Inspection of all the wounds for foreign bodies is imperative to prevent:
   A. Infection
   B. "Tattooing" effect
   C. Improper wound closure (malalignment)
   D. All of the above

15. The primary nursing diagnosis related to Tommy's mechanism of injury is:
   A. Infection, high risk for
   B. Impaired gas exchange
   C. Fluid volume deficit, high risk for
   D. Potential alteration in body temperature

16. Preparation of Tommy's large laceration for suturing includes all of the following except:
   A. Anesthetize the wound prior to cleaning
   B. Shave the eyebrow to remove all surrounding debris
   C. Cleanse with the appropriate solution and rinse thoroughly
   D. Search thoroughly for foreign bodies with a magnification instrument (glasses or lens)

17. Tommy's mother is taught to observe for signs of infection. To evaluate the effectiveness of education, the emergency nurse should:
   A. Have Tommy's mother repeat what she has been taught
   B. Make an appointment for Tommy to return to the emergency department for a wound check
   C. Call Tommy's pediatrician the next day to make sure Tommy's mother has made an appointment for a wound check and suture removal
   D. Make a written referral to the local public health department requesting follow-up information on Tommy

Sinusitis

18. A 46-year-old male comes to the emergency department with a 1-week history of fever, cough, and thick, green nasal drainage. He is now complaining of a severe headache and facial pain. Based on clinical findings the patient is diagnosed with sinusitis. In addition to antibiotics, what other treatments should be prescribed for this patient?
   A. A hand-held inhaler to decrease the possibility of asthma
   B. Lying flat in bed at night to promote sinus drainage
   C. Nasal or systemic decongestants
   D. Fluid restriction to decrease nasal drainage

19. If a nasal decongestant is prescribed, the emergency nurse should caution the patient to not use it longer than 3 days because:
   A. Extended use of topical decongestants decreases sinus congestion
   B. Topical decongestants generally lose their effectiveness after 1 week
   C. The patient will not become dependent on nasal decongestants
   D. The patient may develop an allergic reaction to the nasal decongestant

20. A complete craniofacial separation involving the maxilla, zygoma, orbits, and bones of the cranial base is classified as:
   A. LeFort I
   B. LeFort III
   C. LeFort II
   D. None of the above

ANSWERS

1. **D. Assessment.**[1-3]
2. **A. Assessment.** Obviously, the patient cannot survive without a patent airway. All other assessment parameters are secondary to airway assessment.[3]
3. **D. Assessment.** This is the best method to assess Ms. Green's airway for foreign bodies. The most common are broken teeth, the tongue, and blood. The tongue may obstruct the airway in patients with a decreased level of consciousness. It is important to look for broken teeth and occult bleeding, because fearful patients can easily hide both.[3]
4. **C. Intervention.** Swallowing blood needs to be prevented to keep the patient from vomiting and potentially aspirating.[3]
5. **C. Analysis.** Ms. Green's blood pressure is low and pulse is above average for the normal adult. Both are signs of hypovolemia.
6. **B. Evaluation.** A change in vital signs is a very late indicator of respiratory compromise. Color is a poor assessment parameter in the adult. Frequently patients will exhibit very subtle changes in mental status, such as sudden anger, complaints, or sleepiness, that the alert emergency nurse must be aware of to provide rapid diagnosis and intervention.[3]
7. **C. Assessment.** A blow-out orbital fracture is a depressed fracture of the orbital floor in which the contents of the orbit protrude into the maxillary sinus. Thus the affected eye sinks into the maxillary sinus, producing a lowered pupil position and asymmetry of the eyes. Other common symptoms include conjunctival hemorrhage and eyelid ecchymosis due to blunt trauma, infraorbital nerve paresthesia due to a pinched facial nerve at the fracture site, and diplopia.[1,3]
8. **C. Analysis.** Blow-out orbital fractures alone do not produce impaired thought process, hopelessness, or fluid volume deficit. They do, however, produce severe pain.[1]
9. **C. Evaluation.** Air may build up under pressure in the orbit, producing cessation of blood flow in the central retinal artery.[3,4]
10. **A. Assessment.**[3]
11. **A. Assessment.** Other symptoms of Bell's palsy include rapid onset of symptoms, viral prodrome, lid lag on the affected side when closing the eyes, decreased lacrimation on the affected side, and Bell's phenomenon, which is an upward movement of the eyeball on the affected side when attempting to close the eye.[1]
12. **D. Analysis.** Bell's palsy does not affect the airway, and the patient is unlikely to develop an infectious process. Most patients are extremely anxious due to a lack of knowledge concerning their medical diagnosis.[1]
13. **B. Intervention.** During the recovery phase, Mrs. Jones should be educated to rest and treat her flulike symptoms appropriately. She will also be given eye drops, because of the decreased lacrimation on the affected side, and may require analgesics.[1]
14. **D. Assessment.** Infection, "tattooing," and malalignment may all result from a missed foreign body.[1,3,5]
15. **A. Analysis.** Because Tommy sustained his injury on a gravel road, his potential for infection is high.[3,5-7]
16. **B. Intervention.** Eyebrows should never be shaved. They provide anatomical landmarks to ensure proper alignment of the wound, and they may not grow back.[3,5-7]
17. **A. Evaluation.** A return demonstration or repeat of verbal or written instructions, or both, is the best way to evaluate patient teaching.
18. **C. Intervention.** Nasal and systemic decongestants should be prescribed for the management of sinusitis to keep the sinuses open and decrease the amount of media for bacterial growth.[8,9]
19. **B. Intervention.** Nasal decongestants generally lose their effectiveness after 3 days. Longer or habitual use of nasal sprays can actually cause nasal tissue irritation that will result in increased nasal congestion.[9]
20. **B. Assessment.**
    - LeFort I: transverse maxillary fracture which occurs above the level of the teeth, resulting in a separation of the teeth from the rest of the maxilla
    - LeFort II: Pyramidal maxillary fracture involving the middle facial area
    - LeFort III: Complete craniofacial separation involving the maxilla, zygoma, orbits, and the bones of the cranial base[3]

References

1. Revere CJ: Facial emergencies. In Jordan KS, editor: *Emergency nursing core curriculum*, ed 5, Philadelphia, 2000, WB Saunders.

2. Rahman WM, O'Connor TJ: Facial trauma. In Barkin R, editor: *Pediatric emergency medicine,* St Louis, 1997, Mosby.
3. Emergency Nurses Association: *Trauma nursing core course,* Des Plaines, IL, 2000, Emergency Nurses Association.
4. Gerlock AJ: Facial trauma, *Trauma Q* 2(4):20-34, 1986.
5. Doak SA: Wound care. In Hamilton GC, Sanders AB, Strange GR et al: *Emergency medicine: an approach to clinical problem-solving,* Philadelphia, 2003, WB Saunders.
6. Goldman R: For your eyes only, *Emergency* 19(12):27-29, 1987.
7. Gussack GS, Luterman A, Powell RW et al: Pediatric maxillofacial trauma: unique features in diagnosis and treatment, *Laryngoscope* 97:925-930, 1987.
8. Edlow J, Macnow L: Headache. In Davis M, Votey SR, Greenough PG, editors: *Signs and symptoms in emergency medicine,* St Louis, 1999, Mosby.
9. Olson C: Dental, ear, nose, and throat emergencies. In Newberry L, editor: *Sheehy's emergency nursing: principles and practice,* ed 5, St Louis, 2003, Mosby.

Additional Readings

Kalish MA: Airway management in maxillofacial trauma, *Emerg Med Sci* 18(6):42-44, 1989.

Keresh JW: Ocular and periocular trauma, *Emerg Med Serv* 18(6):46-55, 1989.

Kitt S, Selfridge-Thomas J, Proehl J et al, editors: *Emergency nursing: a physiologic and clinical perspective,* Philadelphia, 1995, WB Saunders.

Lee MJ, Martinez AJ: Focusing on facial and ocular injuries, *J Emerg Med Serv* 17(2):28-42, 1992.

Lower J: Maxillofacial trauma, *Nurs Clin North Am* 21(4):611-628, 1986.

Manson PN, Kelly KJ: Evaluation and management of the patient with facial trauma, *Emerg Med Serv* 18(6):22-30, 1989.

Newberry L: *Sheehy's emergency nursing: principles and practice,* St Louis, 1998, Mosby.

CHAPTER 8

GENITOURINARY EMERGENCIES

REVIEW OUTLINE

I. Anatomy of the genitourinary tract[1]
   A. Kidneys
   B. Ureters
   C. Bladder
   D. Urethra
   E. Renal vessels
   F. Urinary meatus
   G. Adrenal glands

II. Male anatomy
   A. Penis
   B. Glans
   C. Prepuce
   D. Foreskin
   E. Urethra
   F. Scrotum
   G. Testes
   H. Epididymis
   I. Vas deferens
   J. Sexual maturity rating

III. Female anatomy
   A. Mons pubis
   B. Labia majora
   C. Labia minora
   D. Vulva
   E. Clitoris
   F. Posterior fourchette
   G. Fossa navicularis
   H. Vestibule
   I. Hymen
   J. Puberty
   K. Perineum
   L. Urethral meatus
   M. Vagina
   N. Cervix

IV. Function of the genitourinary tract
   A. Management of body fluids
   B. Electrolyte balance
   C. Excretion of metabolic end products
   D. Detoxification of selected products: medications, poisons
   E. Prostaglandin production
   F. Renin production
   G. Insulin degradation
   H. Stimulation of red blood cell production
   I. Metabolic conversion of vitamin D to its active form
   J. Sexual function

V. Assessment and collaborative care of the patient with a genitourinary emergency[1]
   A. History
      1. Onset of problem, sudden or gradual
      2. Last menstrual period
      3. Previous genitourinary diseases or surgeries
      4. Urinary symptoms
         a. Dysuria
         b. Frequency
         c. Urgency
         d. Burning
         e. Nocturia
         f. Hematuria
         g. Dribbling
         h. Incontinence
         i. Difficulty initiating urinary stream
      5. Gynecological related symptoms
         a. Vaginal discharge: color, amount
         b. Vaginal bleeding: color, amount, clots, or tissue
         c. Vaginal itching
         d. Vaginal burning
         e. Sores, lumps
         f. Dyspareunia
      6. Medications
         a. Drugs that may interfere with urination
            (1) Antihistamines
            (2) Anticholinergic agents
            (3) Tricyclic antidepressants
         b. Contraception
         c. Hormone therapy
         d. Erectile dysfunction medications

7. Medical problems
   a. Diabetes
   b. Renal disease
   c. Thyroid disorders
   d. Sexually transmitted diseases
   e. Erectile dysfunction

B. Physical assessment
1. Location of pain and pain patterns
2. Associated signs and symptoms: nausea, vomiting, change in bowel functions
3. Fever, chills
4. Signs and symptoms of septic shock
5. External genitalia
   a. Inflammation
   b. Ulceration
   c. Discharge
   d. Swelling, nodules, lesions
6. Color of urine
7. Amount of urine
8. Evaluation of hematuria
9. Auscultation of bowel sounds
10. Palpation and pelvic examination
11. Palpation and male genital examination
12. Prostate examination
13. Rectal examination, male and female

C. Age-related changes
1. Pediatric patient
   a. Bowel and bladder continence
      (1) Age
      (2) Stage of bowel and bladder training
      (3) Type of diapers used
   b. Tanner's classification of sexual development of the female[1]
      (1) Stage 1: preadolescent, no pubic hair, fine body hair similar to hair on the abdomen
      (2) Stage 2: sparse growth of long, slightly pigmented downy hair mostly along the labia
      (3) Stage 3: darker, coarser hair, beginning to spread
      (4) Stage 4: coarse, curly hair that looks like adult pubic hair, but in a smaller amount than in an adult
      (5) Stage 5: coarse, curly dark hair in the same amount as an adult
   c. Tanner's classification of sexual development of the male[1]
      (1) Stage 1: no pubic hair, and penis and testicles the same size as childhood
      (2) Stage 2: some growth of pubic hair, slight enlargement of penis, testes and scrotum beginning to enlarge
      (3) Stage 3: pubic hair darkening and spreading, penis lengthening, testicles and scrotum continuing to enlarge
      (4) Stage 4: pubic hair as in the adult, but not as much, penis increasing in length and size, glans developing, scrotal skin darkening
      (5) Stage 5: pubic hair in adult quantity, and penis, scrotum, and testicles in adult shape and size
2. Geriatric patient
   a. Bowel and bladder continence
      (1) May experience increase in incontinence
      (2) May experience increase in urgency and frequency
   b. Changes seen once the woman has gone through menopause
      (1) Decrease in amount of pubic hair
      (2) Decrease in size of labia and clitoris
      (3) Shortening of vagina
      (4) Mucosa in the vagina becoming pale, thin, and dry
   c. Changes in the male
      (1) Pubic hair decreases and grays
      (2) Penis decreases in size
      (3) Testicles hang lower in the scrotum

D. Collaborative care
1. Stabilization of ABCs
   a. Airway
   b. Breathing
   c. Circulation

2. Fluid resuscitation
3. Pain management
4. Diagnostic studies or procedures
   a. Complete blood cell count (CBC) with differential
   b. Blood cultures when a fever is present
   c. Electrolytes, blood urea nitrogen (BUN), creatinine
   d. β-Human chorionic gonadotropin in female patients of childbearing age
   e. Type and crossmatch
   f. Urinalysis and urine culture
   g. Urine stone analysis
   h. Urine analysis by reagent strip
   i. Gram stain
   j. Wet mounts
      (1) Saline
      (2) Potassium hydroxide preparation
   k. Cultures and blood tests for sexually transmitted diseases
      (1) Gonococcus culture
      (2) Chlamydia culture
      (3) Rapid plasma reagin for syphilis
   l. Ultrasonography
   m. Intravenous pyelogram
   n. Retrograde urethrogram
   o. Cystogram
   p. Abdominal computed tomography (CT) with or without contrast or magnetic resonance imaging (MRI) of abdomen and selected organs

VI. Collaborative care problems
   A. Anxiety
   B. Body image disturbance
   C. Dysreflexia
   D. Fluid volume deficit, high risk for
   E. Hyperthermia, related to infection
   F. Incontinence, urge
   G. Infection, high risk for
   H. Knowledge deficit
   I. Pain, acute and chronic
   J. Rape-trauma syndrome
   K. Self-esteem disturbance
   L. Urinary elimination, altered
   M. Urinary retention

VII. Genitourinary and gynecological emergencies
   A. Renal trauma
   B. Bladder trauma
   C. Foreign bodies
   D. Kidney stone(s) (urolithiasis)
   E. Urinary tract infection
   F. Urinary retention
   G. Benign prostatic hyperplasia
   H. Pyelonephritis
   I. Hematuria
   J. Renal failure
   K. Testicular torsion
   L. Epididymitis
   M. Priapism
   N. Sexual assault
   O. Foreign body insertion
   P. Sexually transmitted diseases
      1. Syphilis
      2. Gonorrhea
      3. Chlamydia
      4. Herpes simplex
      5. Condyloma acuminatum (venereal warts)
      6. Chancroid
      7. Granuloma inguinale
      8. Lymphogranuloma venereum
      9. Hepatitis B
      10. Human immunodeficiency virus (HIV)

VIII. Selected genitourinary emergencies
   A. Urinary tract infection
   B. Pyelonephritis
   C. Urinary calculi
   D. Testicular torsion
   E. Epididymitis
   F. Genitourinary trauma
      1. Sexual assault
      2. Urethral injury
      3. Renal trauma
      4. Bladder injury
      5. Foreign bodies
   G. Priapism

The assessment and care of the patient who is suffering from a genitourinary emergency begins with obtaining a history of the patient's chief complaint and then performing an evaluation of the patient's back, abdomen, urine, external genitalia, and pelvis. When obtaining information related to urinary tract symptoms, the emergency nurse should include questions about dysuria, frequency, urgency, and hematuria. In addition, the emergency nurse should ask if there are any related symptoms such as fever, chills, nausea or vomiting, or discharge. The age and sexual activity of the patient are additional pieces of information that may shed light on the nature of the patient's problem.

Certain disease processes, such as diabetes, hypertension, gout, and spinal cord injury, leave the patient at risk for developing a genitourinary problem. Trauma to the abdomen, back, or genitals may be a source of injury to the urethra, bladder, or kidneys.

Care of the patient with a genitourinary emergency may include diagnostic studies: CBC, electrolytes, BUN, creatinine, β-human chorionic gonadotropin for female patients of childbearing age, urinalysis, urinary culture, ultrasonography, intravenous pyelogram, and CT or MRI.

Many genitourinary emergencies cause the patient a great deal of pain, and pain patterns may provide clues to the basis of the patient's problem. Pain management may include oral, intramuscular, or intravenous administration of medications, as well as providing the patient with comfort measures such as a warm blanket or a place to lie down. Assisting the patient with pain management will help the emergency nurse determine the cause of the patient's discomfort.

The incidence of sexually transmitted diseases continues to rise despite public awareness and education.[2] A disease such as syphilis, which was not routinely seen in the emergency department, has become more common and now is seen in its secondary and sometimes in its tertiary or neuroleptic stages. Both hepatitis B and HIV are considered sexually transmitted diseases and pose particularly challenging problems for the emergency department, including infection control issues.

The emergency nursing care of the patient with a genitourinary emergency will depend on the origin of the emergency and the patient's response to it.

REVIEW QUESTIONS

Urinary Calculi

A 32-year-old man comes to the emergency department complaining of abdominal and back pain. He states that he has been urinating frequently, but only a small amount of urine comes out. He states that he has seen some blood in his urine.

1. Initial assessment of this patient should include:
A. Palpating the patient's bilateral femoral pulses
B. Determining the pattern of the patient's pain
C. Discovering what type of diet the patient is on
D. Obtaining BUN and creatinine levels to rule out renal failure

2. The most common composition of kidney stones is:
A. Oxalate
B. Magnesium ammonium phosphate
C. Uric acid
D. Calcium oxalate

3. All of the following could contribute to this patient's inability to void except:
A. Ingestion of eight glasses of water
B. Ingestion of 50 mg of amitriptyline (Elavil)
C. Blunt trauma to the bladder
D. A foreign body in the urethra

4. All of the following are nonhematuric causes of red urine except:
A. Eating beets
B. Eating blackberries
C. Taking coumadin
D. Taking rifampin

5. The patient's CT reveals a kidney stone. Because it is a small stone, the patient will be discharged home to attempt to pass it. The patient will be given oxycodone (Percodan) for pain and a strainer to use while voiding. An appropriate nursing diagnosis for the patient's going-home instructions would be:
A. Fluid volume deficit related to renal calculi and potential obstruction
B. Pain related to penile discharge from the catheterization
C. Urinary elimination, altered patterns, related to obstruction from a kidney stone
D. Incontinence, urge, related to renal calculi and the patient's age

6. A nonurgent side effect of oxycodone is:
A. Constipation
B. Anaphylactic reaction
C. Respiratory depression
D. Hypotension

7. When teaching the patient about diet related to the development of renal calculi, the emergency nurse should instruct the patient to avoid which of the following foods?
   A. Orange juice
   B. Red meat
   C. Spinach
   D. Walnuts

8. Quality improvement criteria for the chart of this patient (or any patient who has been treated in the emergency department for renal calculi) should include documentation of:
   A. Hemoptysis
   B. Urinalysis
   C. Hematochezia
   D. CBC with differential

9. Criteria for admission of the patient with renal calculi would be:
   A. Small-diameter stones that can be passed easily
   B. Multiple kidney stones visualized on the CT
   C. Absence of stones in the patient's bladder
   D. Need for intravenous pain management

Testicular Torsion

A 10-year-old boy is brought to the emergency department by his parents. They state that he had been climbing a tree and began suffering severe pain in his groin. The child is alert, diaphoretic, and obviously very uncomfortable.

10. A history that may indicate testicular torsion would include all of the following except:
    A. Age of the patient
    B. Sexual activity
    C. Gradual onset of scrotal pain
    D. Nausea

11. The diagnosis of testicular torsion has been made by the urologist. Manual manipulation of the testicle has failed to reduce the torsion. The emergency nurse will now prepare the patient and his family for:
    A. Care of the testicular torsion at home
    B. Admission to the hospital for observation
    C. A barium enema to reduce the torsion
    D. Surgery for reduction of the torsion

12. The child becomes very upset when he is told that he must go to surgery for repair of the problem with his testicle. He becomes combative and states he will not go. The emergency nurse will plan the care of the patient using the following nursing diagnosis:
    A. Growth and development, altered, related to surgery
    B. Fear related to a potentially threatening situation
    C. Sexual dysfunction, high risk for, related to testicular torsion
    D. Mobility, impaired physical, related to having a surgical procedure

13. The emergency nurse provides the patient and his family with a private place in which to prepare for the surgery and spends time explaining the activities related to the surgery. The emergency nurse might observe which of the following if this intervention is effective?
    A. The patient's pulse rate increases to 150 when the nurse enters the room
    B. The patient turns his back when the nurse enters the room
    C. The patient verbalizes his fear of the surgery
    D. The patient's family takes the child home against medical advice

14. Which of the following positions may be useful when performing a urinary catheterization on a female patient who cannot lie supine?
    A. On her side with her upper leg flexed at the hip and knee
    B. On her abdomen with her hips and knees flexed as much as possible
    C. With her knees flexed and her heels placed as closely as possible to her perineum
    D. In a supine position, because a woman can be catheterized for urine only in this position

15. Suprapubic urine aspiration is indicated in which of the following patients?
    A. Any child older than 2 years who has suspected sepsis
    B. Any patient who is suspected of having a pelvic fracture
    C. A patient less than 2 years of age who has just voided
    D. A child less than 2 years of age who is unable to void

Urinary Tract Infections

An 18-month-old female is brought to the emergency department by her mother. Her mother states that she feels warm, has been drinking only small amounts of fluid, and cries periodically.

16. In children, what symptom may be the only sign of a urinary tract infection?
A. Refusal to drink liquids
B. Fever without other associated symptoms
C. Nausea and vomiting and refusal to eat
D. Complaint of pain with urination and bowel movements

17. Risk factors that contribute to urinary tract infections include which of the following:
A. Estrogen deficiency
B. Carbonated beverage consumption
C. Frequent sexual intercourse
D. All of the above

18. Prescribing a fluoroquinolone to a child under the age of 18 to manage a urinary tract infection is contraindicated because:
A. The primary bacterium that causes urinary tract infections in children is resistant to these antibiotics
B. Children under the age of 18 are frequently allergic to these antibiotics
C. These antibiotics may cause disruption to developing cartilage in children
D. These antibiotics may cause injury to developing teeth in children under 18 years

19. Effectiveness of management of a urinary tract infection can be evaluated by the patient by noting:
A. An increase in urinary frequency 48 hours after treatment
B. A fever of 103° F with chills after 24 hours of treatment
C. A decrease in pain with urination after 24 hours
D. The formation of bruises on the patient's upper extremities

An 80-year-old man is brought to the emergency department by his daughter. She states that he has had a fever and has been incontinent. She also states that he has been more confused than normal. He has a history only of hypertension, which is being managed with atenolol.

20. The initial management of this patient in the emergency department would include:
A. Sending the patient to the radiography department for an abdominal film
B. Obtaining an atenolol level
C. Obtaining a urine specimen to rule out a urinary tract infection
D. Drawing a prostate-specific antigen level to rule out benign prostatic hypertrophy

Sexually Transmitted Diseases

21. A 22-year-old man comes to the emergency department complaining of scrotal swelling and pain. Epididymitis is diagnosed by the emergency physician. The organism that frequently causes epididymitis in sexually active males is:
A. *Trichomonas vaginalis*
B. *Chlamydia trachomatis*
C. *Treponema pallidum*
D. *Escherichia coli*

22. An 18-year-old male comes to the emergency department complaining of a rash on the palms of his hands. He is a runaway and has been sexually active with both men and women to earn money. He has never been treated for a sexually transmitted disease but offers a history of nonpainful sores on the glans of his penis that have disappeared. What is the most likely cause of his rash?
A. Diabetes mellitus
B. Syphilis
C. Gonorrhea
D. Herpes simplex II

23. Recommendations from the Centers for Disease Control and Prevention (CDC) for the management of uncomplicated gonococcal infection include:
A. Intramuscular penicillin G plus azithromycin IM
B. Tetracycline IV plus azithromycin IV
C. Ceftriaxone IM plus azithromycin PO
D. Aqueous penicillin plus azithromycin PO

24. An appropriate nursing diagnosis for the patient who is being treated for a sexually transmitted disease in the emergency department would be:
A. Infection related to *Chlamydia trachomatis*
B. Knowledge deficit related to the etiology and management of epididymitis
C. Sexual dysfunction, high risk for, related to the diagnosis of gonorrhea

D. Violence, high risk for, related to the diagnosis of a sexually transmitted disease

25. Which of the following sexually transmitted diseases may be prevented through vaccination?
A. Hepatitis A
B. Hepatitis C
C. Herpes simplex virus
D. *Chlamydia trachomatis* in infants

26. A 15-year-old boy comes to the emergency department complaining of a yellow penile discharge and burning with urination. He tells the triage nurse he will not stay if she has to call his parents. This emergency nurse assures him that she will not have to notify his parents before he can be treated because:
A. Adolescents in the United States can consent for examination and treatment for a sexually transmitted disease without parental notification
B. A 15-year-old boy is old enough to give his consent if he comes to the emergency department unaccompanied
C. An older brother or sister is allowed to give consent for evaluation and treatment of a sibling if the teenager does not want to notify parents
D. There is no available management for the types of signs and symptoms that he is having

27. When discharging a patient being treated with metronidazole for a trichomoniasis infection, the emergency nurse should emphasize that:
A. His partner does not have to be evaluated and treated if the patient takes all his medication as prescribed
B. He may continue to drink alcohol with all his meals as he did before the medication was prescribed
C. He should be sure that sexual partners use barrier contraception until the person who is infected has been seen again and cleared of infection
D. He should take the medication before he eats any type of food or at any meal

Renal Problems

28. A 78-year-old man was found at home. He fell 3 days earlier and has been lying on the floor since. Upon arrival in the emergency department, he is covered with urine and feces. His right arm and chest are purple from where he has been lying, and compartment syndrome is suspected. The patient is cleaned up, and a urinary catheter is inserted. A small amount of dark yellow urine is obtained and test results are positive for blood. The most probable cause of the blood in his urine is:
A. Benign prostatic hypertrophy
B. Chronic urinary tract infection
C. Hypokalemia from dehydration
D. Rhabdomyolysis from tissue injury

29. Acute tubular necrosis is a cause of:
A. Prerenal failure
B. Postrenal failure
C. Intrarenal failure
D. Urethral stricture

30. A major complication of continuous ambulatory peritoneal dialysis is:
A. Peritonitis
B. Catheter occlusion
C. Renal calculi
D. Rhabdomyolysis

Genitourinary Trauma

An 18-year-old man is brought to the emergency department after having been struck by a car while riding his bicycle. The patient was wearing a helmet. He is alert and oriented, complaining of back and abdominal pain. His vital signs are B/P 80/40, P 140, R 28.

31. A sign of severe injury to the pelvis or bladder is:
A. Coopernail's sign
B. Kehr's sign
C. Homans' sign
D. Chadwick's sign

32. Which of the following would be a contraindication to urinary catheter insertion?
A. The patient has a pelvic fracture
B. The patient complains of lower abdominal pain
C. The patient is unconscious and cannot consent
D. There is blood around the urinary meatus

33. The initial care of this patient would be based on the following nursing diagnosis:
A. Injury, high risk for, related to blunt force to the flank

B. Infection, high risk for, related to catheter insertion
C. Fluid volume deficit related to hemorrhage
D. Anxiety related to potential sexual dysfunction

34. Which of the following interventions may be used to treat a patient with a pelvic fracture in the emergency department?
A. Placing a commercially available pelvic sling on the patient
B. Wrapping a sheet around the pelvis and tying it into a sling
C. Placing pneumatic antishock garments on the patient and inflating all the compartments
D. All of the above

35. Signs and symptoms of a ruptured bladder include:
A. Normal urinary output postabdominal injury
B. Clear urine that was negative for blood per a reagent strip
C. Abdominal distention and pain with palpation
D. Normal distribution of contrast during a cystogram

36. The most serious complication of a human bite to the genitals is:
A. Bleeding from the wound
B. Disfigurement from the wound
C. Inability to reimplant lost tissue
D. Infection from bacterial contamination

37. An indication of renal injury is:
A. Ballance's sign
B. Kehr's sign
C. Grey Turner's sign
D. Cullen's sign

38. A 39-year-old African American man comes to the emergency department with the complaint of a sustained erection. The patient states that he has had this problem in the past. What medical problem may be the cause of this patient's priapism?
A. Sickle cell disease
B. Diabetes mellitus
C. Acute renal failure
D. Systemic lupus erythematosus

39. A common complication of priapism is:
A. Gangrene of the penis
B. Hemorrhagic shock
C. Urinary retention
D. Sexual impotence

40. A 33-year-old mentally retarded male is brought to the emergency department by his caregivers. They state he has a fever of 102° F, a foul-smelling penile discharge, and he is afraid to urinate because of pain. The family states he has never had any sexual contacts. A potential source of his symptoms probably is:
A. Nongonococcal urethritis
B. Foreign body
C. Urinary calculi
D. Pyelonephritis

41. Accidental straddle injuries in the female pediatric patient are usually located:
A. Above the 9 o'clock to 3 o'clock area of the vagina
B. At the 8 o'clock to 2 o'clock area of the vagina
C. Inside the vaginal wall
D. Near the mons pubis

Sexual Assault

A 20-year-old male comes to the emergency department stating that he has been raped. He was hitchhiking and had accepted a ride. The driver hit him in the face and forced him to have anal intercourse. The patient is alert and oriented complaining of pain in his face and rectum.

42. Male victims of sexual assault:
A. Sustain more physical trauma than female sexual assault victims
B. Do not require evidence collection because sexual assault is unlikely
C. Cannot become infected with sexually transmitted diseases
D. Have to be aroused to sustain an erection

43. The most common form of sexual assault in the male patient is:
A. Forced oral intercourse of the assailant
B. Forced genital fondling of the assailant
C. Forced masturbation of the assailant
D. Receptive anal intercourse

Pyelonephritis

A 23-year-old woman comes to the emergency department complaining of fever, chills, dysuria, and pain all over. The patient states that she has never had a kidney or bladder infection.

44. Based on the patient's urinalysis and CBC, the emergency physician makes the diagnosis of acute pyelonephritis. A common physical finding in the patient with pyelonephritis is:
A. Tenderness over the affected flank area
B. Tenderness behind both calves
C. Tenderness in the upper extremities
D. Tenderness over the sinuses

45. The patient is to be discharged from the emergency department. Discharge teaching for the patient diagnosed with acute pyelonephritis should include all of the following except:
A. Rest in bed as much as possible
B. Increase fluid intake to 3500 to 4000 ml per day
C. Take the antibiotics only until feeling better
D. Return if the pain increases

ANSWERS

1. **B. Assessment.** Determination of the location and pattern of the patient's pain will help the emergency nurse discover the origin of the patient's problem. The complaint of inability to void would have alerted the emergency nurse to the possibility of a kidney stone. The location and pattern of pain contributes additional information. The pain may be in different places, depending on the location of the stone. Classic pain patterns for renal stones include pain in the flank area radiating to the groin, pain in the lower quadrant, and low back pain.[3]
2. **D. Assessment.** Seventy-five percent of renal stones are composed of calcium oxalate.[3]
3. **A. Assessment.** All of the answers except ingestion of fluids could contribute to the patient's inability to void. It is important for the emergency nurse to get a detailed history about any problem that could cause the patient to be unable to void. Drugs such as antihistamines, anticholinergic agents, and antidepressants can cause urinary retention. Bladder trauma and the presence of a foreign body in the urethra could also interfere with the patient's ability to void.[2]
4. **C. Assessment.** Several things can cause nonhematuric red or dark red urine. These include food such as beets, rhubarb, and blackberries and drugs such as rifampin.[3]
5. **C. Analysis.** The patient will need to be taught about the use of the strainer while voiding and the use of pain medication and its effect on urinary elimination. The defining characteristics of this nursing diagnosis are dysuria, frequency, urinary retention, and change in amount, color, or odor of the urine.[4]
6. **A. Assessment.** Oxycodone may cause multiple side effects. However, emergent side effects would include an anaphylactic reaction, respiratory depression, and hypotension. Nonurgent side effects are constipation, nausea and vomiting, and drowsiness. The emergency nurse needs to instruct the patient when to return to the emergency department when side effects occur and how to manage other potential side effects such as constipation and nausea and vomiting.[5]
7. **C. Intervention.** Renal stones may form from oxalates. Foods rich in oxalates include tea, cocoa, grapefruit juice, almonds, and greens.
8. **B. Evaluation.** A urinalysis should be obtained on all patients with complaints of urinary symptoms. The color, amount, odor, and presence or absence of blood should be documented on the chart.
9. **D. Evaluation.** A patient who needs intravenous administration of pain medication needs to be admitted so that he can be monitored for complications related to medication administration.[3]
10. **D. Assessment.** History related to testicular torsion includes the age of the patient, which is generally from newborn to 20 years of age, sudden onset of pain, and nausea and vomiting. Sexual activity is related to the risk of epididymitis.[3]
11. **D. Intervention.** To ensure testicular salvage, the torsion needs to be reduced within 6 hours. If manual manipulation is attempted and fails, the patient will need to have surgery performed for detorsion of the testes.[3]
12. **B. Analysis.** Emergency nursing care of this patient would be planned using the nursing diagnosis of fear related to a potentially life-threatening situation, which would be the surgery. The defining characteristics of this nursing diagnosis include terror, fight behavior, flight behavior, and panic.[4]
13. **C. Evaluation.** The patient's ability to verbalize his fears about the surgery would help the

emergency nurse evaluate the effectiveness of the interventions.[4]

14. **A. Intervention.** Women who cannot lie supine can be placed in a side-lying position with the upper leg flexed at the knee and the hip. To insert a catheter in a young female or child, have the patient flex her knees and place her heels as close as possible to her perineum.[6]
15. **D. Intervention.** Suprapubic urine aspiration is indicated in the following situations:
    - A child less than 2 years of age who is unable to void or who cannot void on command
    - A child less than 2 years of age who is suspected of sepsis or fever of undetermined origin and from whom a urine culture is needed

    Routine urine aspiration is not recommended in patients with suspected pelvic fractures. If needed, a suprapubic catheter will be inserted.[6]
16. **B. Assessment.** Many times fever may be the only symptom of a urinary tract infection in young children. Almost 40% of children with urinary tract infections may be asymptomatic.[7]
17. **D. Assessment.** Most common risk factors for urinary tract infections have been divided into physical and behavioral categories. Physical risk factors include congenital abnormalities, urinary obstruction, estrogen deficiency, urogenital surgery, and diabetes. Behavioral risk factors include frequent sexual intercourse, new or multiple sex partners, diaphragm use, spermicide use, recent antibiotic use, and consumption of carbonated beverages.
18. **C. Analysis.** Fluoroquinolones are contraindicated in children under the age of 18 because they may cause disruption in developing cartilage.[7]
19. **C. Evaluation.** Effectiveness of treatment can be evaluated by the patient, who should experience a decrease in symptoms 24 hours after therapy has begun.[3]
20. **C. Intervention.** Urinary tract infections in the elderly manifest themselves with the symptoms of fever, incontinence, decreased appetite, confusion, and lethargy.[7]
21. **B. Assessment.** The most common organism causing epididymitis in a sexually active male patient is *Chlamydia trachomatis.* It may account for over two thirds of the cases of epididymitis.[8,9]
22. **B. Assessment.** Clinical manifestations of secondary syphilis include mucocutaneous lesions that occur in 80% of patients with the disease. The lesions appear on the palate, pharynx, glans of the penis, and vulva. The rashes that occur in secondary syphilis do not itch and can be macular, papular, pustular, or squamous lesions. They frequently appear bilaterally on the palms of the hands or soles of the patient's feet.[2,3,6,10-12]
23. **C. Intervention.** CDC recommendations for the management of uncomplicated gonococcal infections include ceftriaxone 125 mg IM in a single dose, along with azithromycin 1 g orally in a single dose or doxycycline 100 mg orally twice a day for 7 days. There are also recommendations for oral medications in the CDC guidelines. Recently, the CDC issued a warning to practitioners related to the increase of fluoroquinolone-resistant *Neisseria gonorrhoeae* among men who have sex with men. It is important for the emergency nurse to determine with whom the patient has had sexual relations, any history of recent travel and possible exposure to *Neisseria gonorrhoeae* that is resistant to treatment.[9,10]
24. **B. Analysis.** The most important care that the nurse can provide in the emergency department for the patient being treated for a sexually transmitted disease is to give the patient information about the disease process and the treatment regimen to follow to prevent potential problems.
25. **A. Intervention.** Vaccinations are available to prevent hepatitis A and hepatitis B, both of which can be transmitted sexually. Although there is a great deal of controversy about whether hepatitis C is transmitted sexually, the evidence points to a potential that this can be. Research continues on the development of vaccines to prevent herpes simplex virus, human papilloma virus, and HIV.[9]
26. **A. Intervention.** All adolescents in the United States may give consent for a confidential evaluation and for medical treatment of a sexually transmitted disease.[2]
27. **C. Intervention.** When taking metronidazole for trichomoniasis, the patient should not drink any alcohol, should have the partner checked and treated for the disease, should use barrier contraception, and should eat before taking the medication to avoid stomach upset.[2,5]
28. **D. Assessment.** One of the complications of tissue injury, immobility, and dehydration is rhabdomyolysis, which can lead to acute renal failure.[11]

29. **C. Assessment.** Intrarenal (intrinsic) failure is caused by acute tubular necrosis, exposure to nephrotoxins, renal artery or vein stenosis, or thrombosis. A urethral stricture would cause postrenal failure.[3,11]
30. **A. Assessment.** A major complication of continuous ambulatory peritoneal lavage is peritonitis. The patient will come to the emergency department with complaints of diffuse abdominal pain, tenderness, fever, and chills. Gram-positive cocci are the most common cause of infection.[3]
31. **A. Assessment.** The emergency nurse should suspect genitourinary trauma with Coopernail's sign (ecchymosis of the labia or scrotum), Grey Turner's sign (ecchymosis of the flank area), and costovertebral tenderness (fractures of the lower ribs and the vertebrae).[12]
32. **D. Intervention.** Blood at the urinary meatus is an indication of an injury to the urethra. Before the catheter is passed, a urethrogram should be obtained.[3,12]
33. **C. Analysis.** Based on the patient's vital signs on arrival in the emergency department, the initial care of this patient would be directed toward correcting hemorrhagic shock.
34. **D. Intervention.** Acute management of a pelvic fracture would include all of the listed interventions. However, the advent of commercially available devices has been useful for the management of pelvic fractures in the emergency department and during transport.[13,14]
35. **C. Assessment.** Signs and symptoms of a ruptured bladder include inability to void, hematuria, abdominal distention, nausea and vomiting, low or absent urinary output, and extravasation of dye in the pelvis during cystogram.[3,12]
36. **D. Assessment.** Human bites to the genitals can result in serious wound infections because of bacterial contamination from the human mouth. In addition, syphilis, herpes simplex, HIV, and hepatitis may be transmitted through human bites.[2]
37. **C. Assessment.** Grey Turner's sign is an indication of bleeding in the retroperitoneal space.
38. **A. Assessment.** Sickle cell disease, use of psychotropic drugs or anticoagulants, and spinal cord injury are some of the causes of priapism.[2]
39. **C. Assessment.** Urinary retention can occur in 50% of patients with priapism. Sexual impotence is a potential complication, but not a common one.[12]
40. **B. Assessment.** Foreign body placement may be accidental, such as by a patient who does not realize the potential consequences of such behaviors (e.g., a patient with a learning disability or mental retardation). It is important to include this possibility as a differential diagnosis in the care of this patient.[15,16]
41. **A. Assessment.** Accidental straddle injuries typically involve soft tissue injury to the vagina above the 9 o'clock to 3 o'clock line.[15,16]
42. **A. Assessment.** Males who suffer a sexual assault are likely to sustain more physical injuries than female victims. They are at risk of becoming infected with sexually transmitted diseases, require evidence collection, and do not have to be sexually aroused to sustain an erection.[15,16]
43. **D. Assessment.** Receptive anal intercourse is the most common form of male sexual assault suffered. However, a significant number of male victims experience more than one type of nonconsensual sexual contact during an assault.[15,16]
44. **A. Assessment.** Signs and symptoms of pyelonephritis include chills, fever, urinary urgency and frequency, and tenderness over the affected flank area.[3]
45. **C. Intervention.** The patient should be instructed to take all of the antibiotics prescribed.

References

1. Bates B: *A guide to physical examination,* ed 6, Philadelphia, 1995, Lippincott.
2. Kidd P: Genitourinary emergencies. In Kitt S, Selfridge-Thomas J, Proehl J et al, editors: *Emergency nursing: a physiological and clinical perspective,* Philadelphia, 1995, WB Saunders.
3. Barrett-Walters B: Renal and genitourinary emergencies. In Newberry L, editor: *Sheehy's emergency nursing: principles and practice,* ed 5, St Louis, 2003, Mosby.
4. Kim M, McFarland G, McLane A: *Pocket guide to nursing diagnoses,* St Louis, 1993, Mosby.
5. *Mosby's drug consult,* St Louis, 2004, Mosby.
6. Proehl J, editor: *Emergency nursing procedures,* Philadelphia, 2004, WB Saunders.
7. Nicolle L et al: Managing acute uncomplicated cystitis in the era of antibiotic resistance, IMED Communications, 2003, www.medscape.com.

8. Miura B: Scrotal pain. In Davis M, Votey S, Greenough P, editors: *Signs and symptoms in emergency medicine,* St Louis, 1999, Mosby.
9. Centers for Disease Control and Prevention: Sexually transmitted diseases treatment guidelines 2002, *MMWR* 51(RR-6):1-78, 2002.
10. Centers for Disease Control and Prevention: Increase in fluoroquinolone-resistant *Neisseria gonorrhoeae* among men having sex with men—United States, 2003, and revised recommendation for gonorrhea treatment, 2004, *MMWR Morb Mortal Wkly Rep* 53:335-338, 2004.
11. Carriere SR, Elsworth T: Found down: compartment syndrome, rhabdomyolysis and renal failure, *J Emerg Nurs* 24:214-217, 1998.
12. Baxter C: Genitourinary emergencies. In Jordan KS, editor: *Emergency nursing core curriculum,* ed 5, Philadelphia, 2000, WB Saunders.
13. McSwaim N, Frame S, Salomone J: *PHTLS: basic and advanced,* St Louis, 2003, Mosby.
14. Campbell J, editor: *Basic trauma life support,* ed 5, Upper Saddle River, NJ, 2004, Pearson Prentice Hall.
15. Semonin Holleran R, Hutson L: Sexual assault examination. In Proehl J, editor: *Emergency nursing procedures,* ed 3, Philadelphia, 2004, WB Saunders.
16. Girardin B, Faugno D, Seneski P et al: *Color atlas of sexual assault,* St Louis, 1997, Mosby.

CHAPTER 9

MEDICAL EMERGENCIES

REVIEW OUTLINE

I. Anatomy
  A. Immune response system
  B. Genitourinary system
  C. Gastrointestinal system
  D. Neurological system
  E. Hematological system
II. Physiology
  A. Fluid and electrolyte balance
  B. Renin-angiotensin-aldosterone system
  C. Acid-base balance
  D. Renal function
  E. Hepatic function
  F. Glucose metabolism
  G. Blood clotting mechanisms
  H. Immunity
  I. Inflammatory response
III. Assessment of the patient with a medical emergency
  A. Airway
  B. Breathing and ventilatory patterns
    1. Apnea
    2. Hyperventilation
    3. Cheyne-Stokes respirations
    4. Hypoventilation
    5. Biot's (cluster) breathing
    6. Central neurogenic hyperventilation
  C. Circulation
    1. Heart rate and rhythm
    2. Skin color, temperature, and turgor
    3. Capillary refill
    4. Blood pressure
    5. Degrees of dehydration
      a. Mild
      b. Moderate
      c. Severe
  D. Neurological assessment
    1. Level of consciousness
    2. Pupillary response
    3. Sensory response
    4. Motor response
    5. Vital signs
  E. History related to the current medical emergency
    1. Onset of symptoms
    2. Medical history
    3. Medications
    4. Allergies
  F. Risk factors
    1. Lifestyle
    2. Exposure to illness
    3. Splenectomy
    4. Contact with infected materials
    5. Blood transfusions
    6. Recent travel, national and international
    7. Immunization status
    8. Immigration status
IV. Collaborative care of the patient with a medical emergency
  A. Maintenance of airway, breathing, circulation
  B. Diagnostic studies or procedures
    1. Laboratory tests
      a. Complete blood count with differential
      b. Electrolyte levels
      c. Ethanol level
      d. Whole blood glucose value
      e. Creatinine, blood urea nitrogen levels
      f. Urinalysis
      g. Drug screen
      h. Liver function tests
      i. Coagulation studies
      j. Test specific to the suspected disease or problem: thyroid hormone levels, tuberculosis screen, Monospot
      k. Type and crossmatch
      l. Serum uric acid level
      m. Serum ammonia level
      n. Reticulocyte count
      o. Sedimentation rate
      p. Cultures

2. Electrocardiogram
3. Chest radiograph
4. Arteriogram
5. Doppler studies
6. Ultrasonography
7. Computed tomography scan
8. Magnetic resonance imaging

C. Pharmacological agents to manage specific medical emergencies

V. Related nursing diagnoses
A. Airway clearance, ineffective
B. Aspiration, potential for
C. Body temperature, altered, potential for
D. Breathing pattern, ineffective
E. Cardiac output, decreased
F. Diarrhea
G. Fatigue
H. Fluid volume deficit
I. Fluid volume excess
J. Gas exchange, impaired
K. Infection, potential for
L. Injury, potential for
M. Knowledge deficit
N. Pain
O. Anxiety
P. Fear

VI. Selected medical emergencies
A. Infectious and communicable diseases
B. Endocrine emergencies
1. Diabetic ketoacidosis
2. Hypoglycemia
3. Hyperosmolar hyperglycemic nonketotic coma
4. Thyroid storm
C. Fever
D. Rashes
E. Coma (unresponsive patient)
F. Sickle cell disease
G. Hemophilia
H. Fluid and electrolyte imbalances
I. Dehydration
J. Apparent life-threatening events

Medical emergencies may not be as dramatic as a cardiac arrest or multiple trauma, but they certainly can be as life threatening. They may manifest as a cluster of symptoms involving virtually every body system. Many medical conditions overlap with, or cause, other clinical problems. For example, a patient with sickle cell crisis may also have dehydration, fever, and an electrolyte imbalance. Sorting the problem from other related medical emergencies presents the emergency nurse with a unique patient care challenge.

People who have emergent medical problems make up a large percentage of the emergency department patient population. As with any other patient, those with medical emergencies need immediate assessment and stabilization of airway, breathing, and circulation. The emergency nurse needs to have a thorough understanding of the anatomy and physiology of the involved system or systems. A complete history needs to be obtained, along with a complete assessment of the patient's physical state.

Care of the patient with a medical emergency continuously changes as medications and therapies change. This means that the emergency nurse needs to frequently review current literature about the treatment of medical emergencies, such as diabetes and complications related to human immunodeficiency virus (HIV) infection.[1,2]

The cause of the medical crisis may sometimes be as important as the management. The emergency nurse is responsible for coordinating the necessary diagnostic procedures and instituting the appropriate therapy.

REVIEW QUESTIONS

A 19-year-old male comes to the emergency department complaining of fever, general malaise, weight loss, a cough, and a skin rash. He states that he has noticed swellings in his groin. He says he has been living on the street and makes money to live through sexual acts with both males and females.

1. This patient has significant risk factors for:
A. Disseminated gonococcal infection
B. Active *Mycobacterium tuberculosis* infection
C. Acute retroviral syndrome
D. Acute *Giardia lamblia* infection

2. The test used to measure the effectiveness of HIV management is:
A. Enzyme-linked immunosorbent assay test for HIV antibodies
B. HIV RNA (viral load)
C. Complete blood count with differential
D. CD4 (T-cell) counts done monthly

3. Side effects of antiviral medications that may cause patients to come to the emergency department include:
A. Rashes
B. Vision changes

C. Insomnia
D. All of the above

4. An emergency nurse stuck herself in the finger with the needle on a syringe of blood obtained from a patient who is known to have HIV. The needle penetrated her glove. The current basic regimen for occupational exposure to HIV is:
A. Report the incident to the appropriate infectious disease clinical specialist within 24 hours of exposure to a known HIV-positive patient
B. Call an attorney to file a complaint about the unsafe work environment and the lack of a needleless system to provide employee protection
C. Begin treatment with zidovudine (ZDV, Retrovir, AZT) 600 mg in two or three divided doses and lamivudine (Epivir, 3TC) 150 mg twice daily
D. There is no need for treatment, because the risk of infection from this type of exposure is minimal and the side effects are limited on these dosages

Robert B., a 20-year-old foreign exchange student, was transferred to the emergency department from the college infirmary. He was admitted for a sore throat, fever, and malaise. He was transferred to the emergency department when he became short of breath and cyanotic despite high-flow oxygen administration. He had never received any immunizations until he came to study in this country about 3 months earlier.

5. Physical findings that indicate diphtheria include:
A. Dirty gray-white, rubbery membrane covering structures of the pharynx
B. White blisters on the patient's tongue, tonsils, and pharynx
C. Red, blotchy rash on the patient's trunk and lower extremities
D. Trismus with difficulty in pronunciation and chewing

6. The only effective control of diphtheria is:
A. Wearing masks when treating infected patients
B. Washing hands with Betadine after caring for patients
C. Avoiding crowds when an outbreak of the disease occurs
D. Ensuring that everyone has received appropriate immunization

7. Hepatitis A is transmitted by:
A. Fecal-oral contact
B. Blood transfusions only
C. Eating contaminated shellfish
D. Sexual intercourse

8. Persons at high risk for hepatitis B include all of the following except:
A. Health care workers frequently exposed to blood
B. Hemodialysis patients
C. Daycare workers
D. Sexually active individuals

9. The most common infection caused by disseminated herpes is:
A. Hepatitis
B. Meningitis
C. Encephalitis
D. Mononucleosis

10. Which is not a characteristic symptom of the measles?
A. Koplik's spots on the buccal mucosa
B. Projectile vomiting and diarrhea
C. Fever, photophobia, and conjunctivitis
D. Red, blotchy rash over the abdomen

11. Bacterial meningitis is confirmed by a lumbar puncture that reveals:
A. Red blood cells in the fluid too numerous to count
B. White blood cell (WBC) count less than 500, normal glucose and protein levels
C. WBC count up to 20,000, decreased glucose level, increased protein level
D. Viral antibodies in the fluid, decreased protein level

12. Which of the following signs would be evidence of condition improvement in a 3-month-old infant with bacterial meningitis?
A. Takes half of the formula feeding
B. Bulging fontanels
C. Seizure activity
D. Temperature instability

13. Pertussis (whooping cough) primarily occurs in:
A. Long-term smokers who received their childhood immunizations

B. Patients with emphysema or other obstructive respiratory diseases
C. Children under 4 who have not been immunized
D. Young children with asthma who have been immunized

14. A 33-year-old female comes to the emergency department complaining of profuse watery diarrhea and low abdominal pain. The patient states that she just returned from a backpacking trip. She and her friends drank water out of a "clear" stream. Indications of dehydration in this patient would include:
A. Orthostatic vital sign change of an increase in blood pressure of 20 mm Hg or more
B. No changes in resting respiratory rate and rhythm or skin color
C. Orthostatic vital sign change of a decrease in pulse rate of 20 bpm or more
D. Orthostatic vital sign change of an increase in pulse rate of 20 bpm or more

15. The patient is diagnosed with *Giardia lamblia.* Definitive treatment for this infection includes:
A. Metronidazole 250 mg 3 times a day for 7 days and good infection control practice
B. Fluid intake sufficient to decrease the risk of dehydration and reinfection
C. Fluid resuscitation and morphine for the related abdominal pain
D. A bland diet and loperamide (Imodium) until the diarrhea stops

16. A 2-year-old female is brought to the emergency department by her mother with the chief complaint of nausea and vomiting. The child's mother states she has not wet her diaper for over 12 hours. The child is lethargic, breathing at a rate of 42 breaths per minute, and has a heart rate of 140 and a capillary refill time of longer than 4 seconds. Which degree of dehydration does this child exhibit?
A. Mild
B. Severe
C. Moderate
D. None

17. An insulin drip has been initiated to treat a patient whose whole blood glucose is 700 mg/dl. The target glucose level is:
A. 600 mg/dl
B. 250 mg/dl
C. 100 mg/dl
D. 350 mg/dl

18. Which statement, made by the parent of a diabetic child in ketoacidosis, would indicate that more health teaching is needed?
A. "When he gets the flu, I need to take him to the doctor right away."
B. "I can still give him Tylenol when he gets a fever at home."
C. "I can't let him eat anything he wants."
D. "Hopefully he will grow out of this when he gets a little older."

19. The drug of choice for managing hyperglycemia in diabetic ketoacidosis is:
A. Regular insulin
B. Lente insulin
C. Glyburide
D. 70/30 insulin

20. Hyperglycemic hyperosmolar nonketotic coma occurs primarily in:
A. Non–insulin-dependent diabetics
B. Elderly diabetics who do not eat
C. Patients without endogenous insulin
D. New-onset type I diabetes mellitus

Mr. Deaton, a 28-year-old diabetic, was brought to the emergency department by his friends after he fainted while waiting for a table at a local restaurant. He is diaphoretic and lethargic. His whole blood glucose on arrival in the emergency department is 34 mg/dl. Vital signs are B/P 106/70, P 64, R 16, Temp 99.0° F.

21. The next appropriate step would be to:
A. Give orange juice by mouth and have suction available in case he vomits
B. Insert an intravenous line to infuse lactated Ringer's and give one ampule of glucagon IV push
C. Insert an intravenous line to infuse normal saline and give one ampule of dextrose 50% IV push
D. Observe the patient closely and check vital signs every 15 minutes

22. Five minutes after the above action, Mr. Deaton is awake and talking. The next most appropriate step would be to:
A. Discharge the patient from the emergency department

B. Admit the patient to the critical care unit for glucose management
C. Recheck the patient's vital signs every hour
D. Give the patient something to eat and recheck his blood sugar

A 50-year-old woman arrives in the emergency department with symptoms of fever, weakness, nausea with vomiting, and diarrhea. She is tachycardic, hypotensive, febrile, and anxious, and has obvious tremors. Bilateral exophthalmos is present. Medical history is positive for hyperparathyroidism and a two-pack-a-day smoking habit for 20 years.

23. The most probable cause for the above symptoms would be:
A. Acute adrenal insufficiency
B. Adult respiratory distress syndrome
C. Acute alcohol withdrawal
D. Thyroid storm (thyrotoxicosis)

24. The medication used to manage the tachycardia associated with a thyroid storm is:
A. Lidocaine 1 mg/kg IV
B. Verapamil 10 mg IV
C. Propranolol 1 mg IV
D. Adenosine 6 mg IV

25. The nursing diagnosis applicable for a patient who is dehydrated is:
A. Gas exchange, impaired, related to fluid loss
B. Fluid volume deficit related to fluid loss
C. Fluid volume excess related to fluid shift
D. Altered oral mucous membrane related to fluid volume loss

26. A sign or symptom of hyponatremia is:
A. Hypertension
B. Hyperactivity
C. Seizure activity
D. Neck vein distention

27. When caring for patients with abnormal sodium levels, it is important for the emergency nurse to remember that:
A. The similar signs and symptoms of sodium concentration disorders make them virtually impossible to diagnose without laboratory data
B. Abnormal sodium levels are very common in young healthy people and may occur with no apparent cause
C. Sodium is the chief intracellular electrolyte and subject to changes due to fluid shifts
D. Normal sodium levels can range from 110 mEq/L to 160 mEq/L, depending on diet

A 7-year-old boy with hemophilia is brought to the emergency department after falling off his bike and sustaining a 2-cm knee laceration. His bleeding is controlled, and the laceration is sutured. No other injuries are noted.

28. The next appropriate step would be which of the following?
A. Discharge the child to home with his parents for observation
B. Replace missing clotting factor according to protocol
C. Observe the child in the emergency department for 4 hours
D. Admit the child to the pediatric hematology unit for continuous observation

29. If this same boy were to sustain major trauma and be transported to a community hospital emergency department, the staff would be wise to do which of the following?
A. Contact his hemophilia treatment hospital and ask them for guidelines for his care or possible transfer
B. Treat him as any other pediatric trauma patient without consideration of the effects of hemophilia on his injuries
C. Refuse to accept the patient when he arrives, due to the specific treatment needed to stabilize him
D. Ask the parents if they have any factor VIII that the emergency department staff can administer

Mr. Thompson, a 36-year-old African American man, comes to the emergency department in sickle cell crisis.

30. Which of these symptoms should the emergency nurse find most concerning?
A. Bilateral knee joint pain
B. Temperature of 101.4° F
C. Chest pain
D. Anxiety

31. All of the following treatment measures would be used during this crisis except:
A. Factor XIII infusions
B. Intravenous fluids

C. Supplemental oxygen
D. Intravenous analgesics

Mr. McClurg is brought to the emergency department one morning after his friends were unable to wake him after "a night of partying." He is unconscious and responds only to deep, painful stimuli. His vital signs are B/P 108/58, P 60, R 12, Temp 96.0° F rectal, Sao_2 92%.

32. Priorities of care for Mr. McClurg include all of the following except to:
A. Maintain a patent airway
B. Identify injuries
C. Obtain a whole blood glucose level
D. Send him for a routine CT scan

33. The physician orders naloxone (Narcan) 2 mg IV push to be given. What might the emergency department nurse consider before giving this medication?
A. Diluting it with a dextrose solution
B. Applying protective restraints
C. Asking the patient if he has allergies
D. Refusing to give the medication

34. Which of the following patients may be at risk for an allergic reaction to latex?
A. A child with spina bifida or with an allergy that was diagnosed by a physician
B. A patient who has had frequent urinary catheterizations
C. Persons who have frequent occupational exposure to latex products
D. All of the above

Amanda, age 2, is brought to the emergency department for fever and vomiting of 24 hours' duration. Vital signs are B/P 98/50, P 110, R 28, Temp 102.2° F rectal. Acetaminophen (Tylenol) suppository 120 mg was given upon arrival. One hour after arrival she has been assessed by the nurse and examined by the physician, laboratory samples have been drawn, and a chest radiograph has been done. Suddenly her mother screams for help. As you and another nurse enter the room, you note that Amanda is having a generalized tonic-clonic grand mal seizure, which lasts 60 seconds.

35. After determining that her airway is patent and she has a pulse, the next step should be to:
A. Recheck the child's temperature
B. Call for additional help
C. Pad the side rails for patient protection
D. Tell the mother to leave the room

36. A subtle manifestation of seizure activity in a neonate is:
A. Absence of movement or lapses in awareness
B. Unilateral brief muscle contractions of lower extremities
C. Abrupt loss of muscle tone
D. Eye deviation and fluttering, lip smacking

37. In caring for Amanda, you remember that vomiting in children:
A. Is a normal reaction for children in her age group
B. Is an ominous sign of impending cardiopulmonary arrest
C. Is frequently related to a respiratory problem
D. Is commonly a sign of child maltreatment or neglect

38. Amanda's temperature returns to normal and her tests are complete. The diagnosis is a viral illness, and she may now be discharged. After giving her mother discharge instructions, which comment would tell you that more teaching is needed?
A. "If she gets a fever again, I'll give her aspirin every 4 hours until it's back down."
B. "I can let her eat or drink a little at a time as long as she isn't vomiting."
C. "I need to call our doctor and see him tomorrow or the next day."
D. "If she gets worse or has another seizure, I can bring her back here."

39. Based on the above response, the nursing diagnosis applicable to Amanda's mother would be:
A. Knowledge deficit, fever control
B. Feeding self-care deficit
C. Altered health maintenance
D. Health-seeking behavior

40. All of the following may cause an apparent life-threatening event in a pediatric patient except:
A. Seizure disorder
B. Respiratory syncytial virus
C. Munchausen's syndrome by proxy
D. All of the above

41. A common life-threatening complication of uremia is:
A. Pancreatitis
B. Gastric ulcers
C. Hyperkalemia
D. Renal calculi

42. Prophylaxis for the management of hepatitis exposure is available for all of the following except:
A. Hepatitis type A
B. Hepatitis type C
C. Hepatitis type B
D. All hepatitis viruses

43. A 7-year-old male was brought to an outlying emergency department for flulike symptoms. His mother states his pediatrician told her to bring him to the emergency department if he did not feel better. The child is lethargic and pale, with skin cool to the touch. Purpura is noted on both lower extremities. His vital signs are B/P 80/40, P 136 and regular, R 38, Temp 97° F rectal. Which medications may be initiated to maintain the child's blood pressure?
A. Rocephin 1 g intravenously
B. Nipride 0.3 to 0.5 mcg/kg/min
C. Dobutamine 2.5 mcg/kg/min
D. Norepinephrine 2 mcg/min

44. Hypomagnesemia is frequently a cause of which of the following cardiac dysrhythmias?
A. Ventricular bradycardia
B. Complete heart block
C. Torsades de point
D. Asystole

45. A primary skin lesion described as a circumscribed deposit of blood greater than 0.5 cm in diameter is a:
A. Macule
B. Papule
C. Vesicle
D. Purpura

ANSWERS

1. **C. Assessment.** Although it is not confirmed, based on the significant history, risk factors, and symptoms, the nurse should consider acute retroviral syndrome which occurs during the first few weeks after HIV infection, before antibody results are positive. Disseminated gonococcal infections can include septicemia, arthritis, dermatitis, meningitis, endocarditis, and perihepatitis. *Giardia lamblia* and traveler's diarrhea usually does not involve a cough and such profound weight loss.[1-3]
2. **B. Intervention.** CD4 cell counts were the standard that was used by practitioners to evaluate the effectiveness of HIV treatment until 1996, when the Food and Drug Administration approved a test that measured viral load (HIV RNA).[1]
3. **D. Assessment.** The antiviral medications used to manage HIV infection cause multiple side effects that may prompt patients to seek treatment in the emergency department. Some of these can cause serious complications, such as pancreatitis. Examples of possible adverse reactions include insomnia, hepatitis, pancreatitis, neutropenia, changes in dreams, depression, and sores in the mouth.[4]
4. **C. Intervention.** Centers for Disease Control and Prevention recommendations for management of significant HIV exposure include initiating drug prophylaxis as soon as possible.[5]
5. **A. Assessment.** There is a dirty gray-white rubbery membrane covering the pharynx and larynx. The patient may have cutaneous lesions.[6]
6. **D. Intervention.** Diphtheria is contracted by airborne respiratory droplets or direct contact with respiratory secretions. The disease spreads more easily in crowded living conditions. However, the most effective management is to ensure that everyone is appropriately immunized, including booster shots.[6]
7. **A. Assessment.** Hepatitis A is commonly spread via the fecal-oral route. It is found in serum and stool and is infectious 2 weeks before and 1 week after jaundice appears. Hepatitis B is transmitted most commonly by blood and sexual contact. Hepatitis E is an enterically transmitted infection from shellfish and contaminated water.[3,6]
8. **C. Assessment.** Children in daycare and their caregivers are not at risk for hepatitis B. Those at highest risk include health care and public safety workers who have exposure to blood in the workplace, clients and staff at institutions for the developmentally disabled, hemodialysis patients, recipients of clotting factor concentrates, household contacts and sexual partners of hepatitis B carriers, adoptees from countries where hepatitis B is endemic (Pacific Islands and Asia), intravenous drug abusers, sexually

active homosexual and bisexual men, sexually active men and women with multiple partners, and inmates of long-term correctional facilities.[3,6]

9. **C. Assessment.** Encephalitis is the infection most commonly caused by disseminated herpes.[3]
10. **B. Assessment.** Symptoms of the measles usually do not involve vomiting and diarrhea unless a concurrent gastrointestinal problem exists. Patients, especially children, who have measles typically exhibit the following signs and symptoms: fever, Koplik's spots on buccal mucosa, conjunctivitis, photophobia, harsh cough, and a red, blotchy rash that lasts 1 week.[3]
11. **C. Intervention.** Bacterial meningitis is confirmed by a lumbar puncture result that shows WBCs up to 20,000, a decreased glucose level, and increased protein levels. The appearance will be cloudy, and the Gram stain will show that bacteria are present. Viral meningitis will be evidenced by clear cerebrospinal fluid, a WBC count less than 500, normal glucose and protein levels, and no evidence of bacteria. Clinical symptoms are correlated with diagnostic indicators in the diagnosis of any type of meningitis.[3,6-10]
12. **A. Evaluation.** It is usually considered a good sign any time a child begins to eat after a serious illness. A 3-month-old who takes half of his formula is probably improving. Seizure, bulging fontanels, and temperature instability are indications that the infant is still ill.[6,10,11]
13. **C. Assessment.** Pertussis, better known as whooping cough, primarily occurs in infants and children up to 4 years of age who have not been properly immunized, although it may occur at any age.[6]
14. **D. Assessment.** Orthostatic vital sign changes of an increase in pulse greater than 20 beats per minute indicate fluid loss.
15. **A. Intervention.** Giardia occurs all over the world and has become one of the most common causes of diarrhea. Water is the most widespread source of the organism. Management includes hydrating the patient, oral metronidazole, and instructions about good handwashing techniques and appropriate treatment of water, especially when camping.[12]
16. **B. Assessment.** The symptoms of lethargy, increased capillary refill time, and the absence of urinary output indicate severe dehydration and an emergent need for care.[11]
17. **B. Intervention.** For a patient in diabetic ketoacidosis, started on an insulin drip, a goal of whole blood glucose level of 250 mg/dl is desired. If an attempt is made to get the level down to 150 or 100 mg/dl, rebound hypoglycemia may occur quickly, and treating the hypoglycemia may lead to wide fluctuations in the blood glucose level. In other words, conservative treatment of hyperglycemia is recommended to prevent the blood glucose level from "bottoming out."[13]
18. **D. Evaluation.** Children do not outgrow their diabetes. Young adulthood may bring about a more controlled (less brittle) diabetic state, but outgrowing the disease is not seen. The other statements regarding taking the child to the doctor for the flu, continuing to give acetaminophen (Tylenol) for fever, and not letting him eat anything he wants are true.[13]
19. **A. Intervention.** The drug of choice for managing hyperglycemia in diabetic ketoacidosis is regular insulin because of its rapid but short-duration actions. Lente insulin is a longer-acting form of insulin than regular and should not be used. Oral hypoglycemic agents are never used for the initial management of diabetic ketoacidosis.[13,14]
20. **A. Assessment.** Hyperglycemic hyperosmolar nonketotic coma occurs primarily in non–insulin-dependent diabetics and may result in detection of new-onset type II diabetes mellitus cases. It causes profound dehydration due to hyperglycemia and resultant osmotic diuresis. Usually the patient is unable to drink enough fluids to prevent the dehydration. Ketoacidosis does not develop, probably because there is enough endogenous insulin present to inhibit ketogenesis. Usually there is an underlying infection, stroke, or sepsis.[13,14]
21. **C. Intervention.** The priority is to immediately increase the blood glucose level. That would be accomplished by starting an intravenous line to administer normal saline and giving dextrose 50% 1 amp IV push stat. During the initial phase, nothing should be given by mouth due to the patient's impaired level of consciousness. Lactated Ringer's is not the preferred parenteral solution, and glucagon would not be used, either. Simply observing the patient's vital signs is not enough.[13-15]
22. **D. Intervention.** After the dextrose 50% injection, the patient should start to respond within 1 to 2 minutes. This should be followed with an

oral food, especially protein (milk, sandwich, and so on), to prevent rebound hypoglycemia. It would be inappropriate to admit or discharge the patient based on simple hypoglycemia until other problems can be ruled out.[13-15]

23. **D. Assessment.** The symptoms of fever, weakness, nausea, vomiting, diarrhea, tachycardia, hypotension, anxiety, tremors, and exophthalmus all point to thyroid storm or thyrotoxicosis. Additional symptoms that may be seen include abdominal pain, coma, delirium or confusion, rales secondary to congestive heart failure, hepatic tenderness, and periorbital edema. Many of these symptoms resemble those seen in acute alcohol withdrawal, but not in adult respiratory distress syndrome.[16]
24. **C. Intervention.** Propranolol 1 mg IV is given slowly for the tachycardia associated with a thyroid storm.[13]
25. **B. Analysis.** The applicable nursing diagnosis for this patient would be fluid volume deficit. Fluid volume excess is the exact opposite. Impaired gas exchange and altered oral mucous membranes would not apply.
26. **C. Assessment.** Hyponatremia is a well-known cause of seizures. Other signs of hyponatremia include altered mental status, poor skin turgor, sunken fontanels and eyes, dry mucous membranes and skin, flat neck veins, orthostatic vital sign changes, and hypotension and tachycardia. The patient may complain of a recent acute illness, nausea, vomiting, diarrhea, immobility or inability to drink fluids, trauma or burns, lethargy, thirst, confusion, weight changes, muscle cramps, dizziness, fatigue, and headache. Cardiorespiratory arrest and hyperactivity are not normally signs of hyponatremia. A salty taste to the skin may be identified in a patient with hypernatremia or cystic fibrosis.[13]
27. **A. Assessment.** Sodium disorders are difficult to diagnose without laboratory testing to determine the sodium status. Similar symptoms are seen in both hyponatremia and hypernatremia. Sodium, the chief extracellular electrolyte, is normally 135 to 145 mEq/L of plasma. Abnormal sodium levels are common in older people.[16-18]
28. **C. Intervention.** After any type of injury or procedure on a hemophiliac, no matter how minor, the child should be observed for up to 4 hours. Replacement of clotting factors is not done routinely if the wound is minor.[17]
29. **A. Intervention.** Contacting the hemophilia treatment hospital and asking for guidelines on the patient's care is by far the best course of action. Hemophiliacs need very specialized care and treatment, and preparing for transfer to the referral hospital should definitely be considered. Refusing to accept the patient because of his hemophilia status is totally inappropriate and could cost the patient his life.[17]
30. **C. Assessment.** Chest pain, rather than a fever, knee pain, or anxiety, would be of the utmost concern and should receive the highest priority. Patients who are in sickle cell crisis may develop angina, myocardial infarction, pulmonary embolus, high-output cardiac failure, and life-threatening dysrhythmia due to anemia and profound hypoxia. Other complications include hemolytic anemia, cholelithiasis, priapism, renal disease, and infection.[17]
31. **A. Intervention.** Factor XIII infusions are given to hemophiliacs, not to patients in sickle cell crisis. Intravenous fluids, supplemental oxygen, and parenteral analgesics are all appropriate measures.[17,18]
32. **D. Intervention.** Maintaining airway patency, searching for any injuries, and obtaining laboratory specimens should be done in that order.[18]
33. **B. Intervention.** Consideration should be given to applying protective restraints prior to giving naloxone (Narcan). This drug, a potent narcotic antagonist, acts very rapidly. If the patient were suffering from a narcotic overdose, he could awaken quickly and possibly injure himself or the nurse, along with removing IVs, tubes, and so on. An allergy to a narcotic would not prohibit the administration of this drug, nor is it necessary to dilute it with a dextrose solution.[18]
34. **D. Assessment.** All of these persons are at risk of developing an allergic reaction to latex.[19]
35. **A. Assessment.** The child's seizure is probably due to a dramatic rise in her core body temperature. Generally, febrile seizures are due to the speed with which the temperature rises rather than how high. Knowing that the airway is patent and a pulse is present, it would be safe to recheck her rectal temperature at this point and initiate further temperature control measures. Calling for help is not necessary (two nurses are in the room). Padding the side rails is not a priority and can be done later. As long

as the mother is physically and emotionally able to stay in the room, she should be allowed to do so.[11]

36. **D. Assessment.** Newborns may exhibit subtle signs of seizure activity, including eye deviation and fluttering, lip smacking, and "bicycling" movements.[11]
37. **C. Assessment.** Because diaphragmatic irritation and coughing can trigger the gag reflex, infants and children may have a respiratory problem that appears to be a gastrointestinal problem. Many clinicians are confused by these symptoms. Vomiting is not normal for any age group, nor is it an ominous sign or a sign of child neglect.[20]
38. **A. Evaluation.** Aspirin is contraindicated in children because of the risk of Reye's syndrome. Acetaminophen should be used, instead. Giving small sips of fluids and small bites of food if the patient is not vomiting, calling the family physician, and returning to the emergency department for further seizures are all appropriate discharge instructions for the mother to remember.[11]
39. **A. Analysis.** If the mother incorrectly stated that aspirin should be given for a fever, then the applicable nursing diagnosis would be knowledge deficit for fever control. Feeding self-care deficit, altered health maintenance, and health-seeking behavior nursing diagnoses would not apply.
40. **D. Assessment.** An apparent life-threatening event is one that is frightening to the observer of the event and is characterized by a combination of apnea, color change in the child, marked change in muscle tone, choking, and gagging. Sometimes the caregiver actually believes that the child is dead. Differential diagnoses that must be considered include: gastroesophageal reflux disease, respiratory syncytial virus, upper airway obstruction, cardiac disease, breath holding, central nervous system tumors, toxins, child maltreatment, and Munchausen's syndrome by proxy.[11]
41. **C. Assessment.** A common, life-threatening complication of uremia is marked hyperkalemia. This results from the inability of the kidney to excrete potassium and sodium. Hyperkalemia can cause sudden death due to cardiac dysrhythmias.[21]
42. **B. Intervention.** Prophylaxis is available for hepatitis types A and B, including serum globulin, immune globulin, and vaccination.[3,4]
43. **D. Intervention.** Vasoactive support of the child with suspected meningococcemia must be aggressive, and a vasopressor such as norepinephrine (Levophed) will help maintain the child's blood pressure.[11]
44. **C. Assessment.** Ventricular dysrhythmias such as torsades de point, ventricular tachycardia, and ventricular fibrillation are associated with hypomagnesemia.[21]
45. **D. Assessment.** A macule is an area of color change less than 2 cm in diameter that is not palpable, with visible margins, and may be red, brown, yellow, or white in color. A papule is a palpable mass less than 1.5 cm in diameter, which may be red, brown, yellow, or skin colored. A vesicle is a fluid-filled papule less than 1 cm in diameter.[22]

References

1. Klaus B, Grodesky M: HIV in 2000: historical perspective and an outlook for the future, *Nurs Pract* 25(1):103-110, 2000.
2. Sexually transmitted diseases treatment guidelines 2002. Centers for Disease Control and Prevention, *MMWR* 51(RR-6):1-78, 2002.
3. Almeida SL: Infectious and communicable diseases. In Newberry L, editor: *Sheehy's emergency nursing: principles and practice,* ed 5, St Louis, 2003, Mosby.
4. Jones S: Taking HAART: how to support patients with HIV/AIDS, Travel Nursing 2004, *Nursing 2004* June(suppl), 2004.
5. Updated U.S. Public Health Service guidelines for the management of occupational exposures to HBV, HCV, and HIV and recommendations for postexposure prophylaxis. *MMWR* 50(RR-11):1-52, 2001.
6. Peabody SP: General medical emergencies. Part I. In Jordan KS, editor: *Emergency nursing core curriculum,* ed 5, Philadelphia, 2000, WB Saunders.
7. *Mosby's drug consult 2005,* St Louis, 2005, Mosby.
8. Kallenborn JC, Coleman R, Carrico R et al: Occupational exposure: organizing ED care to determine rapid post exposure prophylaxis within hours instead of days, *J Emerg Nurs* 25(6):505-508, 1999.
9. Molitor L: A 15-year-old boy with a rash and fever, *J Emerg Nurs* 24(5):467-468, 1998.
10. Swartz M: Bacterial meningitis. In Goldman L, Bennett J, editors, *Cecil textbook of medicine,* ed 21, Philadelphia, 2000, WB Saunders.

11. Emergency Nurses Association: *Emergency nursing pediatric course,* Des Plaines, IL, 2004, Emergency Nurses Association.
12. Coughlan L: *Giardia lamblia* in adults: a case study, *J Am Acad Nurs Pract* 11(10):431-434, 1999.
13. Miller J: Management of diabetic ketoacidosis, *J Emerg Nurs* 25(6):514-519, 1999.
14. Gisness C: Endocrine emergencies. In Newberry L, editor: *Sheehy's emergency nursing: principles and practice,* ed 5, St Louis, 2003, Mosby.
15. Sengewald J: Update on diabetes medications, *J Emerg Nurs* 25(1):28-30, 1999.
16. Dillman W: Thyroid. In Goldman L, Bennett J, editors: *Cecil textbook of medicine,* ed 21, Philadelphia, 2000, WB Saunders.
17. Janz T, Hamilton G: Disorders of hemostasis. In Marx J, editor: *Rosen's emergency medicine: concepts and clinical practice,* St Louis, 2002, Mosby.
18. Newberry L: General medical emergencies. Part II. In Jordan KS, editor: *Emergency nursing core curriculum,* ed 5, Philadelphia, 2000, WB Saunders.
19. Miller K, Weed P: The latex allergy triage or admission tool: an algorithm to identify which patients could benefit from "latex safe" precautions, *J Emerg Nurs* 24(2):145-152, 1998.
20. Newberry L: Gastrointestinal emergencies. In Newberry L, editor: *Sheehy's emergency nursing: principles and practice,* ed 5, St Louis, 2003, Mosby.
21. Womak K: Fluids and electrolytes. In Newberry L, editor: *Sheehy's emergency nursing: principles and practice,* ed 5, St Louis, 2003, Mosby.
22. Hamilton G, Sanders A, Strange G et al: *Emergency medicine: an approach to clinical problem-solving,* Philadelphia, 2003, WB Saunders.

CHAPTER 10

Mental Health and Behavioral Emergencies

REVIEW OUTLINE

I. General patient assessment
   A. History
      1. Chief complaint
      2. Events that led the patient to seek emergency care
      3. Medical history
      4. Social history
      5. Psychological or psychiatric history
      6. Current medications
      7. Allergies
      8. Previous emergency department visits
      9. History of physical or psychological abuse
      10. History of suicide attempt or suicidal behavior
   B. Physical examination
      1. Primary assessment and critical interventions
      2. Secondary assessment
      3. Signs and symptoms of abuse or maltreatment
   C. Mental status examination
      1. Behavior and general appearance
      2. Speech and speech patterns
      3. Mood and affect
      4. Thought processes or mental content
      5. Perception
      6. Judgment
      7. Cognitive ability
         a. Attention and concentration
         b. Basic knowledge
         c. Abstract reasoning
         d. Orientation: place, time, self
         e. Memory: recent and remote
         f. Thought processes and content
            (1) Hallucinations
            (2) Delusions
            (3) Suicidality
            (4) Homicidal ideation
   D. Assessment of safety and cooperation[1]
      1. Can the patient be directed?
      2. Does the patient appear agitated or irritable?
      3. Is the patient's physical status threatening?
      4. Is behavioral lack of control evident?
      5. Is the patient making threatening remarks?
      6. Was the patient acting erratically before coming into the emergency department?
   E. Diagnostic procedures
      1. Rule out organic causes of altered mental status
         a. Toxicology screen
         b. Whole blood glucose per glucometer
         c. Electrolytes
      2. Electrocardiogram
      3. Radiographic imaging
         a. Computed tomography scan of the head
         b. Magnetic resonance imaging of the head
II. Management of mental health emergencies
   A. Collaborative problems
      1. Altered family processes
      2. Ineffective individual coping
      3. Ineffective family coping
      4. Anticipatory grieving
      5. Dysfunctional grieving
      6. Risk for violence, directed at others
      7. Risk for violence, directed at self
      8. Posttraumatic stress response disorder
      9. Anxiety
      10. Fear
      11. Powerlessness
      12. Sleep pattern, disturbance of
      13. Thought processes, alteration in

B. Collaborative care for mental health emergencies
   1. Management of critical interventions for life-threatening illness or injury
      a. Provision of physical safety for the patient and health care providers
      b. Rule out physical causes of altered mental status and behavioral changes
      c. Physical and chemical restraint
         (1) Chemical restraints
         (2) Physical restraints
      d. Emotional support
         (1) Assess patient's potential for violence
         (2) Allow patient to ventilate
         (3) Set limits
      e. Provide patient and family with follow-up care and options

III. Age-related considerations
   A. Pediatric patient
      1. Appropriate behavior varies with age and psychosocial development
      2. Many pediatric patients may rely on acting-out behavior to express their needs
      3. Must consider child's psychosocial development when observing reactions to specific mental health emergencies, such as grief
   B. Geriatric patient
      1. Always rule out organic causes of altered mental status or behavioral changes
      2. Consider drug interactions as potential source of mental and behavioral changes

IV. Selected mental health emergencies
   A. Panic disorders
   B. Crisis
   C. Depression
      1. Weight gain or loss
      2. Recent significant loss: job, family member
      3. Sleep problems
      4. Inability to make decisions
      5. Physical problems such as headache, nausea, vomiting
   D. Sudden loss and death
      1. Concept of loss
      2. Anticipatory grieving
      3. Loss of bodily functions
      4. Loss of family member or loved one
      5. Loss of belonging
      6. Loss of self-esteem, perhaps from abuse, domestic violence
   E. Grief
      1. Informing the family or significant others
      2. Reactions
      3. Anger
      4. Cultural beliefs
      5. Religious beliefs
   F. Violence
      1. Homicide
      2. Suicide
      3. Threatening behaviors
   G. Psychosis
      1. Increased restlessness
      2. Talkativeness
      3. Impulsiveness
      4. Short attention span
      5. Flight of ideas
   H. Schizophrenia
      1. Disturbance of thought content
      2. Delusions
      3. Hallucinations
      4. Repetitive psychomotor behaviors
      5. Disturbed sense of self
   I. Other emergencies
      1. Anorexia
      2. Bulimia
      3. Munchausen's syndrome
   J. Human abuse or maltreatment
      1. Child maltreatment
         a. Identification of children at risk
         b. Identification of patterns of injury and neglect
         c. History related to the injury
         d. Notification of appropriate authorities
      2. Elderly abuse
         a. Identification of people at risk
         b. Identification of patterns of injury and neglect
         c. History related to the injury
         d. Notification of appropriate authorities
         e. Referral to support systems
      3. Domestic violence
         a. Identification of people at risk
         b. Identification of patterns of injury and threats
         c. Notification of appropriate authorities

V. Joint Commission on Accreditation of Healthcare Organizations guidelines for emergency departments

---

Mental health emergencies encompass a vast expanse of psychological and psychiatric problems and disorders. Sudden loss triggers a cascade of generally normal human responses that emergency nurses must be prepared to deal with in order to provide the care and support patients or their families will need.

The effect of politics on the U.S. health care delivery system is illustrated beautifully in Curry's article published in the October 1993 issue of the *Journal of Emergency Nursing*.[2] The Community Mental Health Centers Act of 1963 essentially shut down many of the psychiatric institutions that provided housing and care for mentally ill patients. Many hospitalized patients were moved to outpatient settings. Over the past 40 years, many of the federal and state funds for outpatient programs have been decreased markedly. Inpatient beds have also been decreased drastically. The emergency department continues to be one of the main sources of care for patients with psychiatric disorders. The patient who is confused, unkempt, homeless, anxious, or violent continues to begin his or her health care journey through the doors of the emergency department.

Any complaint of a mental health or behavioral emergency must be evaluated for an organic cause. Hypoxia, hypoglycemia, and chemical intoxication provide examples of physiological reasons for mental and/or behavioral changes.[3] Management of mental health emergencies involves not just the emergency department, but also the communities these departments serve. Finally, emergency nurses need to recognize the need to care for themselves and their co-workers as well. Stress, grief, depression, and ineffective coping are not just matters limited to the patients and families for whom we care. Care of ourselves provides the energy and dedication needed to continue to care for others.

REVIEW QUESTIONS

1. Ms. Pepper arrives at the triage desk stating, "I know that I am going to die!" She is alert but is shaking. Her skin is cool and diaphoretic. She is complaining of a "choking" feeling in her throat, shortness of breath, and numbness and tingling in both hands. She states that she has been awakened by similar feelings lately. Her family doctor has been unable to find a physical cause to her findings, but she knows something is wrong. Her examination reveals no physical cause of her symptoms. You suspect:
A. Mania
B. Panic disorder
C. Depression
D. Agoraphobia

2. An appropriate nursing diagnosis on which to base Ms. Pepper's plan of care is:
A. Spiritual distress related to her fear of death or impending disaster
B. Knowledge deficit related to problem-solving or coping strategies
C. Self-esteem disturbance related to concern about her stress
D. Potential for violence related to inability to control her anxiety

3. Which of the following are differential diagnoses that may mimic panic disorder?
A. Angina
B. Hyperthyroidism
C. Hypoglycemia
D. All of the above

4. A 15-year-old female comes to triage complaining of insomnia, difficulty concentrating, and thinking about ways to die so that her pain will go away. She states that she moved to this area 6 months previously and had to leave her boyfriend behind. The patient is alert, speaking slowly with a flat affect. She says she came to the emergency department because her teacher felt she needed some help. You suspect:
A. The patient is experiencing normal feelings related to leaving her boyfriend
B. The patient may be experiencing symptoms of depression and may attempt to hurt herself
C. The patient talked to her teacher so that she could be excused from school
D. The patient is trying to make her parents feel guilty because she had to leave her boyfriend

5. Mr. Ivey comes to the emergency department with signs and symptoms of ketoacidosis. He states that 3 weeks ago a mass was found on his neck and he is sure it is cancerous. Since then Mr. Ivey has stopped taking all of his medications. He is very quiet and withdrawn and speaks very softly. He does not make eye contact and relates that he has lost 30 pounds over the last 3 weeks because he has stopped eating. Upon further questioning, Mr. Ivey admits that he stopped taking his medication because he wants to die. Mr. Ivey is displaying signs and symptoms of:

A. Anxiety
B. Depression
C. Psychosis
D. Schizophrenia

6. The priority nursing diagnosis on which to base a plan of care for Mr. Ivey is:

A. Knowledge deficit related to his diabetes
B. Anxiety related to his possible cancer diagnosis
C. High risk for injury related to his depression
D. Sleep disturbance related to his diabetes

7. Mr. Ivey is treated for his ketoacidosis in an area of the emergency department where he can be observed at all times. The nursing staff allows him to ventilate his fears related to cancer. All therapies are aimed at correcting his medical problems while addressing his depression. Evaluative criteria for his plan of care include:

A. Mr. Ivey agrees to hospitalization for further medical and psychological care
B. Mr. Ivey states that he is going to leave the hospital as soon as his blood sugar is under control
C. Mr. Ivey states that he would never go to the local mental health center for help
D. Mr. Ivey states that he would never ask his family for help because they do not understand about his disease

8. Major risk factors for suicide include:

A. Good physical health
B. Married state
C. Alcohol abuse
D. Lack of organized suicide plan

9. The life squad brings Jane, a 16-year-old girl, to the emergency department for superficial lacerations to her wrists. She is crying and states that she hates her mother for making her come to the hospital. Jane states that she cut her wrists because her boyfriend broke up with her. She is alert and oriented and has no history of medical or psychological problems. Your assessment of the lethality of Jane's suicide attempt is:

A. Low risk
B. High risk
C. No risk
D. Acting-out behavior

A 20-year-old male was brought to the emergency department by helicopter after having been pulled out of a running car and suffering carbon monoxide (CO) poisoning. His mother states that he recently returned home from school after a particularly difficult quarter. The patient is intubated, hypotensive, and has a Glasgow Coma Scale score of 3. His initial CO level is 15.

10. In addition to the critical laboratory values that need to be obtained, what other tests should be performed before the patient is released from the emergency department?

A. Computed tomography scan to rule out neurological injury from CO exposure
B. Toxicology screen
C. Abdominal radiograph to evaluate the patient's renal function
D. Liver function tests for potential transplant due to injury from CO exposure

A 16-year-old boy is brought to the emergency department by helicopter after having been shot in the neck by a friend. He arrives in the emergency department in full cardiopulmonary arrest. History of the event reveals that the patient was shot in his basement, but he was able to walk up the stairs and ask his sister for help before he collapsed. His sister, a critical care nurse, administered cardiopulmonary resuscitation until the rescue squad arrived, and the flight team transported him to the hospital. After 20 minutes of additional resuscitation, the trauma team pronounces the patient dead.

11. The emergency nursing assessment of this patient's sister should include:

A. Whether she has a history of allergies so that a sedative can be ordered to ease her grieving
B. Whether her brother had any health insurance coverage so she will not have to worry about his emergency department bills

C. Whether she and her brother had ever discussed a particular funeral home where his remains may be sent
D. Whether she has any family or friends who can come and be with her in the emergency department

12. The most appropriate intervention for the survivors of patients who suffer sudden death in the emergency department is:
A. Providing the family with a sedative to decrease their reaction to grief
B. Providing the family with a room where they can be with other members and make calls as needed
C. Providing the family with the names of local funeral homes so they can begin to make arrangements
D. Explaining to the family that their grief will decrease over time and they will soon forget this experience

13. After being told that her brother is dead, his sister begins screaming and states that she should have done more. Which of the following nursing diagnoses would be most appropriate to provide care for this patient's sister?
A. Powerlessness related to her inability to save her brother's life
B. Fear related to her inability to save her brother's life
C. Anxiety related to inability to save her brother's life
D. Injury, high risk for, related to her inability to save her brother's life

14. One method that the emergency nurse may use to evaluate the effectiveness of her interventions related to the family who has suffered a sudden loss is:
A. Contact the family's chaplain by phone to see how the family is doing since the death
B. Contact the family by phone and ask them how they are doing and if they have any questions the nurse may answer
C. Evaluate the charting that was completed during the resuscitation process
D. Consult the hospital's social service department for ideas related to evaluation of sudden loss

15. A crisis is:
A. The mind's response to a demand or perceived threat
B. An alarm reaction to a demand or perceived threat
C. A sudden unexpected threat or loss of basic resources
D. A stage of exhaustion to a demand or perceived threat

16. Common side effects of conventional antipsychotic agents include each of the following except:
A. Extrapyramidal symptoms
B. Sedation
C. Neuroleptic malignant syndrome
D. Mild hypotension

17. Mrs. Gray, a 44-year-old woman, is transported to the emergency department from the local long-term psychiatric facility. The nurse caring for her states that she has had a sudden mental change and has bilateral upper extremity rigidity. Her vital signs are a B/P 186/102, P 132 and regular, and R 28. All her signs and symptoms developed within the last 4 hours. Her current medications are haloperidol and eye drops. Her symptoms are probably indicative of:
A. A cerebrovascular accident
B. Dehydration from decreased oral intake
C. Neuroleptic malignant syndrome
D. An acute psychotic disorder

18. Mr. Black, a well-kept, articulate 35-year-old man, comes in with a chief complaint of severe lower back pain for the past 2 months. Mr. Black denies trauma but states that his pain began when his new neighbors starting shooting radar beams into his new apartment. Mr. Black is exhibiting symptoms of:
A. Anxiety disorder
B. Acute psychosis
C. Paranoid disorder
D. Dissociative disorder

19. The police bring a 36-year-old male to the emergency department after they were called to a grocery store to subdue him. The man went out of control after he was inadvertently struck by a display of paper towels that fell on him. He began screaming at the top of his voice,

"They're trying to kill me." The police have physically restrained the patient. The patient refuses to communicate with the emergency department staff. This patient is exhibiting symptoms of:
   A. Acute psychosis
   B. Acute social phobia
   C. Acute hysteria
   D. Acute dementia

20. The patient is taken to a quiet room and placed in restraints for safety. When a restraint situation arises, the most important information to document is:
   A. Why the patient needs to be placed in restraints
   B. How the patient is to be restrained
   C. When the patient was placed in the restraints
   D. Where the restraints have been applied

21. Which of the following is a medical condition that may imitate delirium?
   A. Malnutrition
   B. Reaction to steroids
   C. Sepsis
   D. Drug withdrawal

22. Nursing interventions to decrease agitation include:
   A. Shouting at the patient to be sure that he hears you
   B. Allowing the patient time to express himself
   C. Restraining the patient when trying to talk with him
   D. Expecting the patient to answer all of your questions at once

*Mr. White, a 24-year-old man, comes to the triage desk, pounds his fist on the desk, and states, "I need to see a doctor now!" You note the odor of alcohol on his breath. He has several abrasions on his face, and his clothing is soiled and torn. You ask Mr. White what happened, and he tells you "It's none of your *?/ business."*

23. You determine that Mr. White's potential for violence is:
   A. High risk for violent behavior
   B. Low risk for violent behavior
   C. No risk for violent behavior
   D. No relationship to this patient's behavior

24. The triage nurse should:
   A. Tell Mr. White to shut up and sit down until she has time for him because the waiting room is full
   B. Tell Mr. White to leave the emergency department immediately before you hit him
   C. Ask Mr. White to please wait while you place yourself in a safe place
   D. Take Mr. White's hand and ask him if he would like to talk about his anger

Mr. Johnson is a 66-year-old man who is brought to the emergency department by the life squad for uncontrollable behavior. Mr. Johnson reportedly boarded a bus and began yelling at the other passengers. The police were called when Mr. Johnson refused to leave the bus. Mr. Johnson is in restraints and continues to yell, "Let go of me!"

25. Initial emergency nursing interventions should include all of the following except:
   A. Whole blood glucose level
   B. Pulse oximetry
   C. A set of vital signs
   D. Sedation with morphine sulfate

26. Mr. Johnson's whole blood glucose is 40 mg/dl. An intravenous line is inserted and an ampule of 50% dextrose is administered. Mr. Johnson is now alert and oriented and embarrassed about his behavior. He states he is a diabetic and took his insulin, but he did not eat enough for breakfast. Mr. Johnson should remain under observation for:
   A. Continued agitation because of his emergency department admission
   B. Hypoglycemia because he has not eaten properly for several days
   C. Signs and symptoms of increasing intracranial pressure
   D. Potential violence and self-destructive behavior

27. A 16-year-old male is brought to the emergency department after experiencing a "possible seizure." His head and upper torso are twisted to the right. He is having muscle spasms of the face and hands. He reports that he and his friends had taken some "little white pills" they received from a "friend." The paramedics report that they had given him some diazepam

with little effect. The patient has symptoms of:
A. Status epilepticus
B. Acute psychotic reaction
C. Acute dystonic reaction
D. Acute conversion hysteria

28. Reversal of the patient's symptoms will occur with administration of:
A. Diazepam
B. Naloxone
C. Diphenhydramine
D. Etomidate

29. A mother brings her 8-week-old girl to the emergency department. She states that the child has been having vomiting and diarrhea for the past 24 hours. The mother states that the child also fell down the basement stairs. The triage nurse notes that the child has not cried, stares without blinking, and left limbs do not move. Her B/P is 70 by palpation, P 180, R 32. Discoloration is noted around her right eye. When evaluating the history of the child's injuries, the emergency nurse must consider the child's:
A. Growth and development
B. Medical history
C. Immunization history
D. Current medications

30. When child maltreatment is suspected, the emergency nurse must:
A. Notify the parents about the nurse's concerns
B. Report the maltreatment to the appropriate authorities
C. Obtain the appropriate consent for further treatment
D. Consult with an attorney to protect herself from a lawsuit

31. A 5-year-old boy, brought to the emergency department by his teacher, is complaining about his stomach hurting. Initial evaluation reveals a child who will not make eye contact with the emergency nurse, is wearing diapers, and is clinging to his teacher. Of the following, which nursing diagnosis is most appropriate?
A. Functional urinary incontinence
B. Risk for altered parenting
C. Dressing and grooming self-care deficit
D. Caregiver role strain

The life squad brings an 85-year-old man to the emergency department from a nursing home for problems with his urinary catheter. The patient is unable to communicate verbally. The nursing home staff reports that he can become agitated, and they keep soft restraints on his extremities to prevent any injury to the patient or themselves. When the emergency nurse examines the catheter, she finds a large laceration under the surface of the patient's penis. It appears that the catheter has eroded through the urethra and the body of the penis. There is a large amount of bloody drainage coming from the wound.

32. The patient's condition suggests neglect. The secondary survey of this patient must include:
A. Documentation of any belligerent behaviors
B. Patterns of additional injury such as bruising
C. Documentation of blood in the patient's stool
D. Documentation of the patient's level of activity

33. One of the vital emergency nursing interventions for the elderly patient who has suffered abuse or neglect is:
A. Acting as a patient advocate for the elderly
B. Listening to the patient's caregivers
C. Planning for the patient's discharge
D. Teaching others about elderly abuse

34. Because of the large wound caused by the urinary catheter, the most appropriate nursing diagnosis on which to base this patient's care is:
A. Incontinence, functional, related to an ineffective urinary catheter
B. Infection, high risk for, related to the injury caused by the catheter
C. Knowledge deficit related to the patient's ability to care for his catheter
D. Communication, impaired, related to the patient's inability to express what he needs

35. When reviewing documentation related to suspected abuse, charting should reflect:
A. The financial and insurance status of the patient
B. Where the patient receives his primary health care
C. Appropriate referrals related to the abuse

D. The language the patient uses for verbal communication

36. Women who are victims of abuse often visit the emergency department with other complaints that mask the real problem. All of the following are common chief complaints related to battering except:
A. Sexual assault
B. Suicide attempts
C. Alcoholism
D. Positive self-esteem

37. You are caring for a 28-year-old mother of three children, who admits her injuries are the result of battering. She informs you that she will be returning home to her suspected abuser. An appropriate reply to her announcement should be:
A. "I have not heard of anything so stupid in my life! You have wasted our time!"
B. "Have you heard of Nicole Brown Simpson? Maybe you should think about it!"
C. "Well, I am going to call the police and report this for you anyhow even if you will not."
D. "Do you have a plan in mind as to how you will protect yourself and the children if anything should happen?"

38. Complications of bulimia include all of the following except:
A. Electrolyte abnormalities
B. Menstrual regularity
C. Subconjunctival hemorrhage
D. Constipation

39. When documenting information related to an incident of intimate partner violence, the emergency nurse should include:
A. Only information that she feels will make a difference in the patient's case against her partner
B. Record of injuries only if the emergency nurse knows what or who may have caused them
C. Record of all of the patient's injuries on a body map or take pictures of them with descriptions
D. Identification of the location where the patient may go for help so that her partner can find her

40. Psychomotor signs of depression include all of the following except:
A. Tearfulness
B. Memory loss
C. Slowed speech
D. Direct eye contact

ANSWERS

1. **B. Assessment.** A patient who is experiencing a panic attack complains of a feeling of impending doom or death. The patient will manifest physical symptoms of tachypnea, tachycardia, shortness of breath, and numbness and tingling in the extremities related to hyperventilation. These symptoms can lead to physical and psychological dysfunction if the source of the patient's anxiety is not identified and managed.[3]
2. **B. Analysis.** Care of this patient should be directed toward identifying ways to help her cope with her anxieties.[4]
3. **D. Assessment.** Diagnoses that should be considered when a patient has symptoms of panic disorder include:
   - Angina if the patient has chest pain
   - Hyperthyroidism with palpitations, diaphoresis, tachycardia, hypoglycemia, or hyperglycemia
   - Hypoparathyroidism[3]
4. **B. Assessment.** The patient's history suggests that her symptoms have persisted for several months, and she has been unable to find an effective way to cope with the changes in her life. The expression of suicidal thoughts indicates the potential for her to hurt herself.[3]
5. **B. Assessment.** Depression is characterized by alteration in mood, weight loss, insomnia, agitation, and overall negative self-concept. Mr. Ivey is at great risk of causing further injury to himself because he has stopped taking his medications.[5]
6. **C. Analysis.**
7. **A. Evaluation.** The patient's ability to recognize that he needs both medical and psychological care indicates that he has an understanding of his current situation.[6]
8. **C. Assessment.** Major risk factors for suicide include age (less than 19, older than 45), depression, previous attempts, ethanol abuse, loss of rational thinking, lack of social support, organized suicide plan, chronic illness, and no spouse.[6]
9. **A. Assessment.** Jane's suicide attempt ranks low in lethality because of age, sex, and lack of

an organized plan. However, she will need to be watched carefully and taught appropriate coping strategies.[6]

10. **B. Intervention.** Patients who attempt suicide often use more than one method. A drug screen should be performed very early in this patient's evaluation to rule out other causes of his altered mental status and hypotension, because his CO level may not completely explain these.[7]
11. **D. Assessment.** An individual who is facing a sudden loss, such as death of a loved one, will need the support of family, friends, or professional personnel.[8]
12. **B. Intervention.** Providing the family with a private place to be with other family members and make calls or arrangements away from the general distractions of the emergency department is one of the most appropriate interventions for survivors of sudden loss.[9]
13. **A. Analysis.** The nursing diagnosis of powerlessness would be the most appropriate for the care of this patient's sister. Defining characteristics of this nursing diagnosis include verbalization of the feeling that one has no control over a particular situation or its outcome, expression of doubt about one's role performance (particularly in this case, because the sister is a critical care nurse), and expressions of dissatisfaction and frustration over the inability to perform previous tasks or activities.[10]
14. **B. Evaluation.** Families have reported that talking with those who have been a part of the resuscitation and allowing them to ask questions has been of help in assisting them to cope with sudden death.[9]
15. **C. Assessment.** A crisis is a sudden, unexpected threat or perceived threat to or a loss of basic resources or life's goals. Stress is the body's response to a demand, change, or perceived threat. The stress response is divided into three stages: alarm, resistance, and exhaustion.[1-3]
16. **C. Analysis.** Neuroleptic malignant syndrome is a rare, but adverse, effect of antipsychotic medications.[11]
17. **C. Assessment.** The patient whose psychosis is being treated with an antipsychotic medication must be monitored for signs and symptoms of neuroleptic malignant syndrome. The syndrome is characterized by a sudden change in mental status, fever and muscular rigidity, tachycardia, and labile blood pressure. The risk of neuroleptic malignant syndrome is most common in patients receiving haloperidol and may even occur when the patient has been taking it for a long time.[11]
18. **C. Assessment.** Paranoid disorders are characterized by logical, yet bizarre, explanations of medical problems.[5]
19. **A. Assessment.** Acute psychosis is characterized by the patient's inability to recognize reality or communicate. The patient is at great risk for injuring himself or others.[5]
20. **A. Intervention.** The reason for restraining a patient must be documented carefully. The patient's behavior must be described with precision. All patients who are restrained must be monitored closely.[6,11-13]
21. **C. Assessment.** Medical conditions that may cause delirium include head trauma, cancer, sepsis, hypoxia, and sleep deprivation.[12]
22. **B. Intervention.** Interventions to decrease agitation may include approaching the patient in a calm manner, speaking to the patient in a gentle but audible voice, and allowing the patient enough time to express himself.[13,14]
23. **A. Assessment.** Mr. White is exhibiting several signs of potentially violent behavior. He is pounding his fist on the desk, speaking loudly, cursing, has alcohol intoxication, and appears to have been in a fight.[3]
24. **C. Intervention.** Answer A would further irritate Mr. White. Answer B would jeopardize the safety of other staff and patients. Answer D would also irritate Mr. White. You should never touch an angry patient. Answer C is the most appropriate, because your first priority is your own physical safety.[3]
25. **D. Intervention.** The patient's altered mental status and behavioral changes should be evaluated before the patient is given any sedation.[5,15]
26. **B. Assessment.** Mr. Johnson should be observed for a recurrence of hypoglycemia.
27. **C. Assessment.** Dystonic reactions are characterized by prolonged involuntary muscle spasms, usually in the head, neck, and tongue.[15,16]
28. **C. Intervention.** Diphenhydramine is administered intravenously to reverse the effects of haloperidol.[11]
29. **A. Assessment.** Knowledge about growth and development can provide the emergency nurse with important information about whether a child may have been maltreated. In this case study, for example, the history should alert the emergency nurse to the possibility of abuse. An

8-week-old baby who is not ambulatory could not have "fallen down stairs." Signs of abuse include wounds in various stages of healing, specific patterns of injury incompatible with the reported incident, and injuries incompatible with the developmental level of the child.[13,17]

30. **B. Intervention.** In all 50 states, health professionals are required to report suspected child maltreatment and neglect to the children's services boards, department of public welfare, or local authorities.[13,17]
31. **B. Analysis.** The information presented in this question describes a child who is not displaying appropriate growth and development skills. There appears to be potential for problems with the child's caregivers.[4]
32. **B. Assessment.** From the state of the patient's catheter, it appears that there is evidence of neglect. The emergency nurse should perform a secondary assessment focusing on the patient's state of hydration, nutrition, hygiene, mental status, and evidence of any old or new injuries.[3]
33. **A. Intervention.** The most significant emergency nursing intervention that can be provided for this patient is to become the patient's advocate. The emergency nurse has the opportunity to identify patients who are at risk for abuse and neglect, initiate appropriate referrals, and ensure that the patient is safe.[3]
34. **B. Analysis.** The wound from the urinary catheter puts him at high risk for infection and sepsis.
35. **C. Evaluation.** When abuse or neglect is suspected, referral to appropriate authorities and patient care service agencies must be reflected in the nursing documentation.[3]
36. **D. Assessment.** Women who are battered generally suffer from low self-esteem. They may come to the emergency department complaining of sexual assault, attempted suicide, and substance abuse.[3,18]
37. **D. Intervention.** Answers A, B, and C are examples of attempts to manipulate the patient. The patient must be ready to make a change in her life. She also needs to know that options are available.[18]
38. **B. Assessment.** Complications of bulimia include menstrual irregularity, electrolyte abnormalities, gastric or esophageal rupture, and ocular complications such as subconjunctival hemorrhage.[3]
39. **C. Intervention.** Documentation related to intimate partner violence should include:[19]
    - Quote the patient directly using quotation marks
    - Ask the patient the name of the abuser and document it
    - Record the patient's description of the incident
    - Record the patient's injuries on a body map or draw them and describe them
    - Relate injuries to the type of weapon, if possible
40. **D. Assessment.** Psychomotor signs of depression include:
    - Slowed speech, sighs, long pauses
    - Preoccupation
    - Lack of eye contact
    - Tearfulness
    - Memory loss
    - Poor concentration
    - Poor abstract reasoning[3]

References

1. Green G: Guidelines for assessing and diagnosing acute psychosis: a primer, *J Emerg Nurs* 28(6):S1-S6, 2002.
2. Curry JL: The care of psychiatric patients in the emergency department, *J Emerg Nurs* 19(5):396-407, 1993.
3. Weinman S, Newberry L: Behavioral health emergencies. In Newberry L, editor: *Sheehy's emergency nursing: principles and practice,* ed 5, St Louis, 2003, Mosby.
4. McFarland GK, McFarland EA: *Nursing diagnosis and intervention: planning for patient care,* St Louis, 1989, Mosby.
5. Williams D, Dwyer BJ, editors: Safe strategies for recognizing and managing violent patients, *Reports Emerg Nurs* Preview Issue:1-8, 1990.
6. Polli GE, Lazear SE: Mental health emergencies. In Jordan KS, editor: *Emergency nursing core curriculum,* ed 5, Philadelphia, 2000, WB Saunders.
7. Robie D, Edgemon-Hill E, Phelps B et al: Suicide prevention protocol, *Am J Nurs* 99(12):53-57, 1999.
8. Weintraub B: A fatal case of acid ingestion, *J Emerg Nurs* 23(5):414-416, 1997.
9. Fraser S, Atkins J: Survivors' recollections of helpful and unhelpful emergency nurse activities surrounding sudden death of a loved one, *J Emerg Nurs* 16:13-16, 1990.

10. Jacobs BB, Hoyt S, editors: *Trauma nursing core course,* Des Plaines, IL, 2000, Emergency Nurses Association.
11. Daniel D: Recent developments in pharmacotherapy for the acutely psychotic patient, *J Emerg Nurs* 28(6):S12-20, 2002.
12. Pestka E, Billman R, Alexander J et al: Acute medical crisis masquerading as psychiatric illness, *J Emerg Nurs* 28(6):531-535, 2002.
13. George JE, Quattrone MS: Restraining patients: can you be sued? Part II, *J Emerg Nurs* 19(1):408-411, 1993.
14. Allen LA: Treating agitation without drugs, *Am J Nurs* 99(4):36-41, 1999.
15. *Mosby's drug consult 2005,* St Louis, 2005, Mosby.
16. Cahill JJ: A twist of face. Acute dystonic reactions, *J Emerg Med Serv* 18(7):46-54, 1993.
17. Emergency Nurses Association: *Emergency nursing pediatric core course,* ed 3, Des Plaines, IL, 2004, Emergency Nurses Association.
18. Muelleman RL, Feighny KM: Effects of an emergency department–based advocacy program for battered women on community resource utilization, *Ann Emerg Med* 33(1):62-66, 1999.
19. Moore S: Intimate partner violence. In Newberry L, editor: *Sheehy's emergency nursing: principles and practice,* ed 5, St Louis, 2003, Mosby.

CHAPTER 11

NEUROLOGICAL EMERGENCIES

REVIEW OUTLINE

I. Anatomy and physiology[1-3]
  A. Anatomy
    1. Scalp
    2. Skull
    3. Meninges
      a. Dura mater
      b. Arachnoid
      c. Pia mater
    4. Brain
      a. Cerebrum
      b. Diencephalon
      c. Cerebellum
      d. Brain stem
      e. Spinal cord
        (1) Vertebrae
        (2) Ligaments
        (3) Fibrocartilaginous structures
      f. Gray matter
      g. White matter
  B. Physiology
    1. Neurons
    2. Neurotransmitters
      a. Epinephrine
      b. Norepinephrine
      c. Histamine
      d. Insulin
      e. Glucagon
      f. Serotonin
      g. Prostaglandins
      h. Acetylcholine
      i. Angiotensin II
    3. Central nervous system
      a. Frontal lobe
      b. Parietal lobe
      c. Occipital lobe
      d. Temporal lobe
    4. Limbic lobe
    5. Basal ganglia
    6. Pons
    7. Medulla oblongata
    8. Reticular activating system
    9. Consciousness
    10. Spinal cord
      a. Ascending pathways
      b. Descending pathways
    11. Cranial nerves
      a. Olfactory
      b. Optic
      c. Oculomotor
      d. Trochlear
      e. Trigeminal
      f. Abducens
      g. Facial
      h. Acoustic
      i. Glossopharyngeal
      j. Vagus
      k. Spinal accessory
      l. Hypoglossal
    12. Peripheral nervous system
      a. Autonomic nervous system
        (1) Sympathetic
        (2) Parasympathetic
      b. Spinal nerves
        (1) Dermatomes
    13. Circle of Willis
    14. Cerebrospinal fluid
  C. Intracranial pressure (ICP)
    1. ICP-influencing factors
      a. Volume of brain tissue
      b. Volume of blood
      c. Volume of cerebrospinal fluid
    2. Cerebral perfusion pressure = mean arterial blood pressure − ICP
  D. Nutrients of the brain and spinal cord
    1. Glucose
    2. Oxygen
  E. Age-related changes
    1. Pediatric patient
      a. Assessment based on age
      b. Denver Developmental Screening Test
      c. Include parental evaluation of child's behavior

d. Motor assessment of newborn
(1) Normal newborns lie with their limbs semiflexed, legs abducted at the hip, symmetrical posture
(2) Infant reflexes
2. Geriatric patient
a. Changes in hearing, vision, and motor and sensory function will alter neurological findings in the older adult patient
b. Hearing
c. Vision
(1) Loss of accommodative power
(2) Corneal arcus or arcus senilis common
(3) Decreased pupil size
(4) Cataract formation
d. Motor function
(1) Muscular atrophy
(2) Speed of movement decreases
(3) Muscle strength decreases
(4) Development of benign essential tremor
(5) Potentially diminished reflexes
e. Sensory function
(1) Vibratory sense decreases
(2) Position sense may decrease
(3) Altered by chronic diseases such as diabetes
(4) Sensory perception of the extremities may decrease

II. Neurological assessment
A. Level of consciousness
1. Glasgow Coma Scale
a. Eye opening
b. Verbal response (best)
c. Motor response (best)
2. AVPU
a. Alert
b. Verbal stimuli, responsive to
c. Painful stimuli, responsive to
d. Unresponsive
B. Pupillary response
C. Motor response
D. Sensory response
E. Cranial nerves
1. Eye movements (II, III, IV, VI)
2. Speech musculature (VII, IX, X, XII)
3. Protective reflexes
a. Gag reflex (IX and X)
b. Corneal reflex (V and VII)
4. Senses
a. Smell (I)
b. Hearing (VIII)
c. Touch (V)
5. Facial moveme ts (VII)
F. Vital signs, including temperature
G. History
1. Mechanism of injury
2. Medical history
3. Medications
H. Neurological function tests
1. Oculocephalic reflex (doll's eyes)
2. Oculovestibular reflex (cold water caloric)

III. Collaborative care of the patient with a neurological emergency
A. Airway: neurogenic influences, seizure activity, oxygen
B. Breathing: hypoventilation, hyperventilation, cervical spine injury
C. Circulation: normotension, hypotension, hypertension
D. Neurological deficit: baseline neurological assessment
E. Immobilization of the cervical spine
F. History of illness or injury, medical history, current medications
G. Indications of injury or illness
1. Periorbital ecchymosis (raccoon's eyes)
2. Battle's sign
3. Leakage of cerebrospinal fluid
4. Palpable depressions (skull)
5. Hyperthermia
6. Petechiae
7. Purpura
8. Rashes
H. Management of ICP
1. Recognition of the signs and symptoms of increasing ICP
a. Altered level of consciousness
b. Pupillary changes
c. Motor function changes
(1) Decorticate posturing
(2) Decerebrate posturing
(3) Flaccidity
d. Sensory function changes
e. Cushing's response
(1) Widening pulse pressure
(2) Bradycardia
(3) Ataxic respiration
2. Elevation of the head of the bed, decreased stimulation

3. Airway management for oxygenation
4. Medications
   a. Mannitol
   b. Furosemide (Lasix)
   c. Phenobarbital
   d. Phenytoin (Dilantin)
   e. Sedation and pain management
   f. Neuromuscular blocking agents
   g. Neuroprotective agents
      (1) Oxygen free radical scavengers
      (2) Lazaroids
   h. Thrombolytic medications
   i. Steroids for spinal cord injury
   j. Experimental agents

I. Laboratory tests
   1. Toxicology screen
   2. Blood alcohol level
   3. Glucose
   4. Hemoglobin and hematocrit
   5. Complete blood count
   6. Electrolytes
   7. Human immunodeficiency virus status
   8. Lumbar puncture

J. Radiography
   1. Cervical spine evaluation
   2. Computed tomography (CT) scan
   3. Magnetic resonance imaging (MRI)
   4. Carotid Doppler studies

K. Cervical traction

L. ICP monitoring

IV. Related nursing diagnoses[4]
   A. Airway clearance, ineffective
   B. Anxiety
   C. Breathing pattern, ineffective
   D. Fear
   E. Gas exchange, impaired
   F. Grieving, anticipatory
   G. Home maintenance management, impaired
   H. Hopelessness
   I. Hyperthermia
   J. Hypothermia
   K. Infection, high risk for
   L. Injury, high risk for
   M. Knowledge deficit
   N. Pain
   O. Powerlessness
   P. Spiritual distress (distress of the human spirit)
   Q. Swallowing, impaired
   R. Tissue perfusion, altered, cerebral or spinal cord

V. Specific neurological emergencies
   A. Headache
   B. Cerebrovascular accident
   C. Seizure
   D. Coma
   E. Infection
   F. Aneurysm
   G. Bell's palsy
   H. Focal head injury
      1. Scalp laceration
      2. Skull fracture
      3. Contusion
      4. Epidural hematoma
      5. Subdural hematoma
      6. Intraventricular hemorrhage
      7. Subarachnoid hemorrhage
   I. Diffuse brain injury
      1. Mild head injury
         a. Glasgow Coma Scale score: 13 to 15
         b. No focal neurological signs or symptoms
         c. Negative findings on the CT scan
      2. Moderate head injury
         a. Glasgow Coma Scale score: 9 to 12
         b. Focal neurological findings
         c. Positive findings on the CT or MRI scan
      3. Severe head injury
         a. Glasgow Coma Scale score: 8 or less
         b. Neurological findings
         c. Injury noted on the CT or MRI scan
   J. Surface trauma
      1. Scalp laceration
      2. Facial abrasion
   K. Low back pain
   L. Spinal cord injury
      1. Anterior cord syndrome
      2. Posterior cord syndrome
      3. Central cord syndrome
      4. Brown-Séquard syndrome
      5. Complete transection of the cord
      6. Spinal shock

Care of the patient who is suffering from a neurological emergency can be very challenging to the emergency nurse. Many causes of neurological emergencies may be seen in the emergency department, including head and spinal cord injuries, headaches, strokes, infections, and seizures.

One of the most frequent neurological emergencies encountered by the emergency nurse is head trauma. Head injuries account for hundreds of thousands of emergency department visits each year.[5] Head injuries are the most common type of neurological injury seen in both the pediatric and adult emergency patients. Causes of injuries include motor vehicle crashes, falls, assaults, sports injuries, and recreational activities.

One of the most common patient complaints heard in the emergency department is headache. Headaches may result from extracranial causes, such as dehydration, hypoglycemia, glaucoma, allergic reactions, ear infections, and poisonings. Intracranial causes of headache include migraine, tension, trauma, and stroke. Evaluation of headache pain may be one of the most challenging assessments performed in the emergency department.[6]

Initial stabilization and treatment of the patient who has suffered a neurological emergency is based on several factors, including airway and ventilation management to ensure adequate oxygenation, continuous neurological assessment, immobilization of the cervical spine when trauma is suspected, and management of the patient's cerebral perfusion pressure. It is important to review both the physiology and pathophysiology of cerebral perfusion pressure, as well as its management. Several references listed at the end of this chapter are useful for review.

A baseline neurological assessment consists of five components: level of consciousness (Glasgow Coma Scale, Modified Glasgow Coma Scale, AVPU method), pupillary response, motor response, sensory response, and vital signs. Information that can provide additional clues to the patient's neurological status include the patient's medical history, history related to the present illness or injury, and current medications. History of diabetes, drug abuse, or psychiatric problems can help the nurse identify the cause of altered mental status.

Collaborative interventions employed to treat the patient with a neurological emergency include management of the ABCs (all patients with suspected spinal cord injuries should be immobilized), laboratory and radiographic evaluations, medication administration, specific interventions such as bur hole trephination or cervical traction application, and continuous neurological assessment.

REVIEW QUESTIONS

A 53-year-old woman is brought to the emergency department by ground ambulance. She was found on her living room floor. On arrival in the emergency department, the patient is having a generalized seizure and is cyanotic. An intravenous line has been established.

1. What drug should be administered first to control this patient's seizures?
   A. Phenytoin sodium
   B. Lorazepam
   C. Phenobarbital sodium
   D. Lidocaine

2. This patient has a documented history of atrial fibrillation. What other pieces of information are important in determining the cause of this patient's seizure activity?
   A. Medications she is taking to manage her cardiac dysrhythmia
   B. Last time an electrocardiogram was performed on this patient
   C. Family history of partial or generalized seizures
   D. The last time she was seen by her cardiologist

3. When a patient is experiencing a seizure, what is the primary nursing diagnosis on which the emergency nurse should base care?
   A. Swallowing, impaired, related to seizure activity
   B. Thought processes, altered, related to seizure activity
   C. Airway clearance, ineffective, related to seizure activity
   D. Injury, high risk for, related to seizure activity

4. The emergency physician has ordered that the patient be given 500 mg of phenytoin intravenously. The patient is connected to a cardiac monitor, and the infusion is started. What criterion should the emergency nurse use to evaluate the toxic effects of this drug?
   A. No noted seizure activity once the drug begins
   B. Bradycardic dysrhythmia on the cardiac monitor

C. Nausea and vomiting after initiation of the infusion
D. Sinus rhythm on the cardiac monitor

An 18-month-old boy is brought to the emergency department by his parents, who say that the child has been shaking and clenching his teeth for about 15 minutes. They also state that he has not been feeling well for the past 2 days. He has had a fever they have been managing with acetaminophen and fluids.

5. All of the following would suggest that the child is suffering from a febrile seizure except a:
A. Family history of seizures
B. Recent upper respiratory tract infection
C. Fall from his crib striking his head
D. Recent vaccination injection

6. Because of his generalized tonic-clonic seizure activity, an intravenous line cannot be established. What other route would ensure one of the most rapid responses to the anticonvulsant?
A. Oral
B. Intramuscular
C. Subcutaneous
D. Rectal

7. During the child's seizure activity, the emergency nurse observes that the child's lips are cyanotic. What is the most appropriate nursing diagnosis on which the emergency nurse could base care?
A. Injury, high risk for, related to his seizure activity
B. Thought processes, altered, related to his seizure activity
C. Gas exchange, impaired, related to his seizure activity
D. Growth and development, altered, related to his seizure activity

8. The emergency physician has prescribed phenobarbital elixir for the child. What should the parents be taught about the side effects of this drug?
A. The drug will cause drowsiness initially
B. The drug may cause mental retardation
C. The drug may cause overgrowth of the child's gums
D. The drug may discolor the child's teeth

9. After 23 hours of observation, the child is discharged from the emergency department. Which of the following should the emergency nurse instruct the mother to do if the child's fever returns?
A. Dress and wrap the child in wool fabrics to keep him warm
B. Administer aspirin 15 mg/kg for an increase in temperature
C. Sponge the child with tepid water to lower his temperature
D. Sponge the child with alcohol to lower his temperature

A 24-year-old woman comes to the emergency department complaining of severe pain in her head 10/10. She states she has a history of migraine headaches.

10. Common signs and symptoms associated with migraine headaches include:
A. Unilateral pupillary changes
B. Generalized tonic-clonic seizures
C. Photophobia, nausea, and vomiting
D. Multifocal premature ventricular contractions

11. For any patient with the complaint of headache, in addition to an evaluation of the ABCs (airway, breathing, circulation), the following assessment should be performed:
A. Level of consciousness
B. Palpation of peripheral pulses
C. Deep tendon reflexes
D. Abdominal assessment

12. A drug that has been found effective in the acute management of migraine headaches is:
A. Meperidine (Demerol) intravenously
B. Acetaminophen (Tylenol) rectally
C. Naproxen (Anaprox) orally
D. Dihydroergotamine (DHE) intranasally

13. Other emergency nursing interventions that may help relieve the pain of a headache include:
A. Application of a hot pack to the patient's forehead
B. Application of a cold cloth to the patient's forehead
C. Having the patient sit in the waiting room after medication administration
D. Leaving the lights on in the examining room

14. DHE is effective in aborting a migraine headache because:
A. It activates neurotransmitters that respond to norepinephrine
B. It activates serotonin receptors that abort headaches
C. It activates the β-endorphins that control pain
D. It activates corticosteroids that decrease inflammation in the brain

15. A potential common side effect of both DHE and sumatriptan is:
A. Hypertension
B. Feeling of warmth
C. Nausea and vomiting
D. Chest tightness

16. A relevant nursing diagnosis for the emergency nursing care of the patient with a headache would be:
A. Social isolation
B. Tissue integrity, impaired
C. Pain, acute
D. Knowledge deficit

17. The emergency physician has ordered that the patient be given intravenous promethazine hydrochloride for her nausea. An uncommon, but disturbing, side effect of this drug is:
A. Changes in pupillary function
B. Extrapyramidal symptoms
C. Normal muscle movement
D. Diaphoresis and diarrhea

18. A food trigger of migraine headaches is:
A. Oranges
B. Chocolate
C. Tuna fish
D. Lettuce

19. Which of the following headaches would be classified as high risk?
A. Headache associated with motor weakness
B. Headache that occurred after taking nitroglycerin
C. Headache associated with a history of migraine
D. Tension headache related to work and stress

20. Prophylactic management for cluster headaches may include:
A. Morphine sulfate 4 mg intravenously
B. DHE 1 mg orally once a day
C. A short course of oral prednisone
D. Breathing 100% oxygen by mask

A 74-year-old man has been brought to the emergency department by his family, who state that he has been walking "funny," they cannot understand what he says, the left side of his face is drooping, and he is not using his left arm. The onset of his symptoms was within the previous 2 hours.

21. Which cranial nerves control the motor and sensory function of the patient's facial movement?
A. I and II (olfactory and optic)
B. IV and V (trochlear and trigeminal)
C. X and XI (vagus and spinal accessory)
D. V and VII (trigeminal and facial)

22. The National Institutes of Health (NIH) Stroke Scale is used to establish a baseline neurological assessment. When scoring the patient using this scale, the emergency nurse:
A. Should coach the patient to answer questions and perform the tasks correctly
B. Score the patient based on what he actually does, not what she thinks he can do
C. Perform the assessment in whatever order is convenient for her and the patient
D. Allow the patient's family to answer questions when the patient cannot

23. The patient's CT reveals an acute ischemic stroke. The patient is eligible for treatment with tissue plasminogen activator (t-PA). He weighs 100 kg. The initial bolus of t-PA for this patient would be:
A. 90 mg of t-PA intravenously
B. 18 mg of t-PA intravenously
C. 9 mg of t-PA intravenously
D. 9 mg of t-PA intramuscularly

24. One of the common disorders that may be managed with t-PA as an acute ischemic stroke is:
A. Complex migraine
B. Transient ischemic attack
C. Todd' s paralysis
D. Conversion disorder

25. A 57-year-old male comes to the emergency department with an acute headache. The CT scan shows an intracerebral hemorrhage. His

blood pressure is 200/125. Which of the following medications is suggested by the American Heart Association for management of hypertension in acute hemorrhagic stroke?
A. Nitroglycerin paste 2 to 4 inches on the patient's chest
B. Furosemide 10 mg intravenously administered slowly
C. Labetalol 10 mg intravenously over 2 minutes
D. Hydralazine 200 mg orally

26. Bell's palsy can be differentiated from a stroke by the motor involvement of which cranial nerve?
A. V (trigeminal)
B. VII (facial)
C. III (oculomotor)
D. XI (spinal accessory)

27. A nursing diagnosis that the emergency nurse may use to plan care for the patient with Bell's palsy is:
A. Fear related to the patient believing he or she is having a stroke
B. Injury, high risk for, related to the patient's inability to swallow
C. Tissue perfusion, altered cerebral, related to Bell's palsy
D. Thought processes, altered, related to the medications with which the patient will be treated

28. When discharging the patient who is being treated for Bell's palsy, the emergency nurse should instruct the patient to:
A. Keep returning to the emergency department until symptoms subside
B. Remember that symptoms will subside in 2 or 3 days with management
C. Use an artificial tear solution to prevent eye dryness and injury
D. Wear a patch over the affected eye to hide its appearance from the public

A 3-year-old boy is brought to the emergency department by his parents. They state that he has been lethargic, febrile, and vomiting. He was treated recently for an inner ear infection. The patient's vital signs are B/P 70/40, P 160, R 40, and Temp 103° F rectal.

29. During the initial evaluation of the child, the emergency nurse should assess for:
A. Positive Kernig's or Brudzinski's signs
B. Oculocephalic reflex (doll's eyes)
C. Deep tendon reflexes
D. Positive Romberg's test

30. Based on the patient's history and physical examination, the initial care of this patient should include:
A. Preparation for a lumbar puncture
B. Administration of antibiotics
C. Management of hypotension
D. Obtaining a CT scan of the head

31. An arterial blood gas is obtained. The results are pH 7.15, PO_2 60, PCO_2 20, and HCO_3 18. These values indicate:
A. Respiratory alkalosis
B. Metabolic acidosis
C. Respiratory acidosis
D. Metabolic alkalosis

32. The child's blood pressure and pulse indicate that the emergency nurse should base the initial care on which nursing diagnosis?
A. Thermoregulation, ineffective, related to his rectal temperature of 103° F and failure of acetaminophen to decrease his temperature
B. Fluid volume, deficit, related to vasodilation and blood pooling caused by endotoxins
C. Fluid volume, excess, related to reflex hypertension in response to the vasodilation and blood pooling
D. Tissue integrity, impaired, related to systemic hypotension and the response of the body to the shock state

33. A urinary catheter is inserted. What criterion should the emergency nurse use to evaluate adequate urinary output during the fluid resuscitation?
A. Urine output more than 1 ml/kg/hr
B. Urine output less than 1 ml/kg/hr
C. Urine output less than 0.5 ml/kg/hr
D. Urine output more than 0.5 ml/kg/hr

34. For children younger than 5 years, what prevention intervention could the emergency department use to decrease the risk of meningitis?

A. Participate in a community immunization program to decrease the risk of *Haemophilus influenzae* type B infection
B. Instruct pregnant women to have a *Chlamydia* culture performed before delivery to prevent contamination during delivery
C. Discuss with parents the need for vaccine (Heptavax) to be given to young children to prevent hepatitis B
D. Teach parents to wear a mask around their infant children if the parents have a "cold"

35. A clinical indication of meningitis that may be seen in infants, but not older children, is:

A. Headache and altered mental status
B. Vomiting and poor feeding
C. Hyperthermia and hypothermia
D. Bulging anterior fontanelles

36. Who should receive chemoprophylaxis with rifampin for an exposure to *Neisseria meningitidis?*

A. Hospital personnel taking care of an infected child without significant exposure
B. An 18-year-old pregnant woman exposed to the infected child at a daycare center
C. A 4-year-old child who played with the same toys that the ill child did
D. A 4-year-old child who lives in the same neighborhood as the ill child

An 18-year-old man is brought by helicopter to the emergency department after a motorcycle accident. At the scene of the accident, the patient was awake but combative. His initial Glasgow Coma Scale rating was 12. On his arrival in the emergency department, the patient's Glasgow Coma Scale rating is 7. He has abrasions on his face, and both eyes are ecchymotic and swollen shut.

37. Periorbital ecchymosis in a patient with an altered mental status may indicate:

A. Maxillary fracture
B. Basilar skull fracture
C. Mandibular fracture
D. Nasal fracture

38. Which of the following may indicate a skull fracture?

A. Leakage of clear fluid from the nares
B. A fracture of the first rib
C. An eyebrow laceration
D. An intact tympanic membrane

39. Because of the possibility of a skull fracture, the emergency nurse should avoid:

A. Placing a cervical collar on the patient
B. Placing an oral airway in the patient
C. Inserting a nasogastric tube
D. Connecting the patient to a cardiac monitor

40. The emergency physician intubates the patient orally. He is being oxygenated, but his neurological condition does not improve. His pupils are now 6 mm in diameter bilaterally and slow to react. His Glasgow Coma Scale rating has decreased to 5. The emergency physician orders mannitol to be infused. The patient weighs 100 kg. How much mannitol will be infused initially?

A. 100 g
B. 50 g
C. 500 g
D. 25 g

41. ICP is the result of:

A. The volume of brain tissue, plus the volume of blood, plus the volume of cerebrospinal fluid
B. The mean arterial blood pressure minus the mean ICP
C. Adequate oxygenation plus maintaining a whole blood glucose level above 100
D. An increase in mean arterial pressure with use of a vasoactive intravenous infusion

42. In a patient with a severe head injury, the cerebral perfusion pressure should be maintained at:

A. 90 mm Hg
B. 70 mm Hg
C. 10 mm Hg
D. 50 mm Hg

43. Copious amounts of pink, frothy sputum begin to come from the patient's endotracheal tube. The emergency nurse should base the care for this complication on which of the following nursing diagnoses?

A. Cardiac output, decreased
B. Gas exchange, impaired

C. Fluid volume, excess
D. Fluid volume, deficit

44. The rescue squad brings an 18-year-old man who fell from his bicycle to the emergency department. The squad reports that the patient lost consciousness after his fall but was awake, alert, and oriented during transport. Upon arrival in the emergency department, he is unresponsive to verbal stimuli. His right pupil is 6 mm in diameter and unreactive, and his left pupil is 2 mm in diameter and unreactive. With painful stimuli, the patient flexes his arms, and rigidity extends to his lower extremities. What type of posturing is he exhibiting?
A. Flaccid response to painful stimuli
B. Extension (decerebrate) response to painful stimuli
C. Flexion (decorticate) response to painful stimuli
D. Normal motor response to painful stimuli

45. The history of this patient's injury suggests what type of intracranial bleeding?
A. Subdural hematoma
B. Intracerebral hemorrhage
C. Subarachnoid hemorrhage
D. Epidural hematoma

A 2-year-old boy has been brought to the emergency department by EMTs. He was involved in a motor vehicle crash with his parents, at which time he was restrained on his mother's lap by a shoulder harness. On arrival of EMTs, the child was in full cardiac arrest. Cardiopulmonary resuscitation was initiated and a pulse obtained. His vital signs now include B/P 70 by palpation and P 58. He is being ventilated with a bag-valve-mask device.

46. What size endotracheal tube will be needed to intubate this child?
A. 6 cuffed tube
B. 2.5 uncuffed tube
C. 7 uncuffed tube
D. 4.5 uncuffed tube

47. The child's vital signs suggest that the child may be suffering from:
A. Anaphylactic shock
B. Cardiogenic shock
C. Spinal shock
D. Septic shock

48. The collaborative emergency treatment of the patient in spinal shock would include administration of:
A. Ringer's lactate solution until the child's blood pressure is 80/40
B. Packed red blood cells until the child's blood pressure is 80/40
C. An appropriate antibiotic intravenously to prevent meningitis
D. A vasopressor intravenously until vasomotor control is restored

49. The initial emergency nursing care of this patient should be based on which of the following nursing diagnoses?
A. Injury, high risk for
B. Tissue perfusion, altered, spinal cord
C. Growth and development, altered
D. Unilateral neglect

50. Young children are at risk of sustaining a cervical spine injury because:
A. Their heads are small in proportion to the rest of their body surface area
B. Their neck muscles are still undeveloped and initially are stiff
C. Their injuries do not show up on regular radiographic films
D. Their heads are the largest part of their developing bodies

51. An 8-year-old girl who has been diagnosed as having a concussion is going to be discharged from the emergency department. After having been given discharge instructions, her parents should be able to evaluate their daughter for what changes?
A. Changes in blood pressure
B. Changes in level of consciousness
C. Changes in hemoglobin and hematocrit
D. Changes in urinary output

A 27-year-old construction worker fell 3 feet from a ladder, landing on his buttocks, prior to his arrival in the emergency department. He walks into the emergency department, but complains of pain in his lower back that is radiating down his legs. The only obvious signs of trauma are abrasions and bruising on his buttocks.

52. The initial assessment of this patient should include a history of:
A. Loss of consciousness
B. Tetanus immunization

C. Pulmonary disease
D. Type II diabetes

53. An important intervention for the patient who has fallen and sustained a back injury is obtaining a:
A. Blood alcohol level
B. Urinalysis
C. Hepatic profile
D. Drug screen

54. No acute injury was found in this patient. Based on his initial complaint, which of the following nursing diagnoses should the emergency nurse use for basing care?
A. Fluid volume, deficit
B. Pain, acute
C. Cardiac output, decreased
D. Infection, potential for

55. The patient is given discharge instructions for a low back injury. It is important that the emergency nurse question the patient about his understanding concerning which of the following signs of serious complications related to low back injury?
A. Presence of some pain for 7 to 10 days
B. Presence of soreness and stiffness in the lower back
C. Presence of progressive weakness and bladder dysfunction
D. Decrease in pain and stiffness

A 62-year-old man is brought to the emergency department by his caretaker from the state mental facility. His caretakers noted that he suddenly became febrile. Despite management with acetaminophen, his fever has remained at 103° F. His only medication is haloperidol. He is diagnosed with neuroleptic malignant syndrome.

56. Other signs and symptoms of neuroleptic malignant syndrome include all of the following except:
A. Tachycardia
B. Gradual change in mental status
C. Muscular rigidity
D. Hypertension

57. Which of the following medications is used to manage the symptoms of neuroleptic malignant syndrome?
A. Potassium chloride
B. Streptokinase
C. Neuromuscular blocking agents
D. Tricyclic antidepressants

A 16-year-old unrestrained female driver is brought to the emergency department after having been involved in a high-speed crash. Her initial Glasgow Coma Scale score at the scene of the crash was 12. She is now responding only to deep pain (Glasgow Coma Scale score of 7). The emergency physician decides to intubate her using rapid sequence induction for intubation to protect her airway and manage her ICP.

58. Neuromuscular blocking agents:
A. Decrease the success rate of intubation
B. Increase the patient's ICP
C. Control an alert and cooperative patient
D. Manage the hypoxia associated with severe head injury

59. Preparation for administration of rapid sequence intubation for this patient with an acute head injury may include:
A. Lidocaine 100 mg and etomidate 20 mg
B. Atropine 0.02 mg/kg and etomidate 20 mg
C. Midazolam 10 mg and lidocaine 100 mg
D. Atropine 0.02 mg/kg and lidocaine 100 mg

60. A 44-year-old female comes to the emergency department with the "worst headache of her life." A CT reveals a subarachnoid hemorrhage. The emergency treatment of choice for this patient is:
A. Initiation of a heparin drip at 1000 units per hour
B. Administration of t-PA based on a weight-calculated dosage
C. Preparation for insertion of a ventricular catheter for ICP monitoring
D. Administration of nimodipine 60 mg orally every 4 hours

61. A method that may be used to manage a patient's ICP in the emergency department after intubation is:
A. Hyperventilation to maintain the patient's $PaCO_2$ less than 30 mm Hg
B. Administration of neuromuscular blocking agents and sedation
C. Administration of high-dose steroids intravenously
D. Administration of prophylactic anticonvulsant therapy

62. Which of the following methods of administration of anticonvulsant medication has been found to cause fewer adverse affects?
A. Phenytoin intramuscularly
B. Fosphenytoin intramuscularly
C. Phenytoin orally
D. Fosphenytoin orally

63. A patient's gag reflex response is controlled by:
A. Cranial nerve X
B. Cranial nerve IX
C. Cranial nerve V
D. Cranial nerve VII

64. Cerebral hyperemia causes:
A. A decrease in cerebral blood flow and cerebral edema to the injured brain tissue
B. Decreased hydrostatic pressure and disruption of the blood-brain barrier
C. Cerebral edema and decreased cerebral perfusion
D. An increase in the amount of oxygen and glucose to the injured brain tissue

65. An elderly patient is more susceptible to intracranial hemorrhage because of:
A. Decreased ability to regulate body temperature, due to cerebral changes related to age and decreased mobility
B. Increased number of sensory cells, decreasing pain perception in older patients when they strike their heads
C. Increased fragility of cerebral blood vessels, which may result in bleeding from minor head trauma
D. Decreased cerebral blood flow and metabolism, with loss of cerebral cortex neurons

ANSWERS

1. **B. Intervention.** Lorazepam (a benzodiazepine) crosses the blood-brain barrier more quickly than does phenytoin or phenobarbital sodium. The appropriate dose of lorazepam (Ativan) for anticonvulsant therapy is 1 to 2 mg IV, which may be repeated at 10- to 15-minute intervals as needed for a total of not more than 4 mg. Signs and symptoms of respiratory depression must be assessed carefully.[7]
2. **A. Assessment.** Atrial fibrillation is managed with multiple medications. However, some patients are given prophylactic anticoagulants to prevent stroke. It would be important to ascertain if this patient is taking an anticoagulant medication. Seizure activity may be an indication of an intracerebral hemorrhage.
3. **C. Analysis.** Because the patient is having a seizure, she is unable to maintain her airway. Even though the patient is at risk for injury, the emergency nurse's initial care should be directed toward stabilizing the patient's airway. Related factors contributing to this nursing diagnosis include an increase in secretions and cognitive impairment.[4]
4. **B. Evaluation.** The toxic side effects of phenytoin are cardiac dysrhythmia, including bradycardia and heart block.[6,7]
5. **C. Assessment.** A fall indicates that the seizure could be from trauma and not a medical cause.[8,9]
6. **D. Intervention.** When an intravenous line cannot be established, rectal diazepam (Diastat) may be administered.[7,10-14]
7. **C. Analysis.** One of the related factors contributing to this nursing diagnosis is an altered oxygen supply. During the seizure activity, gas exchange may be impaired by airway obstruction and central nervous system depression.[4]
8. **A. Evaluation.** The most common side effects of this drug are drowsiness, lethargy, and depression. It is important to point this out to the child's parents. These effects will generally decrease during continued therapy.[6,7]
9. **C. Intervention.** Tepid water should be used to lower the child's fever. Aspirin is not recommended to manage fevers in young children because of the risk of Reye's syndrome. Using alcohol to sponge the child may cause toxicity, because the alcohol is absorbed into the child's skin. It may also cause shivering, which will only raise the child's temperature.[10]
10. **C. Assessment.** Signs and symptoms associated with migraine headaches are many and varied. Visual disturbances, including homonymous hemianopsia, transient blindness, and photophobia are seen. Other signs and symptoms include nausea and vomiting, vertigo, chills, cold hands and feet, abdominal distention, and cardiac dysrhythmia. However, unilateral pupillary changes and seizures would more likely suggest an expanding lesion.[15]
11. **A. Assessment.** A baseline neurological assessment is imperative in the initial evaluation of a patient who is complaining of a severe headache. It is important to evaluate the patient for focal neurological symptoms that could

indicate an expanding lesion, requiring immediate neurosurgical evaluation and intervention.[15]

12. **D. Intervention.** DHE, a semisynthetic derivative of ergot alkaloid, is effective in the acute management of migraine headaches. Because it is more rapid acting than ergotamine, it can offer the patient quicker pain relief. Meperidine and other opiates are not as effective as dihydroergotamine for pain from severe migraine headaches, because these generally are associated with a depletion of serotonin, a hormone that must be present for opiates to be effective.[7]
13. **B. Intervention.** Application of a cold cloth, along with the prescribed medical regimen, is helpful in the care of the patient with a headache. In addition, a quiet, dimly lit environment can help decrease headache pain.[15]
14. **B. Intervention.** DHE works by activating serotonin-l receptors. The result of this is abortion of the migraine.[7,15,16]
15. **D. Assessment.** A potential side effect common to both DHE and sumatriptan is chest tightness. Hypertension, nausea, and vomiting are more common to DHE use. Sumatriptan may cause tingling and feelings of warmth. Both may cause chest tightness.[15]
16. **C. Analysis.** The emergency nursing care for the patient with a headache would include helping the patient with the management of acute pain. Defining characteristics of pain include a verbal report of intense pain experience, narrowed focus, restlessness, unusual posture, diaphoresis, and increased muscle tension.[4]
17. **B. Evaluation.** Intravenous promethazine hydrochloride can cause many side effects, but some that can be very disturbing to the patient are the extrapyramidal symptoms, including oculogyric crisis, torticollis, and tongue protrusion.[6,7]
18. **B. Assessment.** Foods that can trigger migraine headaches include chocolate, bananas, avocados, nuts, onions, and caffeine.[16]
19. **A. Assessment.** Headaches associated with changes in mental status, lethargy, fever, motor weakness, high blood pressure, rash, or fever should be considered high risk.[17]
20. **C. Intervention.** The acute management of cluster headaches include breathing 100% oxygen by mask, sumatriptan 6 mg subcutaneously, and DHE 1 mg IV or IM. A short course of prednisone has been found effective in preventing cluster headaches.[15]
21. **D. Assessment.** Motor function controlled by the fifth cranial nerve (trigeminal) allows the patient to open and close his jaw. Sensory function of the fifth cranial nerve allows the patient to identify sharp and dull sensations on the forehead and cheek. Motor function controlled by the seventh cranial nerve (facial) allows movement of the face, scalp, and eyelids. The sensory function of the seventh cranial nerve allows the patient taste on the anterior two thirds of the tongue.[18]
22. **B. Intervention.** The NIH Stroke Scale was developed to provide an organized and fairly comprehensive assessment tool for the patient who has suffered a stroke. It also helps to track changes or improvements when specific therapies are initiated to manage an acute stroke. The NIH Stroke Scale should be administered in the order listed, and the patient should not be coached. The emergency nurse needs to score the patient based on what the patient does, not what she believes he can do.
23. **C. Intervention.** The amount of t-PA this patient should receive is based upon the following: 0.9 mg/kg (maximum of 90 mg), with 10% of the dosage given as a bolus over 1 minute. Even though the patient weighs 110 kg, he should not receive a total of more than 90 mg of t-PA.[19,20]
24. **B. Evaluation.** The most common disorder that mimics a stroke is a transient ischemic attack, followed by conversion disorder and Todd's paralysis.[21]
25. **C. Intervention.** The suggested emergency antihypertensive therapy for hemorrhagic stroke is labetalol 10 mg IV.[19]
26. **B. Assessment.** Bell's palsy affects the motor function of the seventh cranial nerve. This results in the patient's inability to wrinkle his or her forehead. Because of crossover of motor innervation of the seventh cranial nerve, the patient with facial symptoms after a stroke will still be able to wrinkle the forehead.[6]
27. **A. Analysis.** Because the symptoms of Bell's palsy are similar to the facial symptoms of a stroke, patients fear that they may be having a stroke. In addition, it generally takes 3 months for the symptoms to disappear. Defining characteristics of fear include apprehension, decreased self-assurance, and sympathetic stimulation.[4]

28. **C. Intervention.** Because Bell's palsy affects the eyelid, it may not close, and blinking will be incomplete. The emergency nurse needs to instruct the patient how to keep the eye from drying out. Symptoms related to Bell's palsy generally take 3 weeks to 3 months to resolve.[6]
29. **A. Assessment.** Because of the history given by the parents and the child's initial vital signs, the emergency nurse should suspect that he might be suffering from meningitis. Positive Kernig's and Brudzinski's signs indicate meningeal irritation. The test for Kernig's sign is performed while the patient is lying flat. The patient's leg is flexed and then extended. If pain is elicited by this maneuver, meningeal irritation is indicated. Brudzinski's sign is elicited by flexing the patient's neck forward. Again, pain with this movement indicates meningeal irritation.[10,15,18]
30. **C. Intervention.** From the initial vital signs obtained, it is obvious that the child is in shock, probably septic shock. Initial care of the child should thus be directed at correcting his shock state. Administration of antibiotics and a lumbar puncture may be indicated later, but the initial emergency nursing interventions need to be based on stabilizing the patient's airway, breathing, and circulation.[22]
31. **B. Assessment.** The child's pH of 7.15 and HCO_3 of 18 indicate metabolic acidosis. In addition, the PCO_2 of 20 indicates that the child is hyperventilating in an attempt to compensate for this metabolic state.
32. **B. Analysis.** Defining characteristics of fluid volume deficit include hypotension, increased pulse rate, narrowed pulse pressure, and decreased urinary output.[4]
33. **A. Evaluation.** Adequate fluid resuscitation for a 3-year-old child would be indicated by a urinary output of greater than 1 ml/kg/hr.[10]
34. **A. Intervention.** Since the development and implementation of the Hib vaccine, the incidence of Hib disease has decreased. One of the most common causes of meningitis in children under 5 years of age is *H. influenzae* type B.[22]
35. **D. Assessment.** An infant's anterior fontanelle remains open until 9 to 18 months of age. When an infant has meningitis and an increase in ICP accompanies the infection, the result is a bulging anterior fontanelle.[3,10]
36. **C. Intervention.** Persons with the most intimate contact with the infected patient should receive antibiotic prophylaxis. Intimate contact includes household, nursery school, and daycare providers, as well as health care personnel who have performed mouth-to-mouth resuscitation or intubation. Rifampin is the drug of choice. Rifampin should never be given to a pregnant woman.[22]
37. **B. Assessment.** Basilar skull fractures occur at the base of the skull. They are not usually seen on radiographic examination but are diagnosed clinically. The signs of a basilar skull fracture are periorbital ecchymosis (raccoon's eyes), rhinorrhea, and otorrhea.[23]
38. **A. Assessment.** Additional indications of a skull fracture include a unilateral or bilateral hemotympanum, mastoid ecchymosis (Battle's sign), conjunctival hemorrhage without evidence of direct trauma to the eye(s), and leakage of cerebral spinal fluid from the ears or nose.[24]
39. **C. Intervention.** When a basilar skull fracture occurs, the cribriform plate of the ethmoid bone may be fractured. This could allow passage of such things as nasogastric tubes directly into the brain.[24]
40. **A. Intervention.** Mannitol is given to the adult patient in dosages of 1 to 2 g/kg body weight. Mannitol generally is infused over a period of 30 to 90 minutes.[7]
41. **A. Assessment.** ICP is a function of the volume of brain tissue, plus the volume of blood, plus the volume of cerebrospinal fluid.[1,2]
42. **B. Intervention.** According to the American College of Surgery (*ATLS Student Manual,* ed 7, Chapter 2, Injuries to the Central Nervous System) the cerebral perfusion pressure should be maintained higher than 60 mm Hg.[23]
43. **B. Analysis.** The appearance of pink, frothy sputum may indicate neurogenic pulmonary edema. These secretions could interfere with the patient's oxygenation. A related factor contributing to this nursing diagnosis is alveolar capillary membrane changes.[4]
44. **C. Assessment.** Flexion response, or decorticate posturing, to painful stimuli is exhibited by arm flexion and adduction. The patient's lower extremities are rigid and extended.[23,24]
45. **D. Analysis.** In 40% of the patients who develop epidural hematomas, a classic history may be collected. This includes a loss of consciousness, followed by a lucid period, and then further neurological changes including altered mental status, lethargy, and unresponsiveness.[24]

46. **D. Intervention.** The formula that can be used to determine the appropriate tube size is 16 plus the age in years divided by 4. This would give an approximate size of 4.5. Other measures that can be used to estimate tube size include looking at the size of the child's little finger or nasal opening. It is important to note that an uncuffed tube should be used for a 2-year-old child.[10,11]
47. **C. Assessment.** Hypotension and bradycardia in a patient after a traumatic injury indicate that the patient may be in spinal shock. In addition, a child will normally be tachycardiac. In this case, the pulse is less than normal for the child's age. Spinal shock results when there is an injury or edema that blocks the sympathetic outflow tract, causing disruption of the vasomotor center, which causes loss of sympathetic tone.[25]
48. **D. Intervention.** Because the patient has suffered an injury that compromises his ability to control vasomotor tone, vasopressors are needed. Drugs that are used include dopamine, norepinephrine, isoproterenol, and dobutamine.[25] High-dose methylprednisolone is an important adjunct in the management of spinal cord injury, used in both adult and pediatric patients. The initial dosage of the drug is 30 mg/kg diluted in normal saline and infused over 15 minutes. Despite the controversy of this management, it remains the standard of care.[26]
49. **B. Analysis.** Initial care of this child should be based on providing both nursing and medical interventions to manage the complications of spinal shock and to prevent further injury. Defining characteristics of this nursing diagnosis include hypotension, decreased capillary filling, and alteration in mental status.[4]
50. **D. Assessment.** The largest part of the young child's body is the head. The neck muscles are weaker than those of an adult. Because of these anatomical differences, young children are more likely to suffer higher cervical spine injuries than are adults.[24]
51. **B. Evaluation.** Because the child has suffered a concussion, her parents need to know the signs and symptoms of possible neurological compromise following injury. The initial symptom is a change in mental status. It is important that the emergency nurse instruct the family on what to look for and to be sure that the family understands the importance of this assessment.[11,24]
52. **A. Assessment.** For any patient who has fallen and sustained possible neurological or spinal injury, a history of whether there was a loss of consciousness should be obtained. This would alert the emergency nurse to the possibility of additional injuries.[25,27]
53. **B. Intervention.** When a patient has sustained a fall resulting in back pain, the possibility of renal injury needs to be evaluated. This is done by obtaining a urine specimen and submitting it for urinalysis, or using a dipstick, to determine the presence of blood.[28]
54. **B. Analysis.** Because of the muscle spasms and tenderness that have resulted from the fall, the patient's care will need to be directed toward relieving the acute pain he is suffering. Pain management may include prescribed medications, hot or cold compresses, and bed rest.[28]
55. **C. Evaluation.** A serious complication of low back injury would be a disk herniation. Signs and symptoms of this complication include progressive weakness and bladder dysfunction.[28]
56. **B. Assessment.** Symptoms of neuroleptic malignant syndrome include a sudden change in mental status, fever, muscular rigidity, and autonomic dysfunction.[29]
57. **C. Intervention.** Neuromuscular blocking agents have been used to manage the muscular rigidity that can lead to rhabdomyolysis.[29]
58. **D. Assessment.** Indications for neuromuscular blocking include:
    - Hypoxia from head injury
    - Status epilepticus
    - Drug overdose requiring gastric lavage for airway protection
    - Status asthmaticus
    - Intubation
    - Struggle against the ventilator
    - Combative patient who needs transport
    - Diagnostic procedures[30-34]
59. **A. Intervention.** Premedication for the patient with a head injury includes lidocaine 1 to 1.5 mg/kg and a medication that produces sedation and amnesia, such as etomidate. Atropine is indicated for premedication of pediatric patients.[30-34]
60. **D. Intervention.** Fibrinolytic therapy is contraindicated in the management of hemorrhagic stroke. Nimodipine (a calcium channel blocker) 60 mg orally can improve outcome after a subarachnoid hemorrhage.[18]

61. **B. Intervention.** Management of ICP includes ensuring that the patient is oxygenated and not agitated. Guidelines published in 1996, entitled *Management of Severe Head Injury,* sponsored by the Brain Trauma Foundation and endorsed by the American Association of Neurologic Surgeons, recommend that hyperventilation, high-dose steroids, and anticonvulsant therapy not be used routinely to manage ICP.[34]
62. **C. Evaluation.** Oral administration of phenytoin is less likely to cause serious side effects such as dysrhythmia, hypotension, pain at the intravenous site, and phlebitis. Fosphenytoin can be administered only intravenously. One disadvantage of oral administration of phenytoin is the amount of time it takes to achieve a therapeutic level.[35]
63. **B. Assessment.** Cranial nerve IX (glossopharyngeal) controls the gag reflex. Swallowing is controlled by cranial nerves IX and X (vagus).
64. **C. Assessment.** Cerebral hyperemia is the body's attempt to react to a severe injury to the brain. However, cerebral hyperemia causes an excess in cerebral blood flow, which actually exceeds the brain's demands. As a result, it causes an increase in cerebral intravascular volume and intravascular pressure. This results in decreasing cerebral perfusion pressure.[36]
65. **C. Assessment.** The increased fragility of cerebral blood vessels that occurs with aging contributes to cerebral hemorrhage, even with minor head trauma. Additionally, many elderly take medications, such as coumadin and aspirin, that increase the risk of bleeding.[36]

References

1. Bickley LS: *Bates' guide to physical examination and history taking,* Philadelphia, 1999, Lippincott.
2. Neff J, Kidd P: *Trauma nursing: the art and science,* St Louis, 1993, Mosby.
3. Engel J: *Pocket guide to pediatric assessment,* St Louis, 1993, Mosby.
4. Kim M, McFarland G, McLane A: *Pocket guide to nursing diagnoses,* St Louis, 1993, Mosby.
5. Howard P: Head trauma. In Newberry L, editor: *Sheehy's emergency nursing: principles and practice,* ed 5, St Louis, 2003, Mosby.
6. Newberry L, Barrett D: Neurologic emergencies. In Newberry L, editor: *Sheehy's emergency nursing: principles and practice,* ed 5, St Louis, 2003, Mosby.
7. *Mosby's drug consult 2005,* St Louis, 2005, Mosby.
8. Adams S, Camarista L, Chadwick L: Neurologic emergencies. In Kitt S, Selfridge-Thomas J, Proehl J et al, editors: *Emergency nursing: a physiologic and clinical perspective,* Philadelphia, 1995, WB Saunders.
9. McQuillan K, Mitchell P: Traumatic brain injury. In McQuillan K, Von Rueden KT, Harstock RL, et al, editors: *Trauma nursing: from resuscitation through rehabilitation,* Philadelphia, 2002, WB Saunders.
10. Kelley J: Seizure emergencies and disorders. In Kelley S, editor: *Pediatric emergency nursing,* Norwalk, CT, 1994, Appleton & Lange.
11. Hazinski M: *PALS provider manual,* Dallas, 2002, American Heart Association.
12. Manley L, Haley K, Dick M: Intraosseous infusion: rapid vascular access for critically ill or injured infants and children, *J Emerg Nurs* 14:63-69, 1988.
13. Seigler RS: The administration of rectal diazepam for acute management of seizures, *J Emerg Med* 8(2):155-159, 1990.
14. Soud T: The febrile child in the emergency department, *J Emerg Nurs* 19:355-358, 1993.
15. Kwiatkowski T, Alagappan K: Headache. In Marx J, editor: *Rosen's emergency medicine: concepts and clinical practice,* ed 5, St Louis, 2002, Mosby.
16. Minirth F: *The headache book,* Nashville, TN, 1994, Thomas Nelson.
17. Gilboy N, Tanabe P, Travers D et al: *The emergency severity index (ESI) implementation handbook,* Des Plaines, IL, 2003, Emergency Nurses Association.
18. Snyder J: Neurological emergencies. In Jordan KS, editor: *Emergency nursing core curriculum,* ed 5, Philadelphia, 2000, WB Saunders.
19. Adams H: Acute ischemic stroke: future options for an unmet medical need. Medscape release date June 30, 2003. Accessed at www.medscape.com, September 27, 2004.
20. Blank SJ, Keyes M: Thrombolytic therapy for patients with acute stroke in the ED setting, *J Emerg Nurs* 26(1):24-30, 2000.
21. Scott PA, Silbergleit R: Misdiagnosis of stroke in tissue plasminogen activator–treated patients: characteristics and outcomes, *Ann Emerg Med* 42(5):611-618, 2003.
22. Fernandez-Frackelton M, Turbiak T: Bacteria. In Marx J, editor: *Rosen's emergency medicine:*

concepts and clinical practice, St Louis, 2002, Mosby.

23. American College of Surgery: Algorithm for the initial management of the patient with severe head injury, www.acssurgery.com. Accessed April 14, 2004.
24. Oman K, Drury T: Head trauma. In Kitt S, Selfridge-Thomas J, Proehl J et al, editors: *Emergency nursing: a physiologic and clinical perspective,* Philadelphia, 1995, WB Saunders.
25. Semonin Holleran R: Head, neck, and spinal cord trauma. In Kelley J, editor: *Pediatric emergencies,* Norwalk, CT, 1994, Appleton & Lange.
26. Nayduch D, Lee A, Butler D: High-dose methylprednisolone after acute spinal cord injury, *Crit Care Nurse* 8:69-78, 1994.
27. Proehl J: The Glasgow Coma Scale: do it and do it right, *J Emerg Nurs* 18:421-423, 1992.
28. Jaworski M, Wirtz K: Spinal trauma. In Kitt S, Selfridge-Thomas J, Proehl J et al, editors: *Emergency nursing: a physiologic and clinical perspective,* Philadelphia, 1995, WB Saunders.
29. Foley J: Recognition and treatment of neuroleptic malignant syndrome, *J Emerg Nurs* 19:139-141, 1993.
30. Walls R: *Course manual national emergency airway management course,* Wesley, MA, 1998, Airway Management Education Center.
31. Munford B: Practical pharmacology of neuromuscular blockade, *J Air Med Trans* 17(4):149-156, 1998.
32. Silverman DG: *Neuromuscular block in preoperative and intensive care,* Philadelphia, 1994, WB Saunders.
33. Vender JS: Sedation, analgesia, and neuromuscular blockade in critical care: an overview, *New Horiz* 2(1):2-7, 1994.
34. Bullock R, Chestnut RM, Clifton G et al: Guidelines for the management of severe head injury, *J Neurotrauma* 13:639-734, 1996.
35. Rudis M, Touchette D, Swadron S et al: Cost-effectiveness of oral phenytoin, intravenous phenytoin, and intravenous fosphenytoin in the emergency department, *Ann Emerg Med* 43(3):386-397, 2004.
36. Emergency Nurses Association: *Course in advanced trauma nursing-II: a conceptual approach to injury and illness,* ed 2, Des Plaines, 2003, Emergency Nurses Association.

CHAPTER **12**

Obstetrical and Gynecological Emergencies

REVIEW OUTLINE

I. Female anatomy
  A. External
    1. Mons pubis
    2. Labia majora
    3. Labia minora
    4. Clitoris
    5. Fourchette
    6. Fossa navicularis
    7. Hymen
    8. Perineum
    9. Urethral meatus
    10. Vagina
  B. Internal
    1. Cervix
    2. Uterus
    3. Ovaries
    4. Fallopian tubes
    5. Bladder
    6. Rectum
II. Physiology
  A. Menstrual cycle
  B. Sexual act
  C. Stages of labor
III. Collaborative care of the patient with a gynecological or obstetrical emergency
  A. Assessment of the pregnant patient
    1. Physiological changes related to pregnancy
      a. Cardiovascular
        (1) Heart rate increases
        (2) Cardiac output increases
        (3) Blood pressure decreases
        (4) Maternal circulation changes
        (5) Electrocardiogram changes
        (6) Anemia of pregnancy occurs
      b. Pulmonary
        (1) Diaphragm elevation
        (2) Respiratory alkalosis
        (3) Oxygen consumption
      c. Anatomical changes
        (1) Pelvic changes
        (2) Pressure on inferior vena cava from gravid uterus
  B. History related to the pregnant patient
    1. Last menstrual period
    2. Estimated date of confinement
    3. Para, gravida, abortions
    4. Abdominal tenderness
    5. Problems with past and present pregnancies
    6. Prenatal care
    7. Maternal medical and surgical history
    8. Medications and allergies
    9. Blood type and Rh factor
  C. Assessment
    1. Abdominal tenderness
    2. Height of the fundus
    3. Vaginal bleeding
    4. Vaginal discharge
    5. Fetal heart tones
  D. Assessment of the nonpregnant female patient
    1. Last normal menstrual period
    2. Sexual activity
    3. Contraceptive method
      a. Oral
      b. Intrauterine device (IUD)
      c. Diaphragm
      d. Condom
      e. Spermicidal agent
    4. History of sexually transmitted diseases
    5. Gynecological symptoms
      a. Vaginal discharge: color, amount
      b. Vaginal bleeding: color, amount, clots, or tissue
      c. Vaginal itching
      d. Vaginal burning

e. Presence of sores, lumps
f. Dyspareunia
6. Medications
a. Prescribed
b. Alternative
7. Medical problems
a. Diabetes
b. Renal disease
c. Thyroid disorders
d. Sexually transmitted diseases
e. Cardiovascular
f. Neurological
8. Associated signs and symptoms
a. Nausea and vomiting
b. Fever, chills
c. Signs and symptoms of sepsis
9. Assessment of external genitalia
a. Inflammation
b. Ulceration
c. Discharge
d. Swelling, nodules, lesions
e. Color of patient's urine
10. Diagnostic studies
a. Laboratory
(1) β-Human chorionic gonadotropin (BHCG) level
(2) Complete blood count with differential
(3) Electrolytes
(4) Blood urea nitrogen and creatinine
(5) Type and crossmatch
(6) Rh factor
(7) Sexually transmitted disease cultures as indicated by the patient's history and signs and symptoms
(8) Urinalysis
(9) Urine culture
(10) Gram stain
(11) Wet mounts
(a) Saline
(b) Potassium hydroxide prep
b. Ultrasonography
(1) Abdominal
(2) Transvaginal
c. Abdominal computed tomographic (CT) scan
E. Interventions
1. ABCs
2. Pelvic examination
3. Abdominal or transvaginal ultrasonography
4. Medications as indicated by the patient's problem
5. Emergency delivery
6. Perimortem cesarean section
7. Apgar scoring
8. Neonatal resuscitation based on pediatric advanced life support (PALS)
9. Measurement of fetal heart tones
10. Dilation and curettage
11. Culdocentesis
12. Emergent surgery
13. Grief counseling
14. Discharge instructions
15. Prevention teaching
IV. Related nursing diagnoses
A. Anxiety
B. Family processes, altered
C. Fluid volume deficit, high risk for
D. Grieving, anticipatory
E. Infection, high risk for
F. Injury, high risk for
G. Pain
H. Spiritual distress (distress of the human spirit)
I. Trauma, high risk for
V. Obstetrical emergencies
A. Ectopic pregnancy
B. Abortion
1. Threatened abortion
2. Incomplete abortion
C. Preterm labor
D. Abruptio placentae
E. Placenta previa
F. Pregnancy-induced hypertension
G. HELLP syndrome
1. Hemolysis
2. Elevated liver function
3. Low platelets
H. Emergency delivery
I. Neonatal resuscitation
J. Maternal trauma
K. Perimortem delivery
VI. Gynecological emergencies
A. Vaginal bleeding
B. Genital trauma
C. Pelvic pain
D. Pelvic inflammatory disease (PID)
E. Sexually transmitted disease
F. Sexual assault

Many women seek care in the emergency department for obstetrical and gynecological problems. These range from management of sexually transmitted diseases to life-threatening difficulties, such as a ruptured ectopic pregnancy or abruptio placentae.

As women continue to work and lead the same lifestyle before and after childbirth, the likelihood that they may become patients in the emergency department will increase. Illness and injury will bring them to the emergency department. Trauma is the most common cause of death for women of childbearing age.[1] A pregnant woman is at risk for both illness and injury that will affect not only the mother, but also the infant.

When caring for the patient who has an obstetrical emergency, the emergency nurse needs to consider several important points. Pregnancy has both a physiological and psychological impact on a woman that will influence her response to trauma and disease states. The pregnant patient will experience changes in her cardiovascular, pulmonary, and nervous systems. Pregnancy may alter the pattern or the severity of trauma or disease states; pregnancy may alter laboratory results; and pregnancy can have its own complications, such as abruptio placentae, amniotic fluid embolism, or eclampsia.[2,3]

An emergency delivery will tend to increase the level of excitement in the emergency department. The emergency nurse should be familiar with the care of the delivering mother, as well as with the initial resuscitation and stabilization of the infant. The PALS course available from the American Heart Association and the Emergency Nursing Pediatric Course developed by the Emergency Nurses Association provide in-depth information related to the resuscitation of the neonate.

Finally, care of the patient who is suffering from an obstetrical emergency can be very stressful for the patient, her family, and the emergency department staff. Unfortunately, many women suffer a miscarriage while in the emergency department, or a woman may lose her child as a result of a traumatic injury. Helping the family to deal with the sudden loss of a child can be very difficult. The emergency nurse needs to be aware of support sources for patient, family, and staff.

When obtaining a history related to a gynecological emergency, questions that should be asked include the date of the patient's last menstrual period and if there were any abnormalities. Information to consider when evaluating a patient's menstrual period involves the age of the patient when her period began, intervals between her periods, duration of her period, and intensity of flow. The type of contraception the patient uses should also be determined.[3]

If the patient is experiencing vaginal discharge, the color and amount should be described and examined. Related symptoms such as fever, chills, nausea, and vomiting may indicate PID. Vaginal discharge may also be a sign of a systemic disease such as diabetes mellitus.

The incidence of sexually transmitted diseases has been on the rise over the past 10 years, and the complications of these diseases are seen more frequently in women. A serious complication from sexually transmitted diseases is PID, which can cause not only sepsis, but also infertility.

Care of an obstetrical or gynecological emergency is based on the particular problem the patient is experiencing. For the patient with an obstetrical emergency, care needs to be appropriate and organized so that both the mother and the child may benefit. Gynecological emergencies must be recognized early and managed, and appropriate follow-up offered.

REVIEW QUESTIONS

Vaginal Bleeding

A 23-year-old woman who is 30 weeks pregnant comes to the emergency department complaining of vaginal bleeding that started 1 hour earlier. She is a gravida 1 and para 0. She states that she is not having any pain or contractions with this bleeding.

1. In the third trimester of pregnancy, the most likely cause of this woman's vaginal bleeding is:
   A. Abruptio placentae
   B. Placenta previa
   C. Ruptured uterus
   D. Incompetent cervix

2. Initial treatment of this patient may include all of the following except:
   A. Insertion of a large-bore intravenous needle for fluid resuscitation
   B. Abdominal ultrasonography to evaluate the fetus
   C. Type and crossmatch for possible blood loss
   D. Pelvic examination by the emergency physician to evaluate cervical dilation

3. The patient with severe vaginal bleeding related to either placenta previa or abruptio placentae is at risk for developing:
A. Disseminated intravascular coagulation (DIC)
B. Adult respiratory distress syndrome
C. Pregnancy-induced hypertension
D. Trauma from a vaginal delivery

4. An 8-week-pregnant female comes to the emergency department complaining of heavy bleeding. The patient's initial vital signs are B/P 80/40, P 120, and R 23. The appropriate nursing diagnosis on which to plan this patient's care is:
A. Airway clearance, ineffective, related to the patient's respiratory rate
B. Fluid volume deficit related to vaginal bleeding
C. Grieving, anticipatory, related to potential loss of pregnancy
D. Infection, high risk for, related to retained products of conception

5. Which of the following lab values would indicate DIC?
A. Hemoglobin level of 14 g/dl
B. Hematocrit of 40%
C. White blood cells in the urine
D. Platelet count of 50,000

6. The number one cause of vaginal bleeding in woman of childbearing age is:
A. Threatened abortion
B. Vaginal infection
C. Cervical cancer
D. Pelvic fracture

7. The greatest fear related to a spontaneous abortion experienced by many women and men is that:
A. The mother will die because of excessive vaginal blood loss
B. The child will not go to heaven unless it is baptized
C. Their families will think they did something to cause the miscarriage
D. The mother will never be able to carry a child to term

Ectopic Pregnancy

A 29-year-old female arrives in triage complaining of moderate abdominal pain, dizziness, and sweating. She states that her symptoms have become progressively worse over the past few days. She has no significant medical history, and her last menstrual period was 8 weeks earlier. She has been trying to get pregnant.

8. The triage nurse places the patient in a pelvic examination room. The primary nurse should perform which of the following interventions during the initial treatment of this patient?
A. Obtain a specimen for serum quantitative BHCG
D. Obtain a chest radiograph, because the patient may go to surgery
C. Insert a gastric tube, because the patient has severe abdominal pain
D. Prepare the patient for an abdominal CT scan with contrast

9. The patient is complaining of pain in her right shoulder. This sign, associated with intraperitoneal bleeding, is known as:
A. Kernig's sign
B. Kehr's sign
C. Cullen's sign
D. Brudzinski's sign

10. Which of the following is a contraindication for performing a culdocentesis?
A. Withdrawal of peritoneal fluid from the cul-de-sac to determine whether a ruptured ectopic pregnancy has occurred
B. Withdrawal of fluid from the cul-de-sac for diagnosis of intraabdominal diseases in a female patient with severe abdominal pain
C. As an alternative to ultrasonography in an acutely ill female patient with a positive history for an ectopic pregnancy in an emergency department without access to ultrasonography
D. Presence of coagulopathy, a pelvic mass, or a nonmobile retroverted uterus, and in late pregnancy because the uterus may be perforated

11. A transvaginal ultrasonogram shows a ruptured ectopic pregnancy. While being prepared for surgery, the patient begins to cry and states that she does not want to lose her baby. The emergency nurse should base the nursing care on which of the following nursing diagnoses?
A. Spiritual distress (distress of the human spirit) related to a lifestyle change

B. Grieving, anticipatory, related to the loss of her baby
C. Grieving, dysfunctional, related to the loss of her baby
D. Thought processes, altered, related to hypotension and tachycardia

12. The patient demonstrates acceptance of the need for surgery, even though there will be a loss, by:
A. Signing out against medical advice, stating that she will be all right once she gets home
B. Refusing to talk to her family when they enter the room
C. Stating that she knows that she may die if she does not have surgery
D. Stating that she will never get pregnant again if she consents to this surgery

13. The most common cause of maternal death in the first trimester of pregnancy in the United States is:
A. Trauma from domestic violence
B. Ruptured ectopic pregnancy
C. Bleeding from placenta previa
D. Bleeding from abruptio placentae

An 18-year-old female comes to the emergency department complaining of irregular vaginal bleeding and mild abdominal pain. She states her last menstrual period was 6 weeks ago. She is sexually active and has not been using contraceptives. A transvaginal ultrasonogram shows an intact ectopic pregnancy.

14. Indications for the medical management of an ectopic pregnancy include:
A. A ruptured fallopian tube
B. Profuse vaginal bleeding
C. Severe abdominal pain
D. No fetal heart activity

15. The patient is given methotrexate 50 mg/m^2. Methotrexate enhances the expulsion of the ectopic pregnancy by:
A. Blocking the ability of the fetal tissue to implant
B. Blocking the effect of progesterone on the fetal tissue
C. Blocking the ability of rapid growth cells to reproduce
D. Blocking the effect of estrogen on the fetal tissue

Pregnancy-Induced Hypertension

The paramedics bring a 34-year-old woman who is a gravida 4 and a para 3 to the emergency department. She has been nauseated, vomiting, and complaining of a headache with blurred vision for 3 days. There have been no problems with her pregnancy until now. Her B/P is 160/120, P 110, and R 20.

16. The diagnosis of pregnancy-induced hypertension (preeclampsia) has been made. The emergency nurse should continually assess this patient for signs and symptoms of:
A. Seizure activity
B. Pulmonary emboli
C. Renal failure
D. Congestive heart failure

17. The patient's blood pressure continues to go up. She is now irritable, complaining of severe pain in her head and in her upper right quadrant. The patient has bilateral clonus. Which of the following medications is used to manage this patient's symptoms?
A. Phenytoin 1 to 5 g in 250 ml of normal saline
B. Lorazepam 3 to 5 mg IV push
C. Magnesium sulfate 4 to 6 g in 250 ml of normal saline
D. Fentanyl 2 to 5 ml IV push

18. A magnesium sulfate infusion is begun. The emergency nurse should evaluate which of the following as a symptom of toxicity?
A. Normal deep tendon reflexes
B. Urinary output greater than 30 ml/hr
C. Magnesium level of 4 to 7 mEq/L
D. Respiratory rate of fewer than 10 breaths per minute

19. The patient is placed in a quiet room with dimmed lights. The side rails are padded and up on all sides of the bed. The patient's room is within sight of the nurse's station. These interventions are derived from which of the following nursing diagnoses?
A. Infection, high risk for, related to a potential for ruptured membranes
B. Thought processes, altered, related to the use of magnesium sulfate
C. Injury, high risk for, related to the potential for seizure activity

D. Knowledge deficit related to the development of eclampsia

20. Magnesium sulfate is used to manage preeclampsia because it:
A. Exerts an antihypertensive action to lower the patient's blood pressure
B. Affects neurotransmission of acetylcholine to decrease seizure activity
C. Exerts a sedative effect so that the patient's headache pain is decreased
D. Affects neurotransmission to prevent diplopia

21. The differential diagnosis of HELLP syndrome includes which of the following?
A. Gastroenteritis
B. Cholecystitis
C. Hepatitis
D. All of the above

Preterm Labor

A 29-year-old woman who is at 28 weeks' gestation comes to the emergency department complaining of regular uterine contractions, back pain, and a bloody vaginal discharge. She has a history of delivering a baby at 26 weeks 2 years earlier who did not survive.

22. Risk factors for preterm labor do not include:
A. Mother's age more than 15 years
B. Use of alcohol and cigarettes while pregnant
C. No or inadequate prenatal care
D. History of uterine bleeding

23. The emergency nurse has the patient lie on a stretcher until the emergency physician can see her. What is the most beneficial position for both the mother and the child while lying down?
A. Flat on her back with a pillow under her lower back
B. On her abdomen with a pillow under her chest
C. In the left lateral recumbent position
D. In the lithotomy position

24. The patient's contractions continue after a fluid bolus is given, and the emergency physician orders a dose of terbutaline 0.25 mg to be administered subcutaneously every hour until her contractions decrease. What common side effect may the patient experience while receiving this drug?
A. Tremors and anxiety
B. Palpitations and tachycardia
C. Hypertension
D. Headache and dizziness

Pregnant Trauma Patient

A 22-year-old woman who is 8 months pregnant has been involved in a motor vehicle crash. She was an appropriately restrained passenger (shoulder and lap belt), whose side of the car was struck by another vehicle going approximately 50 miles per hour. The patient is brought to the emergency department by helicopter with full cervical spine immobilization. Her vital signs are B/P 70/40, P 160, and R 32.

25. The most common type of fracture found in the pregnant trauma patient is:
A. Pelvic fracture
B. Femur fracture
C. Lower rib fracture
D. Cervical spine fracture

26. When the mother has suffered a ruptured uterus as a result of blunt abdominal trauma, the infant may die because of:
A. Abdominal trauma
B. Head trauma
C. Pelvic trauma
D. Chest trauma

27. The primary survey of the pregnant trauma patient includes all of the following except:
A. Airway assessment
B. Ventilatory assessment
C. Abdominal ultrasonography
D. Circulatory assessment

28. In addition to fluid and blood resuscitation, what other intervention could the emergency nurse perform to help raise the patient's blood pressure?
A. Position the patient with her head elevated to 30 degrees
B. Position the patient on her right side with her hips flexed
C. Position the patient in a left lateral position
D. Place the patient in the Trendelenburg position

29. Because the diaphragm is elevated by a gravid uterus and decreases the mother's oxygen reserve, the mother and fetus are at risk for hypoxia. The emergency nurse would base their nursing care on which of the following nursing diagnoses?
   A. Airway clearance, ineffective, related to a full stomach
   B. Gas exchange, impaired, related to ineffective inspiration
   C. Fluid volume deficit, high risk for, related to increased volume
   D. Mobility, impaired physical, related to the size of the fetus

30. The pregnant patient demonstrates knowledge about prevention of blunt trauma during pregnancy by:
   A. Proper use of her lap and shoulder harness throughout her pregnancy
   B. Not wearing her seat belt when she is in her third trimester
   C. Wearing only a lap belt when she is in her third trimester
   D. Not driving at all in her third trimester

31. A pregnant female is at greatest risk for intentional injury from:
   A. Motor vehicle crash
   B. Falling
   C. Drug ingestion
   D. Human abuse

32. A 23-year-old pregnant female suffers a cardiac arrest after a head-on motor vehicle collision. The patient arrives at the hospital 10 minutes after cessation of vital signs. A perimortem cesarean section should be considered only if:
   A. The fundal height is 24 cm
   B. The fundal height is 22 cm
   C. The fundal height is 20 cm
   D. The fundus is above the symphysis pubis

33. When the pregnant woman is injured, factors that do not contribute to fetal death include:
   A. Direct injury to the fetus from penetrating abdominal trauma
   B. Maternal anoxia from traumatic arrest
   C. Fetal head injury from blunt impact to the abdomen
   D. An intact placenta after the injury

34. Indications for a perimortem cesarean section include:
   A. Maternal arrest longer than 15 minutes
   B. Fetal age less than 20 weeks
   C. Unsuccessful closed cardiac massage
   D. Adequate maternal vital signs

Emergency Delivery

35. A 17-year-old teenager called her mother home from work after she delivered a 30-week fetus at home alone. The teenager's mother called the paramedics, who have brought the teenage mother and infant to the emergency department. The mother's vital signs are stable on arrival. The emergency nurse should next assess:
   A. The status of the placenta
   B. Whether the patient has any vaginal tears
   C. Whether the mother wants to breast-feed
   D. The height of the mother's fundus

36. The infant is cyanotic and making little respiratory effort. The paramedics have suctioned the infant, applied oxygen by mask, dried the infant, and attempted tactile stimulation to improve the infant's respiratory function. The emergency nurse should:
   A. Prepare equipment for intubation
   B. Give epinephrine through an umbilical catheter
   C. Perform chest compressions
   D. Ventilate the infant with a bag-mask device using high-flow oxygen

37. Chest compressions should be performed on the newborn:
   A. When the infant's pulse is less than 60 to 80 beats per minute
   B. When the infant's pulse is greater than 90 beats per minute
   C. When the infant's pulse is 160 beats per minute
   D. After the infant has been given atropine

38. A location for emergent vascular access in the newborn is:
   A. Sternal intraosseous space
   B. Umbilical vein
   C. Scalp vein
   D. Femoral artery

Missed Abortion

39. The most common complication of a missed abortion is:
    A. Sepsis
    B. Pulmonary emboli
    C. Clotting abnormalities
    D. Infertility

Gynecological Emergencies

40. A 20-year-old comes to the emergency department complaining of a rash on the palms of her hands and the soles of her feet. She states it does not itch. She states she is sexually active and generally uses a diaphragm for contraception. She reports having had several sexual partners over the last few months, but she has had no symptoms of sexually transmitted diseases in the past few months. What sexually transmitted disease may be causing this rash?
    A. Herpes simplex II
    B. Nongonococcal urethritis
    C. Gonorrhea
    D. Syphilis

41. A 40-year-old female comes to the emergency department complaining of an increase in vaginal discharge, itching, vaginal irritation, and dyspareunia. She states that she has been married for 15 years and has had no other sexual partners. She describes the discharge as white and thick. The most probable cause of her symptoms is:
    A. *Lactobacillus acidophilus*
    B. Vulvovaginal candidiasis
    C. Trichomoniasis vaginalis
    D. *Neisseria gonorrhoeae*

42. Which of the following is a risk factor for complicated vulvovaginal candidiasis?
    A. Multiple sexual partners
    B. Douching every day
    C. Uncontrolled diabetes
    D. Use of an IUD

43. A 22-year-old female arrives in the emergency department complaining about a thin, frothy, malodorous discharge. She states that her last menstrual period was 2 weeks ago and she has recently begun a new relationship. She takes oral contraceptives. The most probable cause of her discharge is:
    A. Bacterial vaginosis
    B. Vaginal trichomoniasis
    C. Urethral chlamydia
    D. Vulvovaginal candidiasis

44. When discharging a patient who has been given metronidazole for vaginal trichomoniasis, the emergency nurse should instruct the patient that:
    A. Her sexual partners do not have to be treated for this sexually transmitted disease
    B. She may continue to drink alcohol with all her meals while taking this medication
    C. Her sexual partners should use barrier contraception until she has been seen again and cleared of all infection
    D. She should always take the medication on an empty stomach because it never causes nausea

45. A 16-year-old girl brings her 10-day-old infant to the emergency department for care. She states that her child has had an eye infection since birth. Both of the infant's eyes are red, and there is white drainage noted along the outside edges of the baby's eyes. The mother states that she did not receive any prenatal care and the baby was born at home. The most likely cause of this child's eye infection is:
    A. Congenital syphilis
    B. Trachomatis
    C. Chlamydia
    D. Candidiasis

46. The child's eye infection should be managed with:
    A. Ceftriaxone 125 mg IM administered in the emergency department for 10 days
    B. Ceftriaxone 1 g ophthalmic ointment placed in the eye for 5 days
    C. Erythromycin 50 mg/kg per day orally, divided into 4 doses, for 10 days
    D. Spectinomycin 2 g IM administered in the emergency department for 10 days

47. Clindamycin cream has been prescribed to a 42-year-old woman for management of bacterial vaginosis. Her discharge instructions should include which of the following information?
    A. Her partner will need to be treated for infection so that she does not become reinfected
    B. Caution should be used when using a condom or diaphragm, because clindamycin cream weakens latex

C. She should not drink any alcohol before or after meals when using clindamycin cream
D. Bacterial vaginosis usually is caused by a gonococcal infection, so her partner should be treated with penicillin

48. Testing and treatment of sexual partners generally is required for all of the following sexually transmitted diseases except?
A. Bacterial vaginosis
B. Chancroid
C. Chlamydia
D. Gonorrhea

49. A 17-year-old girl arrives in the emergency department complaining of severe diffuse lower abdominal pain. Her vital signs are B/P 92/50, P 130 and regular, R 28, and she has an oral temperature of 103.6° F. She is pale, ambulating slowly, and is more comfortable with her hips flexed when she lies down. Which of the following information would assist the emergency nurse to differentiate the cause of the patient's hypotension and tachycardia?
A. History of abdominal surgery
B. Last menstrual period and sexual activity
C. History of urinary tract symptoms
D. Her current diet

50. Risk factors for PID include:
A. Females age 30 to 45 years of age
B. Monogamous sexual relationship
C. Use of an IUD for contraception
D. No history of pelvic surgery

51. In addition to providing care for the patient's infection and administering a fluid bolus, which nursing diagnosis would be appropriate for the care of the patient with PID?
A. Pain, acute, related to PID
B. Sexual dysfunction related to abdominal pain
C. Activity intolerance related to pain experienced with movement
D. Anxiety related to waiting for results of the pregnancy test

52. Which of the following antibiotics are used to treat the patient with acute PID who requires hospitalization?
A. Cefoxitin 2 g IM plus doxycycline 100 mg orally twice a day
B. Cefoxitin 2 g IV plus doxycycline 100 mg IV or orally q 12 hr
C. Ofloxacin 400 mg orally bid for 14 days after discharge from the hospital
D. Aqueous penicillin 4.8 million units IM 3 times a day

53. When counseling the patient who has been treated for PID, the emergency nurse should emphasize which of the following?
A. The emergency department is not where you should be treated for severe abdominal pain
B. Becoming pregnant will decrease your risk of developing PID in the future
C. Follow-up care is not necessary because you were treated in the emergency department
D. Reinfection may recur if your sexual partners are not evaluated and treated

An 18-year-old girl is brought to the emergency department by the police. She states that she had been hitchhiking and was picked up by a man who gave her something to drink. She woke up with her underwear off and she thinks the man had intercourse with her before he left her about 6 hours ago.

54. The initial assessment of a survivor of sexual assault should include:
A. Identification and management of any physical injuries the patient may have suffered
B. The patient's emotional response to the sexual assault
C. How the people with the victim are responding to the sexual assault
D. The amount of time it took for the patient to report the sexual assault

55. Clothing collected as evidence from the survivor of sexual assault should be:
A. Labeled and left outside of the patient's room
B. Labeled and placed in a plastic bag
C. Examined and given back to the patient
D. Labeled and placed in a paper bag

56. The patient stated that she had been given something to drink and has no memory of what has happened to her. Indications that a drug

may have been given to a survivor of sexual assault include all of the following except:
A. Appearance of intoxication with no evidence of alcohol ingestion
B. Explained memory loss related to the incident
C. Unexplained patient drowsiness
D. Complaints of dizziness and confusion

57. Which of the following nursing diagnoses is most appropriate for the treatment of the survivor of sexual assault?
A. Posttrauma syndrome
B. Social isolation
C. Rape-trauma syndrome
D. Powerlessness

58. Before ethinyl estradiol–norgestrel (Ovral) can be administered as postcoital contraception for the survivor of sexual assault, the emergency nurse must:
A. Obtain written consent from the patient and her spouse
B. Be sure that the patient's pregnancy test is negative
C. Determine if the patient is allergic to oral hormones
D. Obtain written consent from the patient

59. The most common cause of gonococcal infection in the preadolescent child is:
A. Sexual experimentation with other children
B. Sexual abuse by a known caregiver
C. Exposure to another infected child
D. There is no known cause

60. A 5-year-old girl is being prepared in the emergency department for a sexual abuse evaluation. What interventions may the emergency nurse use to help decrease the child's anxiety?
A. Separate the child and her caregiver before the examination
B. Tell the child that she is a "big girl" if she does not cry
C. Allow the child to pick which arm the blood may be drawn from
D. Take away all the child's toys before the examination begins

ANSWERS

1. **B. Assessment.** The most likely cause of painless vaginal bleeding in the third trimester of pregnancy is placenta previa. Vaginal bleeding during pregnancy can occur for various reasons, including placenta previa, abruptio placentae, and preterm labor. If the bleeding is associated with pain, boardlike rigidity of the abdomen, and signs and symptoms of hemorrhagic shock, the patient may have abruptio placentae. Painless vaginal bleeding, usually after 28 weeks of gestation, and uterine contractions are symptomatic of placenta previa.[2,4]
2. **D. Intervention.** The patient who has placenta previa or abruptio placentae should not have a vaginal examination unless the appropriate physicians and nursing teams are available to manage the delivery that could be precipitated.[2,5]
3. **A. Assessment.** Because of the potential for the mother to lose a large amount of blood from both of these conditions, the patient is at risk for developing DIC.[2,3]
4. **B. Analysis.** The patient's vital signs indicate that she is suffering from some type of shock. Her vaginal bleeding could be the source of her blood loss. The initial care of this patient needs to be directed toward identifying and managing her shock.[3]
5. **D. Evaluation.** Excessive or sudden blood loss can put the patient at risk for developing DIC. Laboratory values that indicate DIC include a decreased platelet count (normal 150,000 to 400,000), low hemoglobin (normal 12 to 15 g/dl), and low hematocrit (normal 36% to 45%).[2]
6. **A. Assessment.** A threatened abortion is the number one cause of vaginal bleeding in women of childbearing age.[3,4]
7. **D. Assessment.** The greatest fear experienced by both women and men after a spontaneous abortion is that it may recur and the woman will never be able to carry a child to term. The emergency nurse needs to reassure them that even though this is a possibility, 10% to 20% of pregnancies end in spontaneous abortion, and people do go on to carry pregnancies to term.[4]
8. **A. Intervention.** During the initial treatment of this patient, a BHCG level should be obtained to determine if the patient is pregnant and suffering from an ectopic pregnancy. A gastric tube is probably not necessary and a transvaginal ultrasonogram will probably be done before a CT, based on the patient's history.[4]
9. **B. Assessment.** When the patient has significant intraperitoneal bleeding, the resulting

abdominal pain may radiate to either shoulder. This is known as Kehr's sign and is also associated with splenic injury.[3]

10. **D. Intervention.** Even though ultrasonography has made culdocentesis a fairly uncommon procedure, it still may be of value for diagnosis when ultrasonography is not available.[5]
11. **B. Analysis.** The defining characteristics of this nursing diagnosis include the expression of distress because of a potential loss, and the realization or resolution of an impending death or loss.
12. **C. Evaluation.** By acknowledging that she may die if she does not have the surgery, the patient is developing awareness of her loss. The emergency nurse should encourage the patient to continue to discuss her feelings.[1-4]
13. **B. Assessment.** Ruptured ectopic pregnancy is the most common cause of maternal death in the first trimester of pregnancy. Fifteen percent of in vitro fertilizations result in ectopic pregnancy, which makes this an important piece of history to be obtained from any woman complaining of abdominal pain and vaginal bleeding.[7]
14. **D. Assessment.** Indications for medical management of an ectopic pregnancy include unruptured fallopian tube, no active bleeding, and no fetal heart activity.[4,8,9]
15. **C. Intervention.** Methotrexate is a folic acid antagonist, and it blocks the ability of cells to reproduce. It particularly targets cells with a rapid growth rate.[8,9]
16. **A. Assessment.** Because seizures are a frequent complication of preeclampsia, the patient needs to be assessed continually while in the emergency department for signs and symptoms of seizures.[2,3,7]
17. **C. Intervention.** Magnesium sulfate is given in a loading dose of 4 to 6 g as a 10% solution in 250 ml of IV fluid. It is infused rapidly over 15 minutes.[7,9]
18. **D. Evaluation.** Magnesium toxicity can cause respiratory depression. Respiratory failure can occur with magnesium sulfate levels of 12 to 15 mEq/L.[8]
19. **C. Analysis.** One of the goals of the emergency nursing care for this patient would be to prevent injuries that could occur from seizures, a potential complication of preeclampsia.[2,6]
20. **B. Intervention.** Magnesium sulfate directly affects the neurotransmission of acetylcholine to decrease the incidence of seizures.[8]
21. **D. Assessment.** HELLP syndrome is a form of preeclampsia that can cause life-threatening complications, including multiple organ failure. However, the symptoms are similar to other gastrointestinal emergencies including hepatitis, cholecystitis, and gastroenteritis.[3]
22. **A. Assessment.** Risk factors for preterm labor include a mother younger than 15 years, use of alcohol and cigarettes while pregnant, history of uterine bleeding, and inadequate prenatal care.[10]
23. **C. Intervention.** The lateral recumbent position allows the gravid uterus to be displaced from the inferior vena cava, which can increase cardiac output.[2,3,5]
24. **A. Intervention.** Tremors and anxiety are common side effects that patients may experience while being treated with terbutaline. Hypertension, persistent tachycardia, and palpitations are less frequent, and the patient should be monitored closely.[8]
25. **A. Assessment.** The most common type of fracture found in the pregnant trauma patient is a pelvic fracture. The most frequent mechanism of injury in the pregnant patient is the motor vehicle, which generally results in some type of blunt trauma.[1,10,11]
26. **B. Assessment.** When the mother suffers enough impact from blunt trauma to rupture her uterus, fetal death is usually the result of a skull fracture with intracranial hemorrhage.[1,10,11]
27. **C. Assessment.** Saving the life of the mother is the primary objective during the initial treatment of the pregnant trauma patient. If the mother does not survive, the possibility that the fetus may survive—particularly depending on the fetus's gestational age—is limited. An abdominal ultrasonogram should be a part of the secondary assessment.[10-12]
28. **C. Intervention.** Because the gravid uterus compresses the vena cava when the patient is on her back, the patient may experience supine hypotension. Supine hypotension, or vena cava syndrome, is the result of the gravid uterus compressing the vena cava and aorta. The patient should be placed in the left lateral recumbent position as soon as the cervical spine has been cleared. If the cervical spine has not been cleared, a pillow can be placed under the right side of the backboard.[5,10-15]
29. **B. Analysis.** A defining characteristic of this nursing diagnosis is hypoxia. A related factor

contributing to this nursing diagnosis is an altered oxygen supply.[6]

30. **A. Evaluation.** The most common cause of fetal death during pregnancy is death of the mother. Women need to be educated about the proper way to wear safety restraints while they travel. The proper way to wear a restraint while pregnant is as follows: the lap belt is worn across the pelvis, and the shoulder harness is worn between the breasts and off the shoulder.[5,10-13]
31. **D. Assessment.** The incidence of intentional injury from human abuse increases during pregnancy. Connolly and others found a 24% increase, particularly resulting in injury to the fetus.[1]
32. **A. Assessment.** After 20 weeks of gestation, the fundus can be measured in centimeters. The number of centimeters is roughly equal to the age in weeks. Perimortem cesarean section is not recommended for the fetus less than 24 to 26 weeks because of the low likelihood of survival.[3,5,10-15]
33. **D. Assessment.** Factors that contribute to fetal death include maternal death and anoxia, direct injury to the fetus, and fetal head injury.[5,13,14]
34. **C. Intervention.** Indications for a perimortem cesarean section include maternal arrest of 5 minutes or less, fetal age of more than 24 weeks, and inadequate maternal vital signs.[13,14]
35. **A. Assessment.** The status of the placenta should be assessed once the mother's ABCs have been assessed. A lengthening of the cord and a gush of blood indicate the delivery of the placenta. Once the placenta has been delivered, the emergency nurse should place it in a basin or a plastic bag, label it with the patient's name, and send it with the mother to the obstetrical unit.[2,3]
36. **D. Intervention.** Using the inverted pyramid for neonatal resuscitation, the emergency nurse should try bag-mask ventilation with high-flow oxygen. If this should fail to improve the infant's status, chest compressions would be indicated, followed by intubation and medication administration.[16]
37. **A. Intervention.** Chest compressions are performed on a newborn when the pulse rate is less than 60 to 80 beats per minute and when, despite adequate ventilation with 100% oxygen after 30 seconds, the infant's condition does not improve.[16]
38. **B. Intervention.** Locations for emergent vascular access in the newborn include umbilical vein and intraosseous route, such as the proximal tibia or distal femur.[5,16]
39. **C. Evaluation.** Because of the retained products of conception, the patient is at risk of developing hypofibrinogenemia.[2]
40. **D. Assessment.** Clinical manifestations of secondary syphilis include mucocutaneous lesions that occur in 80% of patients with this disease. The lesions appear on the palate, pharynx, glans of the penis, and vulva. Rashes that occur in secondary syphilis do not itch and can be macular, papular, pustular, or squamous lesions. They frequently appear on the palms of hands or the soles of the feet.[17]
41. **B. Assessment.** Based on the signs and symptoms described by this patient, the most probable cause of her discharge is candidiasis. About 25% of vaginal discharge is caused by candidiasis, with signs and symptoms that include white cottage cheese discharge, vaginal irritation, itching, and painful sexual intercourse.[17]
42. **C. Assessment.** Predisposing factors for complicated vulvovaginal candidiasis include debilitating illnesses, immunosuppression, and uncontrolled diabetes.[17]
43. **B. Assessment.** The signs and symptoms of vaginal trichomoniasis include thin, frothy, copious, green-yellow or gray, malodorous discharge. The predisposing factor for this disease is sexual activity.[16]
44. **C. Intervention.** The patient who has been treated for trichomoniasis with metronidazole should avoid drinking alcohol while taking the medication, have the partner checked and treated, use barrier contraception until the disease is cleared, and take the medication with food.[17]
45. **C. Assessment.** Chlamydia is one of the most common causes of conjunctivitis in the newborn less than 30 days of age.[17]
46. **C. Intervention.** The child should be treated with an oral medication, not eye drops, usually erythromycin 50 mg/kg per day orally divided into four doses.[7]
47. **B. Intervention.** Clindamycin cream is oil based and can weaken latex products. Women diagnosed with bacterial vaginosis are the only ones treated, because treatment of male partners has not been found to be of benefit.[16,17]

48. **A. Assessment.** Testing and treatment of sexual partners is recommended for all except bacterial vaginosis. The Centers for Disease Control and Prevention gives specific recommendations for each of the diseases.[17]
49. **B. Assessment.** Differential diagnosis for this patient's hypotension, tachycardia, and abdominal pain include a ruptured ectopic pregnancy or PID. Date and description of the patient's last menstrual period will assist the emergency nurse to identify the possible causes.[7,17]
50. **C. Assessment.** Risk factors for PID include age between 14 and 24; history of PID; previous pelvic surgery; multiple sexual partners; use of cigarettes, alcohol, illegal drugs; and a history of using an IUD for contraception.[7,17]
51. **A. Analysis.** The patient is experiencing acute pain related to the inflammation from her pelvic infection. Defining characteristics of this nursing diagnosis include guarding and protective behaviors, which can make a physical evaluation difficult. The patient's tachycardia may be the consequence not only of infection, but pain as well.[6]
52. **B. Intervention.** Management of acute PID that requires hospital admission is initially IV antibiotics. If the patient can tolerate it, doxycycline should be administered orally, because IV administration is painful.[17]
53. **D. Intervention.** When counseling patients with PID, the emergency nurse should emphasize that if her partner(s) are not evaluated and treated, reinfection is likely to recur. In addition, the nurse should discuss the need to return if the patient experiences increasing abdominal pain. PID during pregnancy can leave both the mother and fetus at risk for serious complications. Finally, the patient needs to follow up to see if her treatment has been effective.[7,17]
54. **A. Assessment.** Initial assessment of any survivor of a violent crime should be focused on the identification and management of any physical injuries that could be life threatening.[3,5,18-20]
55. **D. Intervention.** All evidence that is collected needs to be labeled with the patient's name, date, time of collection, and who collected the evidence. A description of the evidence submitted should also be documented. Evidence such as clothing should be placed in a clean paper bag. Plastic bags retain moisture and may cause destruction of evidence.[5,18-20]
56. **B. Assessment.** Indications of drug ingestion in a sexual assault victim include appearance of intoxication without evidence of alcohol or drugs, unexplained drowsiness, and dizziness and confusion.[20]
57. **C. Analysis.** Unfortunately, sexual assault remains one of our society's major social ills. Nurses interact with the survivors of sexual assault not only in the emergency department, but within the hospital and community, as well. Because of the complex care required by these survivors (females, males, children, young and older adults), specific nursing diagnoses have been developed. These include rape-trauma syndrome; rape-trauma syndrome: compound reaction; and rape-trauma syndrome: silent reaction.[5,6]
58. **B. Intervention.** Before postcoital contraception can be administered, a negative pregnancy test must be documented. Informed consent is necessary before the drug is administered, and only after it is determined that the patient is not pregnant.[18-20]
59. **B. Assessment.** The most common cause of gonococcal infection in preadolescent children (except the neonate) is from sexual abuse by a known caregiver.[17]
60. **C. Intervention.** Allowing the child to have some control over her care in the emergency department will help decrease her anxiety. Keeping everything as simple as possible, including allowing a caregiver to remain with the child as long as possible (obviously not the one responsible for the abuse), holding onto a favorite toy, or in some cases using sedation, will contribute to a less stressful examination for both the child and the emergency department personnel.[18]

References

1. Connolly AM, Katz VL, Bash KL, et al: Trauma and pregnancy, *Am J Perinatol* 14(6):331-336, 1997.
2. Reedy N, Brucker M: Emergencies in gynecology and obstetrics. In Kitt S, Selfridge-Thomas J, Proehl J et al, editors: *Emergency nursing: a physiologic and clinical perspective,* Philadelphia, 1995, WB Saunders.
3. Rita S, Reed B: Obstetric emergencies. In Newberry L, editor: *Sheehy's emergency nursing: principles and practice,* ed 5, St Louis, 2003, Mosby.

4. Carter S: Overview of common obstetric bleeding disorders, *Nurs Pract* 24(3):50-73, 1999.
5. Proehl J, editor: *Emergency nursing procedures,* ed 3, Philadelphia, 2004, WB Saunders.
6. Kim M, McFarland G, McLane A: *Pocket guide to nursing diagnoses,* St Louis, 1993, Mosby.
7. Jordan KS: Obstetrical and gynecological emergencies. In Jordan KS, editor: *Emergency nursing core curriculum,* ed 5, Philadelphia, 2000, WB Saunders.
8. *Mosby's drug consult 2005,* St Louis, 2005, Mosby.
9. Miller J, Griffin E: Methotrexate administration for ectopic pregnancy in the emergency department—one hospital's protocol/competencies, *J Emerg Nurs* 29(3):240-244, 2003.
10. Peterson D: Preterm labor: update on assessment and management, *J Emerg Nurs* 20(5):373-376, 1994.
11. Southard P: The pregnant trauma patient: special considerations in emergency department care, *J Emerg Nurs* 18(3):283-285, 1992.
12. Gerber-Smith L: The pregnant trauma patient. In McQuillan K, Von Rueden KT, Harstock RL, et al, editors: *Trauma nursing: from resuscitation through rehabilitation,* Philadelphia, 2002, WB Saunders.
13. Kloeck W, editor: *ILCOR advisory statements: special resuscitation situations,* Dallas, 1999, American Heart Association.
14. Strong T, Lowe R: Perimortem cesarean section, *Am J Emerg Med* 5:489-494, 1989.
15. Henderson S, Mallon W: Trauma in pregnancy, *Emerg Med Clin North Am* 16(1):209-228, 1998.
16. Hazinski M, editor: *PALS provider manual,* Dallas, 2002, American Heart Association.
17. Centers for Disease Control and Prevention: Sexually transmitted diseases treatment guidelines 2002, *MMWR* 51(RR-6):1-78, 2002.
18. Girardin B, Faugno D, Senski P: *Color atlas of sexual assault,* St Louis, 1997, Mosby.
19. *Sexual assault protocol,* Cincinnati, OH, 2002, University Hospital.
20. Armstrong R: When drugs are used for rape, *J Emerg Nurs* 23(4):378-381, 1997.

CHAPTER 13

OCULAR EMERGENCIES

REVIEW OUTLINE

I. Anatomy and physiology
  A. Anatomical structures
    1. Globe
      a. Sclera
      b. Cornea
      c. Uvea
      d. Retina
      e. Optic nerve
    2. Segments and chambers
      a. Anterior segment
      b. Posterior segment
      c. Retina
      d. Choroid
      e. Vitreous humor
    3. Lens and pupil
    4. Orbit
    5. Eyelids
    6. Lacrimal glands
  B. Physiology
    1. Vision
    2. Accommodation
    3. Extraocular movement (EOM; cranial nerves II, III, IV, VI)

II. Ocular assessment
  A. History of illness or injury
    1. Risk factors for illness and injury
      a. Age of the patient
      b. Environment where patient lives, works, plays
      c. Occupation and hobbies
    2. Mechanism and time
    3. AMPLE history
    4. Change in condition from onset of symptoms to arrival in emergency department
  B. Pain
    1. Provocation
    2. Quality
    3. Radiation
    4. Severity
    5. Time
  C. General appearance of eye
    1. Edema or erythema
    2. Bleeding, tearing, or discharge
    3. Eye movements
  D. Visual acuity
    1. Test with and without glasses or contact lenses
    2. Use a Snellen eye chart, if possible
    3. Determine if patient can see fingers if unable to see eye chart. Start at approximately 10 feet and see if patient can count the number of fingers you are holding up. Continue to move closer to patient until patient can see the fingers. This is recorded as "Counts fingers at X feet." If within 2 to 3 feet and patient still cannot see fingers, determine if patient can see hand motion. Record as "Hand motion at X feet." If patient has only light perception, use a penlight to see if patient can determine which direction light is coming from.
    4. Visual changes include
      a. Blindness
      b. Blurring
      c. Diplopia
      d. Cloudiness or smokiness
      e. Photophobia
  E. Visual fields
    Face the patient. Patient and examiner occlude opposite eyes. Examiner moves to bring his or her hands into the visual field from the periphery. Assess all four quadrants. Absence of vision in any quadrant is recorded.
  F. EOM
    Face the patient. Have patient focus on an object such as a pencil. Move pencil up, down, to the left, and to the right. Observe patient's ability to move the eyes equally in all directions.

G. Pupil reactivity
   Test for direct and consensual pupillary response when light is shined in the eye.
H. Pupil accommodation
   Have the patient focus on a near, and then distant, object. Accommodation causes convergence of the eyes and pupillary constriction.
I. Medical history
   1. Glaucoma
   2. Chronic eye disease or previous eye trauma
   3. Diabetes
   4. Cardiovascular disease
   5. Hypertension

III. Diagnostic methods used for ocular emergencies
   A. Tonometry
   B. Fluorescein staining
   C. Slit lamp examination
   D. Laboratory
   E. Radiology
   F. Visual acuity charts
   G. Eversion of the eyelid
   H. Mydriasis

IV. Related nursing diagnoses
   A. Alteration in comfort, pain
   B. Anxiety
   C. Fear
   D. Knowledge deficit
   E. Tissue perfusion, alteration in, optic nerve
   F. Uncompensated sensory deficit, vision

V. Age-related changes
   A. Pediatric patient
      1. Visual acuity
         a. 200/400 for infants at 2 months, reaching 20/100 by 1 year, and 20/20 by 4 or 5 years of age
         b. Infant vision can be tested by observing the reach for a familiar object and fixation on light sources and objects
         c. Charts and cards for older children include the Allen card, kindergarten test card, and Child Recognition Test
         d. Children are at risk for contagious eye illness because of close contact with others at school, daycare
         e. Children are at risk for injury by running with objects, lack of safety concerns
   B. Geriatric patient
      1. Changes associated with aging, such as a decrease in visual acuity, should be taken into consideration with examination
      2. Medical history and medication history are important when assessing the elderly with an alteration in vision
      3. Globe thins with age and, therefore, is susceptible to rupture with less force

VI. Selected ocular emergencies
   A. Conjunctivitis
   B. Glaucoma
   C. Central retinal artery occlusion
   D. Corneal abrasions
   E. Foreign bodies
   F. Retinal detachment
   G. Chemical burns
   H. Hyphema
   I. Eyelid laceration
   J. Globe rupture

Eye injuries and eye illnesses are common emergencies evaluated and managed in the emergency department.[1] The eyes represent only about 3% of the total body surface area, yet they account for approximately 10% of all bodily injuries.[2] Eye injuries can be a result of blunt or penetrating trauma. Blunt trauma is most frequently the result of physical violence secondary to altercations. Penetrating trauma usually is caused by industrial accidents but can also be the result of an assault. Motor vehicle accidents, sports-related injuries, and falls can cause both blunt and penetrating eye injuries.

Many things, including infection, irritants, and burns, cause conjunctivitis, a common ocular emergency. It is also associated with systemic illnesses such as upper respiratory infections. Millions of Americans suffer from chronic eye disease such as glaucoma. They, too, visit our emergency departments with exacerbation of existing illnesses. Blurred vision may be an indication of an ocular problem or a symptom of disease processes such as transient ischemic attacks or cerebrovascular accidents.[3]

Whether the patient has a traumatic or medical ocular emergency, the emergency nurse must assess and intervene rapidly to prevent permanent visual loss. Patients will be anxious about disfigurement and loss of vision. Therefore, the emergency nurse must be skilled in providing emotional support as well as physical care.

REVIEW QUESTIONS

Match the terms in column A to the definitions in column B.

A	B
1. Blepharitis	A. Inflammation of the cornea that is light sensitive, red, and painful
2. Hordeolum	B. Also known as a stye, infection of the upper or lower eyelid at the accessory gland
3. Chalazion	C. Inflammation of the lid margin, usually caused by *Staphylococcus aureus*
4. Keratitis	D. A sebaceous cyst that forms on the inside surface of the eyelid

Mr. Lord, a 22-year-old construction worker, comes to the emergency department with complaints of pain, redness, and drainage from the left eye, which has worsened over the past 2 days. His visual acuity is normal. He is diagnosed as having conjunctivitis.

5. Upon assessment of Mr. Lord's visual acuity, you would expect to find:
   A. A decrease in visual acuity in the affected eye due to the conjunctivitis
   B. A decrease in visual acuity in both eyes due to the conjunctivitis
   C. No change in the patient's visual acuity due to the conjunctivitis
   D. An improvement in visual acuity in both eyes due to the conjunctivitis

6. An appropriate nursing diagnosis for the patient with conjunctivitis would be:
   A. Sensory-perceptual alteration, input deficit
   B. Infection, high risk for
   C. Alteration in comfort, pain
   D. Tissue perfusion, alteration in, optic nerve

7. Initial nursing interventions for Mr. Lord should be aimed at providing comfort. One method for this would include:
   A. Providing cold compresses to the affected eye
   B. Providing warm compresses to the affected eye
   C. Cleansing the eye with diluted antiseptic solution
   D. Irrigating the affected eye with warm saline until clear

8. Discharge instructions for Mr. Lord should include patient teaching about conjunctivitis being:
   A. Recurring
   B. Contagious
   C. Self-limiting
   D. Nontransmissible

9. The anterior chamber of the eye is that space between the pupil and cornea filled with:
   A. Natural tears
   B. Aqueous humor
   C. Vitreous humor
   D. Interstitial fluid

10. A hyphema is bleeding into the:
   A. Lens of one eye
   B. Posterior chamber
   C. Anterior chamber
   D. Canal of Schlemm

Mr. Gordon, an 18-year-old male, comes to the emergency department with a chief complaint of eye pain as the result of an altercation. Mr. Gordon states his opponent punched him in the eye. Upon medical evaluation, he is diagnosed as having a hyphema. Usually the product of blunt trauma, a hyphema is bleeding from the vessels of the iris into the anterior chamber.

11. Findings associated with hyphema include:
   A. Aching pain in the affected eye
   B. Blood at the top of the anterior chamber
   C. Blindness from the blood in the anterior chamber
   D. No change in visual acuity in the affected eye

12. An appropriate nursing diagnosis for Mr. Gordon would be:
   A. Social isolation
   B. Alteration in comfort, pain
   C. Fluid volume deficit, high risk for
   D. Ineffective airway clearance

13. Interventions for Mr. Gordon include proper patient positioning once his cervical spine has been cleared. Mr. Gordon should:
   A. Lie flat on his abdomen to decrease intraocular pressure

B. Sit with his head elevated to decrease intraocular pressure
C. Sit with head of bed at a 45° angle, turned on the affected side
D. Sit with head of bed at 45° angle, turned on the unaffected side

Mr. Thomas, 66 years old, comes to the emergency department with complaints of a severe headache located along the left eyebrow. He states that he can barely see out of his left eye and when he looks toward the lights, he sees halos around them. Mr. Thomas denies head trauma and states this all began approximately 1 hour ago.

14. You suspect Mr. Thomas has:
A. Corneal abrasion
B. Retinal detachment
C. Central retinal artery occlusion
D. Acute narrow-angle glaucoma

15. As the triage nurse, you would classify Mr. Thomas as:
A. Urgent
B. Emergent
C. Nonurgent
D. Delayed care

16. Several classic findings will assist the emergency medical team in their diagnosis of acute narrow-angle glaucoma. The affected eye's pupil will be:
A. Normal in size and reaction
B. Dilated, yet reactive
C. Constricted, nonreactive
D. Semi-dilated, nonreactive

17. Upon palpation, the affected eye will feel:
A. Normal texture
B. Rock hard
C. Like rubber
D. Soft and mushy

18. The physician may use a tonometer to measure Mr. Thomas's intraocular pressure. The normal reading is 11 to 22 mm. You expect Mr. Thomas's to be:
A. Lower than normal
B. Higher than normal
C. Within normal limits
D. Unable to be determined

19. Mr. Thomas is given an analgesic for pain. Anticipatory care would also dictate that Mr. Thomas be given an:
A. Antibiotic
B. Antiemetic agent
C. Antiinflammatory agent
D. Anticoagulant

20. You also anticipate a medical order for:
A. Miotic eyedrops
B. Mydriatic eyedrops
C. Cycloplegic eyedrops
D. Sublingual nitroglycerin

21. Mr. Thomas is also given 1% pilocarpine. What criteria should the nurse use to evaluate the effectiveness of this drug?
A. An increase in intraocular pressure
B. An increase in visual acuity
C. An increase in blurred vision
D. An increase in halos seen around lights

22. Mr. Thomas is given an osmotic diuretic. The rationale for this therapy for the patient with acute narrow-angle glaucoma is that the diuretic will:
A. Lower intraocular pressure
B. Prevent cerebral edema
C. Raise mean arterial pressure
D. Improve cardiac output

23. Mr. Thomas's "attack" is broken. His vital signs are stable, visual acuity has improved, and pain has subsided substantially. He is given discharge instructions and has an appointment to see the ophthalmologist the next day. Mrs. Thomas begins to cry and expresses fear that her husband has lost his vision forever. An appropriate reply would be:
A. Mr. Thomas's sight can return to normal with appropriate management and compliance with his health care providers' instructions
B. Mr. Thomas will probably go blind in the future, but many social programs can help him adjust to this change
C. Mr. Thomas will probably go blind in the affected eye only, which means only minimal changes in his daily routine
D. Mrs. Thomas should address these concerns with the ophthalmologist tomorrow when her husband's appointment is scheduled

24. Central retinal artery occlusion is differentiated from acute angle-closure glaucoma by:
A. Painless onset of visual changes
B. History of contact lens use
C. Visual acuity unaffected by the disease
D. Gradual unilateral loss of vision

25. Mrs. Rug is a 78-year-old female brought to the emergency department for an eye problem. She states that she tripped on the rug and fell, striking the right anterolateral side of her face on the floor. There was no loss of consciousness. Her vision has decreased progressively in the right eye since the fall. Upon admission to the emergency department, Mrs. Rug states she can see only flashes of light, but mainly sees a curtain effect in her right visual field. You suspect:
A. Acute angle-closure glaucoma
B. Corneal abrasion
C. Retinal detachment
D. Central retinal artery occlusion

26. Your primary interventions for Mrs. Rug are:
A. Bed rest and patches applied to both eyes
B. Measures to increase intraocular pressure
C. Head of bed elevated and patched right eye
D. Application of cold compresses and sublingual nitroglycerin

Mr. Roberts, a 24-year-old carpenter, comes to the emergency department with complaints of pieces of wood in his left eye. Several large foreign bodies are visible. The eye is reddened, tearing, and painful. Visual acuity is normal.

27. Your first nursing intervention for Mr. Roberts would be:
A. To vigorously irrigate the injured eye with dextrose in water
B. Manually remove the larger pieces of wood to prevent blindness
C. Anesthetize the eye with the appropriate eye drops for comfort
D. Test Mr. Robert's intraocular pressure with a tonometer

It is determined that Mr. Roberts has sustained a corneal abrasion secondary to the foreign bodies. The affected eye is patched, and Mr. Roberts is provided with antibiotic ointment, as well as instructions on how to apply the ointment.

28. Mr. Roberts should also be instructed that his eye pain will return. The pain can be relieved by:
A. Application of warm compresses and a metal shield over the injured eye
B. Application of an eye patch and a cool pack to the injured eye
C. Continuous instillation of topical anesthetics to the injured eye
D. Application of over-the-counter eye drops to decrease the pain to the injured eye

29. The legal definition of blindness is visual acuity of:
A. 20/80 or less
B. 20/100 or less
C. 20/160 or less
D. 20/200 or less

30. A life-threatening complication of periorbital cellulitis is:
A. Decreased visual acuity on the affected side
B. A brain abscess
C. Paralysis of extraocular muscles
D. Conjunctivitis

31. A 32-year-old unrestrained driver was involved in a head-on motor vehicle crash. The airbag was deployed. He is now complaining of pain in both eyes. Initial treatment of his eyes should include:
A. Administration of antibiotic ointment to decrease the risk of infection
B. Patching both eyes to decrease movement and allow them to rest
C. Liberal irrigation with large quantities of normal saline solution
D. Administration of cycloplegic and antibiotic eye drops

32. When removing a patient's contact lens, the emergency nurse should:
A. Use as much force as necessary to remove the lens from the eye
B. Instill all eye medications while the contact lens is still in place
C. Use only saline solutions with preservatives when removing a contact lens
D. Look for lost lenses in the upper cul-de-sac of the eye

33. Complications related to eye irrigation include:
A. Corneal abrasion
B. Periorbital edema

C. Fine punctate keratitis
D. All of the above

34. Discharge instructions related to the instillation of eye drops should include:
A. Look down toward the floor when instilling the eye drops
B. Close or blink the eyes gently to spread the medication in the eye
C. Squirt a large amount of solution into the eye to save time
D. Gently pull the lower lid up when instilling the eye drops

35. Which of the following eye injuries should not be patched?
A. Corneal abrasion
B. Hyphema
C. Ruptured globe
D. Chemical burn

ANSWERS

1. **C. Assessment.**[1]
2. **B. Assessment.**[1]
3. **D. Assessment.**[1]
4. **A. Assessment.**[1]
5. **C. Assessment.** The patient with conjunctivitis usually has no change in visual acuity.[4]
6. **C. Analysis.**[4]
7. **B. Intervention.** Warm compresses will provide comfort to the patient with conjunctivitis.[4]
8. **B. Intervention.** Conjunctivitis is contagious, not only to other people, but also to the patient's unaffected eye.[1,2]
9. **B. Assessment.**[3]
10. **C. Assessment.**[4]
11. **A. Assessment.** The patient with a hyphema will have pain and a decrease in visual acuity in the affected eye.[5]
12. **B. Analysis.**[5]
13. **B. Intervention.** The patient with a hyphema should assume an upright position.[5]
14. **D. Assessment.** Mr. Thomas has classic symptoms of acute narrow-angle glaucoma.[3]
15. **B. Assessment.** Mr. Thomas needs emergent therapy and interventions to preserve his eyesight.[3-5]
16. **D. Assessment.**[4]
17. **B. Assessment.** Narrow-angle glaucoma will produce a rock-hard globe on palpation.[4]
18. **A. Assessment.** A tonometer reading reflects the amount of plunger indentation on the eye. Patients with high intraocular pressure produce a low reading, because the plunger cannot indent the eyeball very much. Patients with low intraocular pressure will produce a high reading, because the plunger can indent the eyeball more.[3]
19. **B. Intervention.** Patients with acute narrow-angle glaucoma frequently experience nausea and vomiting. Anticipatory care would dictate the use of an antiemetic to decrease nausea and prevent vomiting.[5]
20. **A. Intervention.** Miotic eyedrops will constrict the pupil to allow for aqueous humor drainage.[3]
21. **B. Evaluation.** The effectiveness of 1% pilocarpine eyedrops can be evaluated by an improvement in visual acuity. Pilocarpine constricts the pupil, pulling the iris away from the cornea and out of the angle, allowing for the free flow of aqueous humor from the posterior to the anterior chamber.[4]
22. **A. Intervention.** An osmotic diuretic for the patient with acute narrow angle glaucoma serves to decrease intraocular pressure. Because diuretics "dehydrate" the body, the amount of aqueous humor produced will also hopefully be decreased, lowering intraocular pressure.[4]
23. **A. Intervention.**[4,5]
24. **A. Assessment.** Central retinal artery occlusion is painless, and can be sudden or gradual in onset. Acute angle-closure glaucoma is usually very painful with a sudden onset. Both conditions are usually monocular, and neither condition is necessarily binocular.[2]
25. **C. Assessment.**[3]
26. **A. Intervention.** Bed rest, bilateral eye patches and, occasionally, a tranquilizer are primary interventions for the patient with retinal detachment. You may also need to prepare the patient for surgery.[3]
27. **C. Intervention.** Providing anesthetic drops is a nursing intervention with the appropriate standing orders. This should be a priority of care, because the patient will then be able to cooperate with other procedures.[4]
28. **B. Intervention.** To alleviate his recurrent pain, Mr. Roberts should be instructed to apply the antibiotic ointment as directed, double patch the eye to achieve a tight eye patch, apply an ice pack, and use over-the-counter analgesics. The purpose of an eye patch is to protect the eye, absorb secretions, and promote comfort. A tight eye patch will act as a pressure dressing and will relieve pain as well as promote

healing. Patients should never be given a bottle of topical anesthetic, because it impairs corneal healing and promotes the development of corneal ulcers. A patient may reinjure the eye without knowing it if a topical anesthetic is used consistently.[5]

29. **D. Assessment.**[6]
30. **B. Assessment.** The most serious complication of periorbital cellulitis is a brain abscess.[3]
31. **C. Intervention.** The gases in an airbag contain sodium hydroxide. Alkali solutions penetrate the eyes more easily than acids and require liberal irrigation with copious amounts of normal saline solution to ensure that the chemical has been removed.[6]
32. **D. Intervention.** When removing a contact lens from a patient's eye, the emergency nurse should never use force. If the eye is dry, instill a few drops of normal saline before attempting to remove the lens. Do not instill medications with the lenses in place, because the lenses could combine with the medication and cause eye damage. Look for the lens in the cul-de-sac if its location is not obvious.[7]
33. **D. Assessment.** All of these are potential complications of eye irrigation.[8]
34. **B. Intervention.** When instilling eye drops:
    - Instruct the patient to look up
    - Gently pull the eyelid down for drop instillation
    - Instill a single drop into the conjunctival sac at the center of the lower lid; more than one drop at a time can cause tearing that can dilute the medication
    - Close or blink the eyes to spread the medication[9]
35. **C. Intervention.** The eye of a patient with a suspected open or ruptured globe should never be patched in order to prevent placing any additional pressure on the injured eye.[5]

References

1. Egging D: Ocular emergencies. In Newberry L, editor: *Sheehy's emergency nursing: principles and practice,* ed 5, St Louis, 2003, Mosby.
2. Barak A, Belkin M: The eyes have it, *Emerg Med Serv* 23(5):50-55, 1994.
3. Epifanio P: Ocular emergencies. In Jordan KS, editor: *Emergency nursing core curriculum,* ed 5, Philadelphia, 2000, WB Saunders.
4. Kitt S, Kaiser J: *Emergency nursing: a physiologic and clinical perspective,* Philadelphia, 1990, WB Saunders.
5. Emergency Nurses Association: *Trauma nursing core course,* Des Plaines, IL, 2000, Emergency Nurses Association.
6. Watts D, Kokiko J: Air bags and eye injuries: assessment and treatment for ED patients, *J Emerg Nurs* 25(6):572-574, 1999.
7. Layman M: Contact lens removal. In Proehl J, editor: *Emergency nursing procedures,* ed 3, Philadelphia, 2004, WB Saunders.
8. Quigley M: Eye irrigation. In Proehl J, editor: *Emergency nursing procedures,* ed 3, Philadelphia, 2004, WB Saunders,
9. Quigley M: Instillation of eye medications. In Proehl J, editor: *Emergency nursing procedures,* ed 3, Philadelphia, 2004, WB Saunders.

CHAPTER 14

ORGAN AND TISSUE DONATION AND POSTTRANSPLANT EMERGENCIES

REVIEW OUTLINE

I. Types of organ donors[1,2]
  A. Nonheartbeating donors: patients who have suffered cardiopulmonary arrest and have been declared dead
  B. Heartbeating donors: patients who have been declared brain dead and whose organs have maintained viability by mechanical ventilation, fluids, and limited and selected medications
II. Organs that may be transplanted
  A. Cornea
  B. Kidney
  C. Skin
  D. Liver
  E. Heart
  F. Lung
  G. Pancreas
  H. Bone
  I. Heart and heart valves
  J. Ligaments
  K. Middle ear
  L. Veins, arteries, nerves
  M. Vertebral bodies, bone marrow
  N. Eyes
  O. Intestines
III. Physiological systems review
  A. Fluid and electrolytic balance
  B. Cardiac system
  C. Respiratory system
  D. Renal system
  E. Hepatic system
  F. Pancreatic system
  G. Neurological system
  H. Skeletal system
  I. Integumentary system
  J. Immunosuppression
IV. Assessment
  A. History related to the cause of death
  B. In-depth head-to-toe physical assessment
  C. Medical history
    1. Risk factors
    2. Current medications
    3. Previous illnesses and injuries
V. Issues related to organ donation
  A. Legislative issues
    1. Consolidated Omnibus Budget Reconciliation Act (COBRA), 1986
    2. Organ Donation Request Act, 1987
    3. Uniform Anatomical Gift Act
    4. State laws
      a. Routine referral
      b. Required request
    5. Hospital policy
    6. Emergency department policy
  B. Brain death
    1. Definition
    2. Criteria
    3. Brain death status
      a. State
      b. Federal
      c. Hospital policy
    4. Coroner's cases
  C. Nonheartbeating donors
VI. Identification of potential organ and tissue donors
  A. Respiratory and circulatory functions artificially maintained
  B. Tissue donation: either respiratory-maintained and circulatory-maintained brain-dead patients or patients who have died of cardiorespiratory arrest (nonheartbeating donors)
  C. Identification of potential donor
    1. Medical history
    2. History of precipitating injury or condition
    3. Present physiological condition
    4. Contraindications
    5. Brain death

- D. Donor eligibility rule (Food and Drug Administration, 2004): additional tissue that must now be tested before donation
  1. Reproductive tissue
     a. Semen
     b. Ova
     c. Embryos
  2. Hematopoietic stem cells from circulating blood sources
     a. Cord blood
     b. Peripheral blood sources
  3. Cellular therapies and other innovative products
- E. Organ procurement organization
  1. Protocols
  2. Role of coordinators
     a. With emergency department
     b. With families
     c. With donors
- F. Brain death
  1. Definition
     a. Generally accepted (Harvard brain death criteria)
     b. State
     c. Hospital policy
  2. Role of ethics committee
- G. Criteria for organ donor suitability
  1. Vary according to organ or tissue involved
  2. Time frames for retrievability
- H. Exclusionary criteria for donor identification
  1. Untreated septicemia
  2. Human immunodeficiency virus
  3. Viral hepatitis
  4. Active tuberculosis
  5. Malignancy, except primary brain tumor
  6. Disease of the donated organ or tissue
  7. Chronic systemic disease

VII. Donor maintenance management
- A. Goal: ensure organ viability
  1. Maintain optimal hydration
  2. Maintain adequate oxygenation
  3. Maintain hemodynamic stability
     a. Maintain adequate fluid hydration (central venous pressure 8 to 12 cm H_2O)
     b. Maintain urine output (more than 100 ml/h)
     c. Maintain systolic blood pressure at over 100 mm Hg
     d. Maintain electrolyte balance and blood glucose level
     e. Maintain normal body temperature
     f. Prevent and manage infection
- B. Basic principles of donor treatment
  1. Resuscitation
  2. Organ perfusion
  3. Hydration
  4. Diuretics
  5. Avoidance of infection

VIII. Approaching families of potential donors
- A. Establishing legal next of kin
  1. Spouse
  2. Adult brother or sister
  3. Guardian
  4. Any other person who is responsible for the disposal of the patient's body
- B. Approach to family, intervention
  1. Obligations to approach
  2. Dignified, professional manner
  3. Positive attitude
  4. Knowledgeable
  5. Offer emotional support
  6. Answer questions, allow expression of feelings
  7. Accept and support decision of family
- C. Involvement of others
  1. Physician
  2. Social worker
  3. Clergy
  4. Medical examiner or coroner
  5. Organ procurement coordinator
- D. Answers to most commonly asked questions
  1. No cost
  2. No disfigurement
  3. No disruption of funeral arrangements
  4. Confidentiality maintained
  5. Donated organs always given to those in great need
  6. Religious leaders support organ donations
  7. Family can visit patient's body

IX. Specific emergency nursing considerations
- A. Completion of physical assessment
- B. Collection of history
- C. Awareness of organ and tissue donation inclusion and exclusion criteria
- D. Knowledge of appropriate ways to approach families
- E. Knowledge of brain death criteria
- F. Awareness of role of organ procurement coordinator

G. Awareness of other support services, personnel, and referral agencies
H. Knowledge about donor management protocols
I. Awareness of legal next of kin
J. Coordination with intensive care unit
   1. Donor maintenance
   2. Documenting, reporting
   3. Following policy or procedures
K. Legal issues
   1. Legal next of kin
   2. Hospitals must contact organ procurement organizations in a timely manner
   3. Only designated requesters can approach family, once recognized by the hospital staff
   4. Witnessed telephone consent
   5. Documentation

X. Related nursing diagnoses
A. Breathing pattern, effective
B. Cardiac output, decreased
C. Coping, family, ineffective
D. Fluid volume deficit, high risk for
E. Gas exchange, impaired
F. Grieving, anticipatory
G. Infection, high risk for
H. Skin integrity, impaired
I. Spiritual distress (distress of the human spirit)
J. Tissue perfusion, altered
K. Urinary elimination, altered patterns

XI. Posttransplant emergencies
A. Patient assessment
   1. Location of the transplanted organ
   2. Differences in symptoms
      a. Chest pain different in the patient who has received a heart transplant because of denervation of the donated heart
      b. Electrocardiogram may show two P waves, because parts of both the donor's and recipient's hearts are kept
B. Immunosuppression
   1. Drug reaction
      a. Bone marrow suppression
      b. Hepatic dysfunction
      c. Leukopenia
C. Infection
D. Rejection
   1. Fever
   2. Fatigue
   3. Irregular cardiac rhythm
   4. Jaundice
   5. Edema
   6. Decreased appetite
E. Diagnostic tests
   1. Complete blood count with differential
   2. Culture and sensitivity
   3. Cardiac enzymes
   4. Liver enzymes
   5. Electrolytes
   6. Blood urea nitrogen and creatinine

Many advances in technology, surgical techniques, and immunosuppression make transplantation increasingly successful. Organ donation has continued to take on both a national and international focus over the past 10 years. The supply of organs for transplant, however, remains a major limiting factor, and thousands of people await transplants each year. Many continue to die each year while waiting.[2] Two particular pieces of legislation mandate that hospitals and medical personnel inform all families of their option of organ and tissue donation. A brief overview of these laws is presented here. A discussion of the vital role emergency nurses play in identifying and maintaining potential donors follows.[3,4]

The first legislation, COBRA, was passed in 1986 and has been revised several times over the past 2 decades. The first law became effective on October 1, 1987, and made provisions requiring all hospitals receiving Medicaid or Medicare reimbursement to do the following:

1. Have written protocols for donor identification
2. Inform families of their option of organ and tissue donation
3. Observe discretion and sensitivity
4. Notify organ procurement organizations of potential organ or tissue donors[1-5]

The federal government also enacted a second piece of legislation, the Organ Donation Request Act (the "required request" act), in January 1987, because health care professionals had demonstrated reluctance in asking families for organ and tissue donation. This act outlined the following provisions:

1. The next of kin must be asked for consent
2. Consent may be secured by the attending physician
3. Deference should be paid to the donor's religious beliefs

4. Notification must be made to the organ procurement organization
5. No sanctions are imposed for hospital noncompliance, but funding may be withheld[3]

These legislative acts make it clear that hospitals must comply with the provisions outlined, or Medicare and Medicaid reimbursement may be withheld. "Required request" laws now exist in all states and require hospitals to notify the nearest organ procurement agency when brain death is diagnosed and also require a request for organ and tissue donation when the deceased meets specified criteria.

Local procurement agencies play a large role in assisting the emergency department nurse to comply with these laws. The local organ procurement agency is linked with the United Network for Organ Sharing System and, by way of a national computer system, connects with current information on all potential recipients and all available organs. This system ensures that those with the greatest need receive organs or tissues first. The organ procurement agency serves a vital role in providing information and guidance to the emergency department nurse.

Because emergency department nurses are frequently the first health care professionals to identify a potential donor, they must be diligent in their efforts to identify and treat potential donors to help meet the increasing demand for organs and tissues. Although organ donors are usually transferred to the critical care unit for care until brain death has been declared and consent obtained from the family, the emergency department nurse provides emotional support for the family and provides proper nursing care of the patient prior to transport. Tissue donors may be identified and maintained in the emergency department, because no ventilatory or cardiovascular support is necessary. After it is determined that the patient meets the criteria for organ or tissue donation, the emergency department nurse should follow the established protocol quickly and notify the local organ procurement organization.[6]

Nurses can facilitate the decision making of families who are considering donation, and they can work with the health care team to introduce the concept of organ donation to families who have not considered it at all. This is important because, although many families would be willing to donate organs for transplantation, most families will not think of donation unless someone cares enough to let them know about this opportunity. The family's willingness to donate organs can be enhanced by allowing them to participate as much as possible in the end-of-life decision making and by identifying ways to help the family cope with their feelings of helplessness and powerlessness.[7,8]

It is crucial that emergency department nurses know their state laws and hospital and departmental policies regarding organ and tissue donation. They must be able to identify potential donors, know the role of the organ procurement agency, know the interventions to be used in the care of donors, know how to approach families, and know the nursing diagnoses related to the care of these patients. Efforts to increase the number of available donor organs and tissues are underway to meet the steadily increasing demand. In addition, the emergency department nurse must become comfortable with approaching a family and making a request. Increasing public awareness through education regarding the need to consider donation remains a role of the emergency department nurse.

With the advent of more effective immunosuppressive agents and an increase in the number of hospitals that perform organ and tissue transplantation, patients are living longer and more active lives than did those in the past.[5] Because of this, emergency nurses may find themselves faced with the challenge of caring for a patient who is having a posttransplant complication. One of the most common complaints that brings posttransplant patients to the emergency department is fever, which may be a sign of infection or potential organ rejection.

The emergency nurse needs to be aware of the anatomical, physiological, and psychological impact that organ and tissue transplantation makes on patients' lives. The transplanted organ may be in a different anatomical location, such as the transplanted kidney that is placed lower in the pelvic cavity. Because of physiological differences in the transplanted heart, the patient will not experience chest pain, or may have a cardiac dysrhythmia considered normal for that patient.[1-3]

Finally, the drugs that are used to prevent rejection may contribute multiple problems, including hepatic, renal, and infectious complications.[1-4]

REVIEW QUESTIONS

The rescue squad brings a 56-year-old man to the emergency department. He was on a construction site and fell from a bridge into a river. He has suffered severe head injuries and has fixed, dilated pupils. Cardiopulmonary resuscitation (CPR) was begun at the scene. The patient is brought to the emergency department under full CPR. After a brief period of additional resuscitation efforts, the patient is pronounced dead by the trauma team.

1. How would the emergency nurse determine whether this patient is a potential organ donor?
   A. Completing a physical examination and obtaining a detailed history
   B. Calling the organ procurement agency with a potential referral
   C. Asking the family's consent for potential organ and tissue donation
   D. Notifying the coroner that the patient is a potential organ or tissue donor

2. Federal and state laws require that:
   A. Families of all potential donors must be asked about donation
   B. Only families of medically suitable donors be asked about donation
   C. Catholic families should not be approached about organ donation
   D. Families should never be asked about donation while they are still in the emergency department

3. The emergency department nurse finds the deceased patient's driver's license among his belongings. The patient had signed the donor card. When the family is approached about organ donation, the patient's relatives vehemently oppose the idea. The Uniform Anatomical Gift Act allows for:
   A. The individual's decision to override the wishes of relatives
   B. Hospitals to create their own policies about organ and tissue donation
   C. The family's decision to override the patient's request
   D. The need to contact a judge before any decision can be made

4. When the family is told that CPR was ineffective and that the patient has died, the family members begin to yell and scream. One of them attempts to hit the emergency physician and states, "You did not do enough!" The nursing diagnosis on which the emergency nurse would base care is:
   A. Coping, ineffective family, related to the suddenness of the patient's death
   B. Family processes, altered, related to the patient's sudden death
   C. Grieving, anticipatory, related to the suddenness of the patient's death
   D. Injury, high risk for, related to the family attempting to strike the emergency physician

5. Based on the family's reaction to the news of the loss of their family member, the best approach for the emergency nurse to use concerning organ or tissue donation would be to:
   A. Refrain from asking about organ donation because the family is too upset to make the decision at this time
   B. Ask the family, and if they do not agree, try to convince them that they should donate because it is what the patient wanted
   C. Provide emotional support, such as from a chaplain, and when the family is calmer, offer them the option of donation
   D. Tell the family it is the nurse's job to ask them about organ donation, and they have to sign a paper saying the nurse did ask them

6. The major goal of organ donation management is to:
   A. Reassure family members that the organs of the deceased are donated to the person of their choice
   B. Ensure organ viability so that the organs can be used effectively in the patient who is to receive them
   C. To make sure the religious beliefs of the family are explored and respected by the organ procurement team
   D. Notify the appropriate agencies so that the organs can be transported by either air or ground to the receiving facility

7. A recommended method of maintaining fluid volume in the patient who is a potential organ donor is to:
   A. Slowly infuse dextrose 5% in water with 20 mEq of potassium to maintain adequate organ perfusion until donation can be completed
   B. Perform vigorous fluid resuscitation with crystalloids, colloids, and blood products to maintain organ perfusion

C. Transfuse the patient with packed red blood cells only to maintain adequate organ perfusion
D. Begin a dopamine drip to maintain a systolic blood pressure of 150 mm Hg to maintain adequate organ perfusion

8. If adequate fluid replacement therapy has been attempted and is unsuccessful, the best choice of vasopressors to maintain a systolic blood pressure of more than 100 mm Hg is:
A. Dopamine
B. Norepinephrine
C. Dobutamine
D. Azathioprine

9. A patient may be declared brain dead when which of the following criteria has been met?
A. The patient exhibits conjugate eye movements in response to a caloric test
B. The pupillary light reflex is intact and the patient has dilated pupils bilaterally
C. All functions of the brain have ceased irreversibly, including those of the brain stem
D. Cerebral angiogram that shows filling above the level of carotid bifurcation

10. A 35-year-old single woman has been deemed an appropriate candidate for organ donation. The nurse approaches the waiting room and finds 12 of the patient's relatives there. The sister of the patient has become the spokesperson for the family. The emergency department nurse needs to determine who is the legal next of kin. Of the following, the nurse should obtain consent from the:
A. Patient's sister, because she is the spokesperson for the family
B. Patient's boyfriend, because he was the last to speak to her
C. Mother of the patient
D. Woman who states she is the patient's closest friend

11. All of the following organs or tissues must be tested for human immunodeficiency virus, hepatitus B, and hepatitus C before donation *except:*
A. Embryos
B. Cord blood
C. Bone marrow
D. None of the above

12. Candidates for organ donation who are victims of a drowning or, in the case of severe burns, who require prolonged ventilatory support, have been thought to be less suitable for organ donation because of which of the following nursing diagnoses?
A. Fluid volume deficit, high risk for, related to prolonged ventilatory support
B. Infection, high risk for, related to prolonged ventilatory support
C. Poisoning, high risk for, related to prolonged ventilatory support
D. Breathing pattern, ineffective, related to ventilatory support

13. A 5-year-old child who had a heart transplant 6 months earlier is brought to the emergency department by her parents. They state that the child has had a fever of 102°F and has been nauseated and vomiting. The child was recently exposed to chickenpox by one of her cousins. Her parents state that she has received the human varicella zoster immune globulin but now has lesions on her abdomen. Which medication will the child need on an emergent basis?
A. Tacrolimus
B. Ceftriaxone
C. Acyclovir
D. Gentamicin

14. A serious side effect of cyclosporine (Sandimmune) is:
A. Vomiting
B. Hepatotoxicity
C. Tremors
D. Oral candidiasis

15. Patients who have received a heart transplant generally do not:
A. Develop congestive failure
B. Develop cardiac dysrhythmias
C. Develop immunosuppression reactions
D. Experience angina

ANSWERS

1. **A. Assessment.** A thorough history and physical examination are essential to the initial assessment for donor suitability. A number of

underlying conditions immediately exclude the potential donor from further consideration.[1-5]

2. **A. Intervention.** The law requires that all potential donors (or their families) be approached. Families may wish to have their relative's bodies donated for research if they are not suitable for organ or tissue donation. Sometimes, as in the case of patients with cancer, middle ears may be suitable for donation. The patient may be mistakenly considered "medically unsuitable" for donation.[1,2,5]
3. **A. Assessment.** If the patient had complied properly with the provisions of the Uniform Anatomical Gift Act of the state in which he or she was a resident, the request of the patient to be an organ donor would take precedence over the wishes of the patient's family. The gift takes effect immediately on death and is, therefore, binding on relatives. Thus, technically, the decision of an individual to donate an organ is legally binding on the family. In practical terms and as a matter of policy, however, few hospitals go against the wishes of family members if they choose not to proceed with donation. A common practice is to obtain consent for organ and tissue donation from the donor's next of kin.[1,2,4-6]
4. **A. Analysis.** The family is exhibiting an inability to cope with the tragic news of their family member's death. Although individuals react differently to a family member's death, violent and threatening behavior is not acceptable behavior. This family needs a lot of support, and a referral should be made to a member of the clergy or to a social worker.
5. **C. Intervention.** The timing of when organ or tissue donation is requested, and the way a family is approached, are key issues in obtaining consent for organ donation. Physicians and nurses may be reluctant to discuss organ donation with potential donor families, fearing that this will cause the families more distress. However, it has been found that organ donation may actually bring consolation to a grieving family.[5-8]
6. **B. Evaluation.** Ensuring organ viability is the primary goal in organ donor treatment. This is accomplished by maintaining optimal hydration, oxygenation, and hemodynamic stability.[1,3,5]
7. **B. Intervention.** Maintaining hemodynamic stability is mandatory in order to maintain adequate tissue perfusion. Fluid resuscitation with crystalloids, colloids, and blood products should be employed to maintain the patient's blood pressure. Dopamine may be used once adequate fluid resuscitation has been achieved.[9]
8. **A. Intervention.** Dopamine is the vasopressor of choice for restoring autoregulatory control. Norepinephrine should be avoided, because it raises the body's oxygen demands and can constrict the vessels supplying major organs. Large doses of vasopressors should be avoided whenever possible to prevent vasoconstriction, which can also produce decreased organ perfusion.[9]
9. **C. Analysis.** Brain death may be declared when a person has sustained either irreversible cessation of circulatory and respiratory function or irreversible cessation of all functions of the brain, including the brain stem.[2,10]
10. **C. Intervention.** The legal priority of individuals from whom consent can be obtained for a patient's organ or tissue donation are, in this order, the patient's spouse, an adult son or daughter, either parent, an adult brother or sister, a guardian, or any other person authorized or under obligation to dispose of the body.[1-3,5-11]
11. **D. Assessment.** All of the above tissues need to be screened, based on the May 20, 2004 rule, from the Food and Drug Administration. The list has been expanded to include reproductive tissues, hematopoietic stem cells, cellular therapies, and other innovative products. This rule has been expanded to keep up with the advances in technology that have occurred related to organ and tissue donation.[11]
12. **B. Analysis.** Exposure to foreign substances such as soot, a chemical, or water, which may contain debris or bacteria, increases the patient's potential to develop infection.
13. **C. Intervention.** If the child has received the human varicella zoster immune globulin and still develops chicken pox, she needs to be treated with intravenous acyclovir. The drug will need to be continued for 7 to 10 days.[4]
14. **B. Assessment.** A serious side effect of cyclosporine therapy is hepatotoxicity. Other side effects include nausea and vomiting, diarrhea, oral candidiasis, pancreatitis, rash, tremors, and headache.[12]
15. **D. Assessment.** When the patient's heart is removed for transplant of the donor's heart, the

parasympathetic and sympathetic innervation is severed and the patient no longer experiences angina.[13]

References

1. Cosby C: Organ and tissue donation. In Jordan KS, editor: *Emergency nursing core curriculum,* ed 5, Philadelphia, 2000, WB Saunders.
2. www.unos.org. Accessed September 30, 2004.
3. Lewis D, Valerius W: Organs from non-heart-beating donors: an answer to the organ shortage, *Crit Care Nurse* 19(2):70-74, 1999.
4. Rowland DJ: Organ and tissue donation in the emergency department. In Kitt S, Selfridge-Thomas J, Proehl J et al, editors: *Emergency nursing: a physiologic and clinical perspective,* Philadelphia, 1995, WB Saunders.
5. Bernardo LM, Bove M: Care of the pediatric organ transplant recipient. In Kelley S, editor: *Pediatric emergency nursing,* Norwalk, CT, 1994, Appleton & Lange.
6. Pedersen M: Tissue and organ donation. In Newberry L, editor, *Sheehy's emergency nursing: principles and practice,* ed 4, St Louis, 1998, Mosby.
7. Riley L, Collican M: Needs of families of organ donors: facing death and life, *Crit Care Nurse* 19(2):53-59, 1999.
8. Roark D: The need for increasing organ donation among African Americans and Hispanic Americans: an overview, *J Emerg Nurs* 25(1):21-27, 1999.
9. Holmquist M, Chabalewski F, Blount T, et al: A critical pathway: guiding care for organ donors, *Crit Care Nurse* 19(2):84-100, 1999.
10. Sullivan J, Seem DL, Chabalewski F: Determining brain death, *Crit Care Nurse* 19(2):37-46, 1999.
11. www.fda.gov/bbs/topics/news/2004/NEW01070.html Accessed September 30, 2004.
12. Bush WW: Overview of transplantation immunology and the pharmacotherapy of adult solid organ transplant recipients: focus on immunosuppression, *AACN Clin Issues* 10(2):253-269, 1999.
13. Rourke T, Droogan M, Ohler L: Heart transplantation: state of the art, *AACN Clin Issues* 10(2):185-201, 1999.

CHAPTER 15

ORTHOPEDIC EMERGENCIES

REVIEW OUTLINE

I. Anatomy and physiology[1,2]
   A. Function of the musculoskeletal system
      1. Support
      2. Protection
      3. Movement and leverage
      4. Storage of mineral salts and fats
      5. Red blood cell production
   B. Components of musculoskeletal system
      1. Bones
      2. Nerves
      3. Vessels
      4. Muscles
      5. Tendons
      6. Ligaments
      7. Joints
   C. Range of motion
   D. Neurovascular status affected by orthopedic injuries
      1. Circulation
      2. Sensory perception
      3. Motor function
II. Orthopedic assessment
   A. History
      1. Chief complaint
         a. Mechanism of injury
         b. Position of limb when injured
         c. Ability to use body part since injury
         d. Time of injury or onset
         e. Swelling, deformity
         f. First aid or treatment since onset
         g. Associated injuries
      2. Medical history
         a. Previous injury to same site
         b. Current medications
            (1) Steroids
            (2) Anticoagulants
            (3) Chemotherapy
         c. Allergies
         d. Immunization status
         e. Chronic diseases
            (1) Osteoporosis
            (2) Cancer
            (3) Diabetes
            (4) Cardiovascular disease
   B. Physical examination
      1. Overview
         a. Position of the injured limb or limbs
         b. Degree of distress
         c. Skin color, moisture, and temperature
         d. Vital signs
      2. Affected part
         a. Deformity
         b. Swelling
         c. Ecchymosis
         d. Loss of function
         e. Abnormal position or mobility
         f. Point tenderness
         g. Lack of skin integrity
         h. Five Ps
            (1) Pain
            (2) Pulse
            (3) Paresthesia
            (4) Paralysis
            (5) Pallor
         i. Range of motion
   C. Neurological assessment, motor and sensory
      1. Median nerve
      2. Ulnar nerve
      3. Radial nerve
      4. Tibial nerve
      5. Peroneal nerve
   D. Reflexes
      1. Biceps
      2. Brachioradialis
      3. Triceps
      4. Patellar
      5. Ankle reflexes

E. Age-related characteristics[2,3]
  1. Pediatric
     a. Epiphyseal, or growth, plate is present until maturity
     b. Bones are more porous, more susceptible to injury
     c. Periosteum is thicker and more vascular, with faster healing
     d. During adolescence, growth occurs, legs elongate, hips and chest widen, and shoulders broaden
     e. Fractures may indicate intentional abuse and injury
  2. Geriatric
     a. Loss of height with aging
     b. Development of kyphosis with aging
     c. Decrease in muscular strength and range of motion
     d. Chronic disease states such as osteoporosis may contribute to changes in aging

F. Diagnostic studies or procedures
  1. Skeletal radiographs
  2. Computed tomography scan
  3. Arteriograms
  4. Magnetic resonance imaging
  5. Complete blood cell count with differential
  6. Electrolytes
  7. Type and crossmatch
  8. Coagulation studies
  9. Urinalysis
  10. Uric acid level
  11. Wound cultures
  12. Compartment pressure measurement

III. Related nursing diagnoses
  A. Activity intolerance
  B. Anxiety
  C. Body image disturbance
  D. Fear
  E. Fluid volume deficit, high risk for
  F. Infection, high risk for
  G. Injury, high risk for
  H. Knowledge deficit
  I. Mobility, impaired physical
  J. Pain
  K. Posttrauma response
  L. Powerlessness
  M. Self-care deficit
  N. Skin integrity, impaired, high risk for
  O. Tissue perfusion, altered peripheral

IV. Collaborative care of the patient with an orthopedic emergency[4]
  A. Airway maintenance
  B. Bleeding control
  C. Blood and fluid replacement
  D. Cardiac status monitoring
  E. Amputated part preservation
  F. Pharmacological interventions
     1. Analgesics
     2. Antibiotics
     3. Antiinflammatory agents
        a. Steroidal
        b. Nonsteroidal
     4. Muscle relaxants
     5. Local or regional anesthesia
  G. Immobilization
     1. Splinting
     2. Casting
     3. Traction
        a. Skin
        b. Skeletal
     4. Serial reassessment
     5. Local comfort measures
        a. Positioning
        b. Cold
        c. Heat
     6. Wound care
     7. Mobilization
        a. Crutches
        b. Walker
        c. Cane
     8. Compartment pressure monitoring
     9. Emotional support
     10. Patient and family teaching

V. Selected orthopedic emergencies
  A. Sprains, strains
  B. Fractures
  C. Dislocations, subluxations
  D. Inflammatory conditions
     1. Bursitis
     2. Tendonitis
     3. Joint effusion
  E. Carpal tunnel syndrome
  F. Amputations
  G. Complications
     1. Hemorrhage
     2. Compartment syndrome
     3. Fat embolus

Orthopedic emergencies are responsible for a considerable number of patient visits to emergency departments. Motor vehicle and bicycle crashes, falls, industrial equipment accidents, and sports activities are all contributors to bone, joint, tendon, and muscle problems.[5]

The musculoskeletal system is made up of 206 bones and skeletal muscle equaling 40% to 50% of body weight.[2] It has two major functions, the first of which is to provide a framework for the body. In doing so, the musculoskeletal system provides support and protection for the vital organs. The second purpose is to provide for leverage and movement of the various body parts and of the body as a whole. In considering the anatomy and physiology of this system, it is important to note that veins, arteries, and nerves follow the course of long bones and that damage to the bone may include or cause injury to any of these structures. Also, injury to long bones such as the femur places the patient at great risk of significant blood loss. For example, a unit of blood may be lost with a closed femur fracture.

The musculoskeletal system undergoes changes from birth until death. Pediatric musculoskeletal differences include the presence of the epiphyseal or growth area, bones that are more porous, and a thicker periosteum. During adolescence, growth changes lead to adult development.

The geriatric patient's musculoskeletal changes include shortening of bones, ligaments, and tendons, a decline in muscular strength, and a decrease in range of motion.

Musculoskeletal injuries may also be a sign of intentional injury. Because both children and some elderly persons are in dependent situations, abuse may manifest itself in fractures. The mechanism of injury should match the type of injury being managed.

The most important nursing measure in the initial phase of caring for the patient who has an orthopedic emergency is to assess the whole patient immediately. Compound fractures, dislocations, and severe deformities have a dramatic appearance but are not life threatening. Stabilization of airway, breathing, and circulation is essential and should not be overlooked or delayed. An important axiom to remember is that the most obvious may not be the most severe.

In obtaining a history of the chief complaint, careful scrutiny is given to the mechanism of injury. Factors such as force involved, trajectory, position of the limb when injured, time elapsed since the incident, activity or ability to use the body part since injury, and any first aid prior to seeking care all contribute to understanding the clinical picture. In addition, this information assists in discovering associated injuries, of which the patient may be unaware. A history of any previous similar injury, as well as a review of current medications, use of alcohol or other drugs, and any significant medical history will be helpful. Special considerations of the elderly, infants, and children include the possibility of abuse and complications such as hypothermia and dehydration.

An objective assessment of the patient with an orthopedic emergency includes observing the affected area for abnormalities such as deformity, swelling, discoloration, loss of function, and abnormal position or movement. Palpation may reveal point tenderness or crepitus. Neurovascular status distal to the site is assessed initially and serially.

Interventions appropriate to the treatment of a patient with an orthopedic emergency include stabilizing the injured part as soon as possible. Open wounds are covered with sterile saline dressings. Splinting is performed, using whatever device will immobilize the part and still allow access for circulatory checks. It is important to remember to pad the splint well and to immobilize the joint above and below the injury.

Pain control is an important facet of care. Local comfort measures of ice and elevation decrease venous congestion and reduce swelling, a major factor contributing to pain. In addition, pharmacological agents are indicated. Concurrent skin defects are cleansed and dressed as indicated. The potential for infection can be significant and requires administration of antibiotics.

An orthopedic emergency of life-threatening proportion is a fractured pelvis. Significant pelvic fractures are incurred in incidents involving severe, direct force. Tears in pelvic and lumbar vessels can result in rapid, massive blood loss. With pelvic fractures it is common to have injuries in other systems as well, especially the genitourinary and gastrointestinal systems. Interventions in this instance include aggressive fluid resuscitation, application of the pneumatic antishock garment (PASG) for stabilization and tamponade effect, and rapid identification and management of associated injuries.

REVIEW QUESTIONS

1. A 34-year-old woman comes to the emergency department complaining of right wrist pain of 1 week's duration that is gradually becoming worse. She has no history of direct trauma to

the extremity. Vital signs are B/P 116/82, P 84, R 16, and Temp 97.8° F. Pertinent subjective assessment obtained by the nurse includes:
A. Family history of arm pain
B. Activity prior to the onset of pain
C. Current use of contraceptives
D. Allergies to food or animals

2. The appropriate nursing diagnosis on which to base care for this patient is:
A. Mobility, impaired physical, due to pain with movement
B. Infection, high risk for, related to the presence of pain
C. Skin integrity, impaired, high risk for, related to the presence of pain
D. Tissue perfusion, altered peripheral, related to limited movement due to pain

3. The physician prescribes ibuprofin 800 mg three time a day for this patient. The nurse recognizes this drug as a:
A. Synthetic narcotic, analgesic
B. Salicylate derivative
C. Tricyclic antidepressant
D. Nonsteroidal antiinflammatory drug

4. When discharging this patient, the emergency nurse instructs her to be rechecked by her physician in 1 week if she is not better. What specific instructions should the nurse give this patient for taking her medication?
A. Take medication before meals so that it is absorbed completely
B. Watch for signs of gastrointestinal bleeding such as dark stools
C. Take the medication with meals to prevent gastrointestinal upset
D. Ingestion of more than three glasses of wine a day will not interfere with the medication.

5. An evaluative criterion to determine whether this patient's treatment is working is:
A. The patient develops gastritis from taking the ibuprofen
B. The patient regains full range of motion
C. The patient continues to complain of pain
D. The patient requires physical therapy for the rest of her life

The rescue squad brings a 32-year-old man to the emergency department after being involved in a head-on motor vehicle crash. He was a restrained front-seat passenger who required some extrication. He is fully immobilized, awake, alert, and complaining of pain in both legs. He has some minor abrasions of the face, the left knee has a deep laceration with crepitus, and the right ankle is obviously deformed. Vital signs are B/P 122/72, P 106, R 24, and Temp 98.4° F.

6. The emergency nurse's initial intervention upon receiving this patient should be to:
A. Immobilize the cervical spine with a soft collar to make him more comfortable
B. Apply a splint to the right ankle for comfort and limited movement
C. Assess and manage the patient's airway, breathing, and circulation
D. Inquire if others injured in the accident will be brought to this facility

7. While performing this patient's assessment, the nurse notes that pulses are absent in the right foot. An appropriate intervention for this physical finding would be to:
A. Splint the extremity above the knee so that no further harm may be done
B. Expedite portable radiographs of the right lower extremity to identify injury
C. Attempt to straighten the deformity and apply a hare traction splint for comfort
D. Notify the physician at once about this significant physical finding

8. The mechanism of injury and the presence of left knee injury alert the nurse to what possible associated injury?
A. Left hip or acetabular injury
B. Lumbar spine injury
C. Left os calcis fracture
D. Left lower tendon rupture

9. The physician orders intravenous antibiotics. Which nursing diagnosis is reflected in this order?
A. Pain related to multiple fractures
B. Infection, high risk for, related to an open fracture
C. Tissue perfusion, altered peripheral, related to an open fracture
D. Anxiety related to the patient's immobility

10. A 4-year-old girl fell down the steps before arrival in the emergency department. Her only complaint is that she cannot move her right

forearm. A radiograph of her arm shows a right ulnar fracture involving only one side of the bone. This type of fracture is described as a:
A. Barton's fracture
B. Galeazzi's fracture
C. Colles' fracture
D. Greenstick fracture

A 55-year-old male who was a restrained driver struck a telephone pole at 60 miles per hour. The patient was entrapped for over 45 minutes. Upon arrival in the emergency department, the patient is alert and oriented, B/P 80/40, P 140, R 30, and Temp 94° F rectal. The only obvious sign of trauma is a swollen left thigh and a large laceration on the inner aspect of his left thigh. The patient has been fully immobilized.

11. Pelvic radiography shows an avulsion of the ischial spine and a total disruption of the soft tissues on the left side of his pelvis. The patient is to be transferred to a level I trauma center by ground. What may the emergency nurse do to stabilize the patient's pelvis for transport?
A. Apply a pelvic sling or make one out of sheets and leave the patient on the backboard to ensure that he remains immobilized during the transport
B. Take the patient off the backboard and place him on a soft mattress to decrease the pain that may occur with transport
C. Place pillows between the patient's legs, use cravats to stabilize the patient's legs, and leave him on the backboard for transport
D. Place bilateral hare traction splints on both of the patient's femurs to stabilize the patient's pelvis, and use the backboard to stabilize the traction splints

12. Based on the patient's injury and current vital signs, what nursing diagnosis should the emergency nurse use to plan his care?
A. Injury, high risk for, related to the movement required to evaluate the patient and transfer him for further care
B. Infection, high risk for, related to the wound on his left thigh and the need to transfer the patient for further care
C. Fluid volume deficit related to active loss of body fluid secondary to bleeding from his pelvic injury
D. Mobility, impaired, related to the patient's ability to assist in moving him from the emergency department stretcher to the transport stretcher

13. Signs and symptoms of an open pelvic fracture include all of the following except:
A. Paresis of the lower extremities
B. Blood from the urethra or vagina
C. Ecchymosis in the flank area
D. Low-riding prostate on rectal examination

14. An early complication of an open pelvic fracture is:
A. Coagulopathy
B. Exsanguination
C. Paraplegia
D. Multiple organ failure

15. The patient has been given 9 L of crystalloid fluid and 5 units of packed red blood cells. Which of the following laboratory values should the emergency nurse monitor during aggressive fluid resuscitation to avert further complications?
A. Cardiac enzymes
B. Blood urea nitrogen and creatinine
C. Coagulation studies
D. Liver function tests

16. The expected outcome for the patient being medicated for pain from a fractured ankle is:
A. Absence of pain after the administration of the medication
B. Decrease in the amount of swelling after the administration of the medication
C. Tolerance of the pain after administration of the medication
D. No change in pain after administration of the medication

17. A 26-year-old man is brought to the emergency department by the rescue squad. He is complaining of a sudden onset of shortness of breath, and he is restless and somewhat cyanotic. Vital signs are B/P 102/60, P 138, R 44, and Temp 102.8° F. The nurse's first intervention in caring for this patient is to:
A. Start high-flow oxygen by means of a nonrebreathing mask
B. Draw arterial blood gases from the patient's radial artery

C. Attach a cardiac monitor and obtain a 12-lead electrocardiogram
D. Establish an intravenous access and give a fluid bolus of normal saline

18. Further assessment reveals that the patient sustained fractures of his right tibia and fibula 2 days earlier in a soccer game. The nurse recognizes that this puts the patient at risk for:
A. Embolus secondary to deep venous thrombosis
B. Adult respiratory distress syndrome from his injury
C. Air embolus from an open fracture
D. Fat embolus from the lower extremity fracture

19. The initial blood gases on this patient reveal a pH of 7.21, P_{CO_2} of 66, P_{O_2} of 60, and bicarbonate level of 26. The nurse recognizes these values as:
A. Respiratory alkalosis
B. Metabolic acidosis
C. Respiratory acidosis
D. Metabolic alkalosis

20. Based on the initial evaluation, the most appropriate nursing diagnosis is:
A. Airway clearance, ineffective, related to shortness of breath
B. Cardiac output, decreased, related to change in blood pressure and pulse
C. Anxiety related to returning to the emergency department
D. Gas exchange, impaired, related to a fat embolus

21. The physician orders a heparin infusion. He orders 25,000 units of heparin in 500 ml of dextrose 5% in water to infuse at the rate of 1000 units per hour. The flow rate in milliliters per hour is:
A. 12 ml per hour
B. 24 ml per hour
C. 20 ml per hour
D. 6 ml per hour

A 17-year-old youth comes to the emergency department complaining of left leg pain after being struck by an automobile and pinned against a wall. His lower left leg is deformed and markedly contused. He has no other apparent injury. Vital signs are B/P 128/86, P 98, R 20, and Temp 98.4° F.

22. The nature of this patient's injury alerts the emergency nurse to the possibility of his developing:
A. Osteomyelitis
B. Deep venous thrombosis
C. Compartment syndrome
D. Secondary skin infection

23. An external cause of compartment syndrome is:
A. Black widow spider bite of the hand
B. Prolonged entrapment of an extremity
C. Electrical burn of a lower extremity
D. Open fracture of the lower extremity

24. Nursing assessment of this patient's lower leg should include:
A. Observation for skin discontinuity
B. Palpation of the posterior popliteal pulse
C. Palpation of the dorsalis pedis and posterior tibial pulses
D. Check for movement, sensation, and capillary refill of the toes

25. This patient is given fentanyl 150 mcg IV for pain, and a long-leg splint is applied. Thirty minutes after medication administration, he continues to complain of severe pain in his left leg, which increases with movement of his toes. Sensation and capillary refill remain intact. An appropriate nursing intervention at this time would be to:
A. Notify the physician immediately so further interventions can be initiated
B. Adjust the splint until the patient says he is more comfortable and the pain goes away
C. Reposition the patient's leg on some soft pillows to make the patient more comfortable
D. Administer a second dose of the fentanyl at one half of the original dose intravenously

26. Compartment syndrome is managed by:
A. Administering high doses of pain medication until the pressure equalizes itself in the extremity
B. Insertion of a drain to relieve the pressure in the effected extremity
C. Elevating the injured extremity above the level of the patient's heart
D. Preparing the patient for immediate fasciotomy in the operating room

27. Evidence of compartment syndrome may be reflected in which other system?
A. Pulmonary
B. Cardiac
C. Renal
D. Gastrointestinal

28. The nursing diagnosis that best reflects the problems of compartment syndrome is:
A. Pain, acute, related to decreased blood flow to the extremity
B. Gas exchange, impaired, related to decreased blood flow to the extremity
C. Skin integrity, impaired, high risk for, related to decreased blood flow
D. Tissue perfusion, altered peripheral, related to decreased blood flow

29. A 12-year-old male caught his right hand in a corn picker while attempting to clean it. He has suffered an amputation of the first four digits. The life squad transports the patient and his digits to the emergency department. Detriments to the possibility of reimplantation of his digits include:
A. Length of time of less than 12 hours since the amputation
B. Availability of a qualified reimplantation team at the receiving facility
C. Crush- or avulsion-type injuries to the amputated extremities
D. Upper-extremity amputations such as fingers and forearms

30. A 17-year-old male with a severe ankle sprain has been given crutches for ambulation. Appropriate fitting of these crutches includes:
A. Each hand piece should be fitted so that the elbow is flexed at 60 degrees
B. Crutches should fit so that each arm piece is two finger widths below the axilla
C. Crutches should fit so that all the weight of the upper body is on the axilla
D. Tips of the crutches should be placed 12 inches to the front of the patient

31. Initial emergency nursing interventions for the management of a joint dislocation include:
A. Apply firm traction to reduce an abnormally deformed joint dislocation
B. Leave any distal constricting jewelry in place for patient comfort
C. Immobilize the joint below the level of injury only for patient comfort
D. Immobilize the joint and extremity in a position of comfort

32. A 23-year-old male patient came to the emergency department complaining of swelling, redness, tenderness, and excessive warmth in his left elbow. The patient states he has no history of medical problems. He is diagnosed with a septic joint. The pathogen that most commonly causes a septic joint is:
A. *Streptococcus*
B. Gonococcus
C. *Clostridium*
D. *Staphylococcus*

33. An ankle radiograph should be obtained when:
A. The patient is able to bear weight on the ankle upon admission to the emergency department
B. The patient does not have bone tenderness over the posterior edge or tip of the lateral malleolus
C. The patient does not have bone tenderness over the posterior edge or tip of the medial malleolus
D. The patient is unable to bear weight on the injured extremity immediately after injury and in the emergency department

34. When assessing a patient who has sustained a knee dislocation, which nerve should be evaluated for potential damage?
A. Radial
B. Ulnar
C. Peroneal
D. Median

35. When applying a splint to an injured extremity, the emergency care team should:
A. Record sensation and circulation to the injured extremity only after the splint has been applied
B. Pad joints and hard spots carefully, ensuring that splints are padded well to prevent skin injury
C. To avoid complications, immobilize only the injured area, never the joint above or below a fracture
D. Always reduce a deformed extremity, even if sensation and circulation are intact before transport

ANSWERS

1. **B. Assessment.** The most beneficial information concerning this patient's problem can be derived from learning what the patient was doing before the pain began. Most often the nurse will discover some repetitive activity involving the affected joint, in this case the wrist.[4]
2. **A. Analysis.** The goal in management of tendonitis is to reduce irritation by immobilizing the affected area. In addition, local application of cold alternating with heat may be beneficial.[5,6]
3. **D. Intervention.** Nonsteroidal antiinflammatory medications are first-line agents for inflammatory conditions such as tendonitis. The action of these drugs is related to inhibition of prostaglandin synthesis; however, the exact mechanism of action is not known.[7]
4. **B. Intervention.** A serious side effect of the nonsteroidal antiinflammatory drugs is gastrointestinal bleeding. Even though it is not a common side effect, it can occur, so patients need to be warned about the side symptoms of a gastrointestinal bleed, such as dark tarry stool. Ibuprofin may be taken with or without food, and it is not recommended for children under 18 years of age.
5. **B. Evaluation.** Pain relief and the ability to use the extremity as before would indicate that management is working.
6. **C. Intervention.** Evaluating the status of airway, breathing, and circulation should be the automatic first response to every patient. The appearance of deformed limbs should never divert the nurse from a basic primary assessment.[4]
7. **D. Intervention.** Initial and serial reevaluation of circulation distal to the injury is a nursing responsibility. A pulseless extremity is a serious emergency and should be brought to the physician's attention at once so that appropriate collaborative interventions can be initiated.[4]
8. **A. Assessment.** In a front-end collision, the patient sustains a blow to the knee while it is in the flexed position. This energy is transmitted up the femur to the flexed hip joint, causing hip fracture, acetabular fracture, or posterior hip dislocation. Careful evaluation of this patient's left hip and pelvis is indicated.[8]
9. **B. Analysis.** Compound fractures, such as this patient's left knee injury, are prime targets for serious infection. Vigorous prevention of this complication is begun early in the patient's stay.[4,5]
10. **D. Assessment.** A greenstick fracture is a longitudinal fracture that involves only one side of the cortex of the bone. Because the periosteum is thicker in children, the fracture may not go completely through the bone. Barton's fracture is a radial fracture associated with dislocation of the carpal bones and the hand. Galeazzi's fracture involves the middle to distal third of the radius associated with radioulnar subluxation. Colles' fracture involves the distal radius with volar angulation, along with a Salter type II epiphyseal fracture of the ulnar styloid.[4]
11. **A. Intervention.** Immobilization of a possible or confirmed fractured pelvis for transport can be accomplished by applying PASG, "sheeting" the pelvis, or using a commercially available pelvic sling.[9]
12. **C. Analysis.** Blood loss from a pelvic fracture can range from 750 to 6000 ml. Emergency care should be directed toward replacing the patient's lost volume and monitoring the effects of the resuscitation.[6,8]
13. **D. Assessment.** An open pelvic fracture results in a direct communication between the fracture and the vagina, perineum, groin, or rectum. Signs and symptoms of an open pelvic fracture include paresis, ecchymosis of the perineum, groin, and flanks, blood from the urethra and vagina, and a high-riding prostate.[10,11]
14. **B. Assessment.** Because of the large vessels located in the pelvis, the most serious early complication of an open pelvic fracture is exsanguination.[10,11]
15. **C. Evaluation.** Patients with open pelvic fractures have a high mortality of between 40% and 60%. The major cause of early death is exsanguination. Late death from open pelvic fractures is associated with multiple organ failure and sepsis.[10,11]
16. **C. Evaluation.** Pain medication will only help the patient tolerate pain. Until the ankle is appropriately treated and healing begins, the pain will persist.
17. **A. Intervention.** All of the interventions listed are indicated in the early care of this patient; however, the first priority is to provide supplemental oxygen. Tachypnea, restlessness, and cyanosis are clear-cut signs of respiratory distress and must be addressed immediately.[8]

18. **D. Assessment.** A serious complication in patients who have sustained long-bone fractures is fat embolus. This phenomenon is characteristically seen 12 to 48 hours after injury. The embolization is thought to be a result of fat and marrow break-off directly related to the fracture, as well as a result of changes in circulating lipids secondary to stress.[8]
19. **C. Assessment.** Interpretation of the ABGs should begin with the pH. Normal pH is 7.35 to 7.45. Because this patient's pH is 7.21, he is in a state of acidosis. Next, note the PCO_2. This reflects the respiratory side of the acid-base equation. Normally the value should be 35 to 45 mm Hg. A value of 66 mm Hg indicates retained carbon dioxide. A normal bicarbonate level is 22 to 26 mEq/L and represents the metabolic, or buffer system, component. The patient's value of 26 falls within the normal range. This patient's blood gases demonstrate a respiratory acidosis.[10]
20. **D. Analysis.** The respiratory compromise this patient is experiencing is at the alveolar-capillary level, where carbon dioxide–oxygen exchange occurs. Because emboli have obstructed vessels in the lungs, there is a decreased area in which gas exchange can take place.[6]
21. **C. Intervention.** 25,000 units in 500 ml is 50 units/ml. To determine the number of milliliters per hour, divide what is desired (1000 units) by what you have (50 units) to arrive at the correct amount of 20 ml/h.[7]
22. **C. Assessment.** Compartment syndrome is a real possibility in orthopedic injuries in which the mechanism of injury is a crushing force. The most common site of development is the anterior compartment of the lower leg.[8] The forearm may also be affected.
23. **B. Assessment.** There are both external and internal causes of compartment syndrome. Internal causes include crushing injuries, burns, spider and snake bites, and prolonged hypotension and ischemia. External causes of compartment syndrome include prolonged application of PASG, prolonged entrapment of an extremity, skeletal traction, or lying in the same position for an extended period.[8]
24. **D. Assessment.** Compartment syndrome develops when tissue pressures within a limited space, the muscle compartment, exceed the intraarterial hydrostatic pressure, causing collapse of capillaries and venules, and subsequent tissue necrosis. Loss of a pulse distal to the affected area is a late sign. Initial and frequent checks for motion, sensation, and capillary refill are most valuable in detecting this complication early.[5,12]
25. **A. Intervention.** A hallmark sign of developing compartment syndrome is severe pain, not relieved by narcotics, that increases with muscle stretching. This finding needs to be reported immediately, so that proper medical intervention may ensue.[5,12]
26. **D. Intervention.** The patient needs to be prepared to go to the operating room for a complete fasciotomy to normalize elevated compartment pressure.[12]
27. **C. Evaluation.** When this complication advances to the stage of muscle death, myoglobinuria and subsequent renal complications may develop.[12]
28. **D. Analysis.** This diagnosis is defined as a decrease in oxygenation and nutrition at the cellular level due to a deficit in capillary blood supply.[6] This is an accurate physiological description of what happens in compartment syndrome.
29. **C. Assessment.** The possibility of reimplantation decreases with the amount of damage done to the amputated parts, lack of availability of an experienced reimplantation team, and the amount of time that has elapsed since the injury. Generally, longer than 24 hours decreases the chances of a successful reimplantation.[9]
30. **B. Intervention.** When fitting patients with crutches, the arm piece should be 2 inches or two finger widths from the axilla; no weight should be placed on the axilla, because nerve damage may occur; the tips of the crutches should be placed 6 inches to the side and to the front; and the elbows should be flexed at 30 degrees.[13]
31. **D. Intervention.** The joint and extremity should be immobilized in position of comfort initially unless there is neurovascular compromise. If there is neurovascular compromise, only gentle traction should be applied until the pulse returns. Constricting jewelry should be removed to prevent further damage.[12]
32. **B. Assessment.** The pathogen that most commonly causes a septic joint, particularly in a young person, is the gonococcal organism.[13]
33. **D. Assessment.** Evidence-based research has demonstrated that ankle radiographs are not always necessary to rule out a fracture. The

Ottawa ankle rules state that a radiograph should be obtained when:

- The patient is unable to bear weight on the ankle immediately after injury or in the emergency department
- The patient has bone tenderness at the posterior edge or tip of the lateral malleolus
- The patient has bone tenderness at the posterior edge or tip of the medial malleolus[14,15]

34. **C. Assessment.** The peroneal nerve should be evaluated when there is a tibia or fibula fracture or dislocation of the knee. Radial, ulnar, and median are upper extremity nerves.[14]
35. **B. Intervention.** Circulation and sensation should be checked before and after any manipulation; the joint above and below should be immobilized when splinting an extremity; and padding is important to prevent any skin injury.[9]

References

1. Walker J: Orthopedic emergencies. In Jordan KS, editor: *Emergency nursing core curriculum,* ed 5, Philadelphia, 2000, WB Saunders.
2. Bickley LS: *Bate's guide to physical examination and history taking,* Philadelphia, 1999, Lippincott.
3. Thomas TO, Bernardo L, Herman B: *Core curriculum for pediatric emergency nursing,* Boston, 2003, Jones and Bartlett.
4. Phelan A: Musculoskeletal trauma. In Kelley S, editor: *Pediatric emergency nursing,* Norwalk, CT, 1994, Appleton & Lange.
5. Jagmin MG: Musculoskeletal emergencies. In Kitt S, Selfridge-Thomas J, Proehl J et al, editors: *Emergency nursing: a physiologic and clinical perspective,* Philadelphia, 1995, WB Saunders.
6. Kim MJ, McFarland GK, McLane AM: *Pocket guide to nursing diagnoses,* St Louis, 1993, Mosby.
7. *Mosby's drug consult 2005,* St Louis, 2005, Mosby.
8. Walsh CR: Musculoskeletal injuries. In McQuillan KA, Von Rueden KT, Harstock RL, et al, editors: *Trauma nursing: from resuscitation through rehabilitation,* ed 3, Philadelphia, 2002, WB Saunders.
9. Campbell J, editor: *BTLS for paramedics or other advanced providers,* ed 5, Upper Saddle River, NJ, 2004, Pearson Prentice Hall.
10. Cwinn AA: Pelvis. In Marx J, editor: *Rosen's emergency medicine: concepts and clinical practice,* ed 5, St Louis, 2002, Mosby.
11. Ziglar M, Parrish R: An 18-year-old male patient with multiple trauma including an open pelvic fracture, *J Emerg Nurs* 20:265-270, 1994.
12. Geiderman JM: General principles of orthopedic injuries. In Marx J, editor: *Rosen's emergency medicine: concepts and clinical practice,* ed 5, St Louis, 2002, Mosby.
13. O'Steen D: Orthopedic and neurovascular trauma. In Newberry L, editor: *Sheehy's emergency nursing: principles and practice,* ed 5, St Louis, 2003, Mosby.
14. Proehl J: Compression syndrome, *J Emerg Nurs* 14:283-290, 1988.
15. Selfridge-Thomas J: *Emergency nursing: an essential guide for patient care,* Philadelphia, 1997, WB Saunders.

CHAPTER 16

PAIN MANAGEMENT

REVIEW OUTLINE

I. Definition of pain
   A. From the Greek word *poine,* which means penalty or punishment
   B. Historical perspectives[1,2]
      1. Pain management was provided with rituals, magic, physical maneuvers
      2. Egyptians believed spirits of the dead caused pain
      3. Buddhists believed there was a relationship between emotion and pain
      4. In China pain management was through pharmacopoeia and acupuncture
      5. Ancient Greeks used opium
         a. Aristotle believed that pain originated in the heart
         b. Hippocrates believed that pain was a manifestation of a disequilibrium of the humors of blood, phlegm, and yellow or black bile
      6. Sixteenth to nineteenth centuries
         a. Application of cold for pain management
         b. Morphine isolated from opium
         c. Ether
         d. Aspirin
         e. Physical therapy
      7. Twentieth century
         a. Chronic pain
         b. Pain centers
         c. Pain societies
         d. Pain legislation
         e. JCAHO standards
   C. Pain[1]
      1. A sensory experience associated with actual or potential tissue damage, as well as physiological and psychological responses
      2. A personal experience and may be whatever the patient says it is
      3. Manifested in both verbal and nonverbal behaviors, physiological responses, and emotional and spiritual responses
   D. Acute pain
   E. Chronic pain

II. Sources of pain in the prehospital, transport, and emergency department environments
   A. Pain from the illness or injury
   B. Pain from procedures
      1. Intravenous insertion
      2. Gastric tube insertion
      3. Blood draws
      4. Chest tube insertion
      5. Cardiopulmonary resuscitation
   C. Environment
      1. Noise
      2. Light
      3. Excessive heat or cold

III. Perception and response to pain
   A. Patient's previous experience with pain
   B. Source of pain
      1. Physical
      2. Emotional
      3. Spiritual
   C. Caregiver reactions to the patient's pain
   D. Response to pain learned and influenced by
      1. Age
      2. Socioeconomic status
      3. Gender
      4. Ethnicity
      5. Cultural beliefs
      6. Values
   E. Behavioral response to pain, varies by age
      1. Vocalization
      2. Facial expressions
      3. Body movements
      4. Coping strategies

IV. Barriers to pain management in the prehospital, transport, and emergency department environment
   A. Lack of knowledge about pain management
   B. Lack of knowledge about pharmacology of pain medications
   C. Fear of addiction
   D. Respiratory depression and hypotension
   E. Concentrating on life-threatening illness and injury
V. Physiology of pain
   A. Nociceptors
   B. A fibers
   C. C fibers
   D. Spinal cord
   E. Neurons
      1. Medial
      2. Lateral
   F. Afferent pathways
   G. Efferent pathways
VI. Theories of pain
   A. Gate theory of pain
   B. Pattern theory of pain
   C. Neurotransmitters
VII. Pain assessment
   A. Source of the pain
   B. Level of the pain: pain rating
      1. FACES pain rating scale
      2. Numerical pain scales
      3. Visual analog scales
      4. Word graphic rating scale: no pain to worst possible pain
   C. Patient's response to the pain
      1. Physiological
      2. Emotional
      3. Spiritual
   D. Cultural and gender differences related to pain[3]
      1. Gender orientation
      2. Cultural boundaries
      3. Behavioral responses
   E. Related nursing diagnoses
      1. Pain
      2. Pain, chronic
VIII. Pain management
   A. Patient's past experiences
   B. Conscious sedation
   C. Pain management pharmacology
      1. Opioid analgesics
      2. Dissociative agents
      3. Benzodiazepines
      4. Nonopioid analgesics
      5. Sedative-hypnotic agents
      6. Local anesthetics
      7. Other medications
IX. Patient assessment and management
   A. Monitoring of airway, breathing, circulation
      1. Respiratory rate
      2. Pulse oximeter
      3. Carbon dioxide monitoring
   B. Circulation
      1. Cardiac monitor
      2. Blood pressure
      3. Pulse
   C. Neurological status
      1. Protect patient from injury
      2. Orient patient
      3. Decrease outside stimulation
   D. Dosage-related patient response
   E. Availability of appropriate antagonists
   F. Sedation scale
   G. Additional methods to manage pain and enhance pharmacological management
      1. Cutaneous stimulation
         a. Hot
         b. Cold
      2. Distraction
      3. Relaxation
      4. Proper positioning
      5. Soaking
      6. Comfort measures
      7. Therapeutic presence
      8. Therapeutic touch
      9. Music
      10. Therapeutic listening
      11. Acupressure
      12. Acupuncture
      13. Imagery
      14. Breathing techniques
      15. Other methods
X. Medication abuse
   A. Undermanagement of pain
   B. Physical tolerance
   C. Prescription medications
   D. Patterns of abuse
      1. Specific drugs
         a. Hydrocodone
         b. Dextromethorphan
      2. Medication and alcohol
   E. Management in the emergency department[4]
      1. When was the last time you were seen for this condition?

2. When was the last time you were seen by any health care provider (including emergency departments, minor emergency centers, clinics)?
3. What was the last medication, including narcotic, prescription that you filled? Where? When?

REVIEW QUESTIONS

1. Chronic pain is:
A. Limited to a duration of 0 to 7 days
B. Persistent over a period of time, usually 6 months or longer
C. From a known or unknown cause, usually a fixable event
D. Always perceived through input from the peripheral nervous system

2. Reasons why pain management is not always given high priority in patient care in the prehospital setting include:
A. Prehospital providers are well versed about the pharmacology of pain management and alternative methods to manage pain in the prehospital environment
B. Administration of a dissociative agent in the prehospital environment may cause significant respiratory depression
C. Prehospital providers are not concerned about the patient becoming addicted to the sedation and analgesic agents used in the field
D. Prehospital providers are more focused on the patient's illness or injury, and pain management is not a primary concern

3. A 3-month-old infant is brought to the emergency department by his parents. The parents state that he has not stopped crying. He has a firm, distended abdomen. The diagnosis of peritonitis and sepsis is made. There are many myths related to the management of pain in pediatric patients. Which of the following is an appropriate expectation?
A. Children respond the same as adults to most pain medications
B. Children's nervous systems are immature, and they perceive pain differently
C. It is easier to hold small children down (brutaine) than to medicate them
D. Children will experience respiratory depression more quickly than adult patients

4. Reliable indicators of pain in the neonate include all of the following except:
A. Squeezing their eyes shut
B. Palmar diaphoresis
C. No change in heart rate
D. Nasolabial furrow

5. Stimulation of the nociceptors causes the release of:
A. Histamines
B. Endorphins
C. Enkephalins
D. Gamma-aminobutyric acid

6. Pain medications used in the prehospital and emergency department environment should:
A. Possess multiple side effects
B. Have a long duration of action
C. Produce multiple complications
D. Provide sedation as well as analgesia

7. The medication propofol is classified as:
A. An opioid analgesic
B. A sedative-hypnotic
C. A local anesthetic
D. A nonopioid analgesic

8. A 42-year-old male was given fentanyl and midazolam intravenously for conscious sedation to reduce his fractured ankle. A splint has been applied and he is to be referred to his orthopedic physician for follow-up. The emergency nurse may determine that the patient is ready to be discharged when:
A. His family is ready to take him home by car
B. He falls back to sleep easily when not stimulated
C. He can ambulate using his crutches
D. When his oxygen saturation ranges between 85% and 90%

9. The transport team is called to a referring facility to transport a patient who has been involved in an all-terrain vehicle rollover. He is awake and alert, but in acute respiratory distress because of a severe pulmonary contusion and multiple rib fractures. His oxygen saturation is 90% on high-flow oxygen. Because of the length of the transport, the patient is intubated using rapid-sequence intubation for oxygenation. He is given vecuronium to facilitate his oxygenation. During the 3-hour transport,

which medications will the patient require for comfort?
A. Midazolam and vecuronium for sedation and amnesia during the period of transport from the referring to the receiving facility
B. Fentanyl and vecuronium for sedation and analgesia during the period of transport from the receiving to the referring facility
C. Morphine sulfate and vecuronium for analgesia and to facilitate oxygenation during the period of transport from the referring to the receiving facility
D. Fentanyl, midazolam, and vecuronium for sedation, amnesia, and analgesia, and to facilitate ventilation and oxygenation

10. Massage may be effective in relieving pain in selected situations because:
A. It decreases the blood flow to the injured area
B. It causes retention of the toxins to only the injured area
C. It releases the patient's endorphins through relaxation
D. The patient wants it to no matter what others may say

11. A 23-year-old male comes to the emergency department complaining of dental pain. This is his third visit within 7 days for the same complaint. Which of the following patient characteristics may indicate drug-seeking behaviors?
A. This is the patient's first visit to the emergency department for this complaint
B. The patient states that only oxycodone can take away his persistent dental pain
C. The patient has no allergies to any pain medications
D. The patient regularly visits a dentist for preventive dental care

12. Which of the following is observed in Latino patients as a cultural response to pain?
A. High pain threshold
B. No fear of addiction
C. Pain is a punishment
D. Limited family ties

13. A 3-year-old child suffered a deep forehead laceration after hitting her head against the edge of a coffee table. There was no loss of consciousness and the patient's Pediatric Coma Score is 15. Which of the following medications would be most appropriate for short-acting sedation, analgesia, and wound repair?
A. Morphine sulfate
B. Propofol
C. Midazolam
D. Lidocaine

14. Which of the following statements about pain management in the emergency department is most accurate?
A. Because many elderly patients are on numerous medications, there is an increased risk of drug-drug interactions with sedative and analgesic agents
B. Previous experience with pain such as immunizations does not increase a child's physiological and psychological responses to painful procedures in the emergency department
C. Patients who repeatedly visit the emergency department asking for pain medication do not have a true medical reason for pain and are only drug seeking
D. Health care providers are not held legally accountable for adequately managing patients' pain when dealing with end-of-life care

ANSWERS

1. **B. Assessment.** Chronic pain is described as having duration of longer than 6 months, unknown or nonspecific cause or causes, mild to severe character, and no known peripheral pain receptors (nociceptors).[1,2,4]
2. **D. Intervention.** Explanations for not providing pain management in the prehospital and emergency care environment include:
   - Lack of knowledge about pain management and pain medications
   - Fear of causing addiction, both the patient and the care provider
   - Possibility of respiratory depression and hypotension with some pain medications
   - Focus on the patient's illness or injury[2]

   The risk of adverse effects of pain medications in the pediatric patient is directly related to the rate of drug administration, total dosage, and combination with other medications.[4]
3. **A. Assessment.** Myths about children and pain management include:
   - Children perceive pain differently than adults because they have immature nervous systems

- Children are more sensitive to pain medication than are adults and may suffer a respiratory arrest if given pain medication
- It is easier to hold a small child down (brutaine) than to administer pain medication[3,4]

4. **C. Assessment.** Indicators of pain in the neonate include:
   - Changes in heart and respiratory rates, including both bradycardia and tachycardia
   - Palmar sweating
   - Vagal tone
   - Nasolabial furrow
   - Crying[5-7]
5. **A. Assessment.** Stimulation of the nociceptors causes the release of histamines, serotonin, bradykinins, prostaglandins, potassium, and acetylcholine.[5]
6. **D. Intervention.** Pain medications that are used in the prehospital and emergency department environments should:
   - Cause minimal side effects
   - Possess uniform efficacy
   - Have a short and controllable duration of action
   - Possess few contraindications
   - Produce both a sedative and analgesic affect; to do this most effectively, combinations of medications generally need to be administered
7. **B. Assessment.** Propofol is classified as an ultrashort-acting general anesthetic, sedative-hypnotic agent, which is not related to either benzodiazepines or barbiturates.[2]
8. **C. Evaluation.** The patient who has undergone a procedure that required conscious sedation should be awake, able to ambulate (this patient would need to demonstrate this with crutches), and drink and swallow.[1]
9. **D. Intervention.** The patient will require medications that provide sedation, amnesia, and analgesia and assist in facilitating ventilation and oxygenation.[8,9]
10. **C. Intervention.** Massage therapy may be useful in decreasing patient pain in selected situations because:
    - It causes the release of endorphins through relaxation
    - It releases toxins from the injured area
    - Touch helps with pain management
    - It increases blood flow to the injured area[10]
11. **B. Assessment.** Consistently documented characteristics of drug-seeking patients include objective physical findings not correlating with the subjective complaint, asking for or demanding a specific pain medication, aggressive behavior if demands are not met, doctor and emergency department shopping, stealing prescription pads, and history of forgery or fraud related to medications.[4]
12. **C. Assessment.** One of the fastest growing ethnic groups and cultures in the United States is the Latino population. Cultural responses to pain include strong family ties; patients may desire family members to stay with them during treatment. They express their pain, have strong spiritual beliefs (including the belief that prayer may heal), fear addiction, use heat or cold for management, and prefer oral and intravenous routes of drug administration.[2]
13. **B. Intervention.** Morphine will provide analgesia and sedation but will require longer recovery time; midazolam provides sedation but no analgesia. Propofol is classified as a short-acting nonopioid, nonbarbiturate, sedative-hypnotic agent. It has several advantages for use in the emergency department. Its clinical effect is immediate after intravenous administration, it can produce analgesia and sedation for very painful procedures, and recovery time is generally short—between 5 and 15 minutes. Disadvantages are that patient safety requires a physician remain in attendance, greater depth of sedation is achieved, administration can be painful, and respiratory depression and hypotension occur.[11-15]
14. **A. Assessment.** Pain management in the emergency department is an important component of patient care. Physiological and pharmacological differences in age groups need to be recognized and included when selecting pain medications. It is also important to be aware of potential drug interactions. Patients with multiple visits to the emergency department complaining of pain need to be evaluated for a preexisting painful condition. Children who have had painful experiences may undergo both physiological and psychological changes in anticipation of another painful experience. Finally, public awareness and JCAHO standards are causing an increased awareness of the consequences of inadequate pain management, especially related to end-of-life care.[3]

REFERENCES

1. Albrecht S, Bernardo L: Pain management. In Jordan KS, editor: *Emergency nursing core cur-*

riculum, ed 5, Philadelphia, 2000, WB Saunders.

2. St Marie B: *Core curriculum for pain management,* Philadelphia, 2002, WB Saunders.
3. Rupp T, Delaney K: Inadequate analgesia in emergency medicine, *Ann Emerg Med* 43(4):494-503, 2004.
4. Roscoe M: The drug-seeking patient: undertreated pain or underhanded motives? *Clin Rev* 14(2):51-58, 2004.
5. Selbst M, Clark M: Analgesic use in the emergency department, *Ann Emerg Med* 19(9):1010-1013,1990.
6. Woolard D, Terndrup T: Sedative-analgesic agent administration in children: analysis of use and complications in the emergency department, *J Emerg Med* 12(4):453-461, 1994.
7. Prevention and management of pain and stress in the neonate, *Pediatrics* 105(2):454-461, 2000.
8. Semonin Holleran R, editor: *Air and surface transport: principles and practice,* St Louis, 2003, Mosby.
9. Krupa D, editor: *Flight nursing core curriculum,* Park Ridge, IL, 1997, Road Runner Press.
10. Morse J: The science of comforting, *Reflections* 22(4):6-10, 1996.
11. Trautman D: Pain management. In Newberry L, editor: *Sheehy's emergency nursing: principles and practice,* ed 5, St Louis, 2003, Mosby.
12. Barsan W, Jastremski M, Syverud S: *Emergency drug therapy,* Philadelphia, 1991, WB Saunders.
13. Green S, Krauss B: Propofol in emergency medicine: pushing the sedation frontier, *Ann Emerg Med* 42:792-797, 2003.
14. Coll-Vincent B, Sala X, Fernandez C et al: Sedation for cardioversion in the emergency department: analysis of effectiveness in four protocols, *Ann Emerg Med* 42:767-772, 2003.
15. Bassett K, Anderson J, Pribble C et al: Propofol for procedural sedation in children in the emergency department, *Ann Emerg Med* 42:773-782, 2003.

CHAPTER 17

RESPIRATORY EMERGENCIES

REVIEW OUTLINE

I. Anatomy and physiology[1]
  A. Anatomy
    1. Nasal cavity
    2. Oropharynx
    3. Mucous membranes
    4. Larynx
    5. Epiglottis
    6. Vocal cords
    7. Cricothyroid membrane
    8. Trachea
    9. Bronchi
    10. Bronchioles
    11. Alveoli
    12. Lung parenchyma: right three lobes, left two lobes
    13. Pleura
    14. Mediastinum
    15. Sternum
    16. Manubrium
    17. Xiphoid process
    18. Sternal angle
    19. Scapulae
    20. Clavicles
    21. Ribs
    22. Thoracic vertebrae
    23. Esophagus
    24. Heart
    25. Diaphragm
    26. Intercostal muscles
    27. Accessory muscles
    28. Expiratory muscles
    29. Aorta
    30. Nerves associated with respiration
  B. Physiology
    1. Oxygen transport, gas exchange
    2. Ventilation: inspiration, expiration
    3. Tidal volume
    4. Nervous system innervation
    5. Positive-negative pressure flow system

II. Assessment[1-3]
  A. Inspection
    1. Airway patency
    2. Work of breathing
      a. Use of accessory muscles
      b. Level of consciousness
      c. Respiratory rate and depth
      d. Skin color
      e. Cyanosis
      f. Flaring of nares
      g. Sternal retraction
      h. Patient's posture
    3. Tachypnea
    4. Bradypnea
    5. Apnea
    6. Splinting
    7. Audible wheezing
    8. Inspiratory stridor
    9. Productive cough, sputum
    10. Wounds, scars, impaled objects
  B. Palpation
    1. Pain, tenderness
    2. Crepitus
    3. Skin temperature
  C. Assessment landmarks
    1. Anterior chest
      a. Midsternal line
      b. Anterior axillary line
      c. Midaxillary line
    2. Posterior chest
      a. Posterior axillary line
      b. Scapular line
      c. Vertebral line
  D. Percussion
    1. Flatness
    2. Dullness
    3. Resonance

4. Hyperresonance
5. Tympany

E. Auscultation
1. Evaluate all lung fields
2. Inspiration, expiration
3. Normal breath sounds
   a. Vesicular
   b. Bronchovesicular
   c. Bronchial
   d. Tracheal
4. Adventitious breath sounds
   a. Wheezes
   b. Rhonchi
   c. Crackles
5. Absence of breath sounds

F. Age-related characteristics[1-3]
1. Pediatric
   a. Pediatric airway smaller and shorter than that of adult
   b. Tongue large and may easily block the airway
   c. Cricothyroid membrane narrow, forming an anatomical cuff
   d. Chest rounded in children younger than 6 years of age
   e. Infant's sternum pliable and may appear to be "caving" in with inspiration
   f. Use of diaphragm for breathing in children younger than 7 years of age
   g. Chest wall thinner in younger children
   h. Ribs and sternum more cartilaginous and flexible in younger children
   i. Respiratory rates faster in infants and young children
2. Geriatric
   a. Vital capacity decreases
   b. Skeletal changes of aging may result in kyphosis or "barrel chest"
   c. Gag reflex diminishes, leaving elderly adult at greater risk for aspiration

G. History
1. Onset of symptoms
2. History of trauma, mechanism of injury
3. Pain on inspiration or expiration
4. Cough
   a. Onset
   b. Sputum
   c. Related symptoms
   d. Time of day
5. Fever, chills
6. Smoking history
7. Medical history
8. Productive cough, sputum
9. Work history (e.g., "black lung")
10. Environmental history
11. Date of last tuberculosis test, chest radiograph
12. Human immunodeficiency virus (HIV) status
13. Recent international travel: China, Southeast Asia
14. Recent travel in southwestern United States, or hiking and staying in an enclosed space where rodents may live
15. Associated diseases: heart disease, emphysema, asthma, allergies

H. Diagnostic studies or procedures
1. Chest radiograph studies
2. Blood gases
   a. pH
   b. PCO_2
   c. PO_2
   d. HCO_3
   e. Arterial
   f. Capillary
   g. Venous
3. Pulse oximetry
4. End-tidal carbon dioxide monitoring
5. Electrocardiogram
6. Sputum evaluation
7. Laboratory tests
   a. Complete blood count with differential
   b. Electrolytes
   c. Amylase
   d. Liver function tests
   e. Levels of prescribed medications
8. Computed tomography of the chest
9. Magnetic resonance imaging of the chest
10. Ultrasonography of the chest
11. Esophagogram
12. Lung scan (ventilation-perfusion scan)

III. Related nursing diagnoses
A. Airway clearance, ineffective
B. Anxiety
C. Aspiration, high risk for
D. Breathing pattern, ineffective
E. Fatigue

- F. Fear
- G. Gas exchange, impaired
- H. Infection, high risk for
- I. Knowledge deficit
- J. Pain

IV. Collaborative care of the patient with a respiratory emergency
- A. Airway management
  1. Airway adjuncts
  2. Oxygen delivery
  3. Intubation
  4. Alternative airways
  5. Airway management medications
- B. Ventilation
  1. Bronchodilators
  2. Humidification
  3. Ventilators
- C. Cardiac monitor
- D. Antibiotics
- E. Thoracentesis
- F. Autotransfusion
- G. Chest tube insertion
- H. Thoracotomy, open and closed

V. Specific respiratory emergencies
- A. Chest pain differentiation
- B. Chronic obstructive pulmonary disease (COPD)
- C. Pneumonia
- D. Acute respiratory distress syndrome
- E. Pulmonary embolus
- F. Epiglottitis
- G. Croup
- H. Bronchiolitis
- I. Foreign body aspiration
- J. Rib fractures
- K. Flail chest
- L. Pneumothorax
- M. Tension pneumothorax
- N. Hemothorax
- O. Pulmonary contusion
- P. Ruptured diaphragm
- Q. Tracheal trauma
- R. Respiratory infections

No matter what the origin of the respiratory emergency, the nursing assessment must begin with an evaluation of the patient's airway and its patency, effort and effectiveness of ventilation, and the level of oxygenation. A pulse oximeter reading during triage can provide a "spot" check on the status of the patient in respiratory distress.

The amount of data that is collected in relation to the patient's respiratory distress will depend on the patient's history and ability to provide information. Many patients with chronic respiratory problems, and their families as well, are quite well versed in the management of their disease and can be a good source of information concerning what they need.

The cause of shortness of breath (dyspnea), chest pain, cough, and cyanosis may be difficult to determine quickly. Chest pain may be pulmonary, cardiac, or abdominal in origin. Cyanosis may be the result of poor perfusion or a sign of poisoning.[4] Just as with other body systems, the respiratory system may be the source of the disease or injury, or simply where the symptoms manifest.

Chest Pain

Assessment of the patient with chest pain can cause some difficult problems for the emergency nurse. There are numerous causes of chest pain, including those that require immediate interventions and those that may require little, if any, nursing or medical care.

The origins of chest pain include asthma, acute and chronic bronchitis, COPD, pneumonia, pulmonary embolus, or a traumatic injury to the chest, which may result in rib fractures, pulmonary contusion, pneumothorax, or hemothorax.

Asthma

Asthma is a response of the lung to various stimuli that cause narrowing of the airways. These stimuli may include allergens, such as dust and molds, stress, or intoxicants.[4] Even though asthma can be successfully managed in the emergency department, the death rate from acute asthma has been increasing. Reasons for this increase may include lack of access to care and that increased use of bronchodilators may mask a worsening respiratory status. The National Heart, Lung, and Blood Institute has issued Guidelines for the Diagnosis and Management of Asthma. These guidelines were updated in 2002. They can be used as an algorithm for the treatment of asthmatics in the emergency department and offer one of the few ways patients may receive evidence-based care.[5]

Chest Trauma

Chest trauma accounts for approximately 25% of deaths related to trauma.[6] The patient with chest trauma requires a rapid and organized emergency nursing assessment so that injuries and potential threats to life, such as a tension pneumothorax, can be identified rapidly and appropriate interventions provided.

It is important to keep in mind that trauma to the chest may not result in injury to the chest alone. Contained in the thoracic cavity are the heart, great vessels, and sometimes abdominal organs. Injuries to any of these vessels or organs can be life threatening.

Pediatric Respiratory Emergencies

The most common cause of cardiopulmonary arrest in the pediatric patient is interference with the child's airway and ventilation.[3,7,8] The child's airway is different from the adult airway. It is smaller in diameter and shorter. The tongue is larger and may easily obstruct the airway. The narrowest part of the pediatric airway is the cricothyroid ring, which forms a physiologic cuff. These differences require that the emergency nurse be familiar not only with the impact of these differences, but also with how the pediatric airway should be managed.

Signs and symptoms of pediatric respiratory distress include increased respiratory rate, decreased respiratory rate, apnea, fatigue, head bobbing, stridor, prolonged expiration, grunting, retractions, nasal flaring, altered mental status, and cyanosis.[3,7,8]

Pulmonary Diseases

Emergency departments are called upon to manage various pulmonary disorders that may be entities in and of themselves or symptoms of other disease states. One of the most common pulmonary diseases seen in the emergency department is COPD. The American Thoracic Society has released definitions of COPD, described as a preventable and manageable disease state that is characterized by airflow limitation that is not fully reversible. The airflow limitation is usually progressive and is associated with an inflammatory response by the lungs to noxious stimuli, such as cigarette smoke. COPD affects not only the lungs; it can also cause systemic problems. Diseases such as chronic bronchitis, emphysema and, in some patients, asthma may be a cause.[10]

Community-acquired pneumonia is another common cause of visits to the emergency department. One major problem with this disease is that many practitioners use multiple medications to manage it. Currently, there is an important focus on the use of evidenced-based medicine to manage this disease in the emergency department.[11]

The patient who is positive for HIV may also have a viral or fungal type of pneumonia. Organisms causing pneumonia seen in HIV-infected patients include *Pneumocystis carinii*; the fungi responsible for histoplasmosis and cryptococcosis; *Legionella*; and *Nocardia.*[12]

There has been a significant increase in the number of patients with tuberculosis in recent years in the United States. Many of these patients seek care in the emergency department, which poses particular challenges to emergency nursing practice.[13] Some of these challenges include early identification of the disease, appropriate triage and isolation of infected patients, and methods to decrease the emergency department staff's risk of infection.

Finally, because of the emergence of unfamiliar diseases, such as the hantavirus and severe acute respiratory syndrome (SARS), or the reemergence of diseases thought conquered, such as pertussis, emergency nurses need to keep up to date on information that protects both their patients and themselves.[14]

REVIEW QUESTIONS

Asthma

A 30-year-old man comes to the emergency department complaining of shortness of breath. The patient states that he has been treated for asthma in the past and has not taken any medication for over a month. He is alert, oriented, and barely able to speak. His color is pale and his skin is diaphoretic.

1. What specific physical signs may indicate acute respiratory distress in the adult asthmatic patient?
A. Paroxysmal coughing
B. Sternocleidomastoid retractions
C. Audible wheezing
D. Nausea and vomiting

2. This patient has a peak expiratory flow (PEF) of 85 L/min. This is an indication of:
A. Moderate obstruction
B. No obstruction
C. Severe obstruction
D. Minor obstruction

3. After assessment of this patient's lung function, what intervention should the emergency nurse initiate?
A. Administration of a corticosteroid
B. Administration of theophylline

C. Administration of a bronchodilator
D. Administration of an antibiotic

4. An initial nursing diagnosis for the patient having an acute asthmatic attack may be:
A. Health maintenance, altered, related to the diagnosis of asthma
B. Fluid volume excess related to his fluid intake
C. Activity intolerance related to the diagnosis of asthma
D. Anxiety related to the inability to breathe

5. The emergency physician orders a dose of methylprednisolone for the patient. The most effective way to administer the drug to this patient is:
A. Orally
B. Inhaler
C. Intramuscularly
D. Intravenously

6. An indication that the asthmatic patient may need to be intubated would include all of the following except:
A. A change in mental status, such as confusion, agitation, or unresponsiveness
B. Respiratory arrest from work of breathing and fatigue
C. Blood gas results of pH 7.35, Po_2 100, and Pco_2 40
D. Pco_2 continues to increase despite therapy

7. A trigger of pediatric asthma in an urban setting is:
A. Soy bean pollen
B. Cockroaches
C. Pigeon feathers
D. Horse dandruff

8. An ominous sign that indicates marked airflow obstruction in the asthmatic patient is:
A. Expiratory wheezing
B. Expiratory stridor
C. Paroxysmal coughing
D. "Silent chest"

9. The most effective method of administering a bronchodilator to a patient in severe distress is:
A. Administration of a nebulized β-agonist agent every hour
B. Continuous administration of nebulized β-agonist agent
C. Two to three puffs of a β-agonist agent in a metered-dose inhaler (MDI) one time
D. Administration of a β-agonist agent intravenously

10. When teaching the patient with asthma how to use an MDI, the emergency nurse should give the following instruction:
A. Clean the mouthpiece daily with soap and water and dry it thoroughly
B. Soak the mouthpiece for 20 minutes daily in chlorine bleach (Clorox) to prevent infection
C. Store the canister in the freezer to keep the drug potent
D. Use the MDI as often as the patient thinks it's needed before cleaning it

11. All of the following may cause wheezing in a patient except:
A. Anaphylaxis
B. Pulmonary embolus
C. Pertussis
D. All of the above

Pneumonia

The paramedics bring a 52-year-old man to the emergency department. He generally lives outside, but the weather has been cold and he was forced to enter the local shelter. Today, he arrives with fever, chills, and a productive cough of blood-tinged yellow sputum. A chest radiograph reveals a right lower lobe pneumonia. He states that he has smoked 1 to 2 packs per day for 40 years and has not received any preventive health care for 5 years.

12. Pneumonia, an acute infection of the lung parenchyma, may be caused by all of the following except:
A. *Mycoplasma pneumoniae*
B. *Legionella pneumophila*
C. HIV
D. *Streptococcus pneumoniae*

13. An important emergency nursing intervention for the patient being treated for pneumonia is:
A. Ordering the appropriate antibiotic to manage the infection
B. Providing the patient with fluids and obtaining a sputum specimen

C. Deciding when the patient should be intubated
D. Ordering a blood gas analysis to evaluate oxygenation

14. One method that can measure the ventilatory status of this patient is to connect him to a:
A. Pulse oximeter with a disposable probe
B. Cardiac and apnea monitor
C. Side-stream carbon dioxide monitor
D. Noninvasive blood pressure monitor

15. Factors that may limit the usefulness of a pulse oximeter include:
A. Limited ambient light
B. Carbon monoxide poisoning
C. Normovolemia
D. Limited patient movement

16. Atypical infiltrates are also noted on this patient's chest radiograph. Active tuberculosis is diagnosed in addition to pneumonia. This patient should:
A. Remain in the treatment room
B. Be discharged to the homeless shelter for care
C. Be admitted to an open ward on the floor
D. Be moved to a negative-airflow room for isolation

17. Outpatient treatment of patients diagnosed with pneumonia should include:
A. Drawing two sets of blood cultures before the patient is discharged
B. Administering the first dose of antibiotics in the emergency department
C. Asking the patient to return every 12 hours for an arterial blood gas analysis
D. Instructing the patient to not complete the course of antibiotics when feeling better

Chest Pain

A 30-year-old woman comes to the emergency department with severe chest pain, shortness of breath, and diaphoresis. She states that the pain began suddenly and is crushing. Her B/P is 80 by palpation, the cardiac monitor shows sinus tachycardia, and her respiratory rate is 48.

18. When obtaining a history from this patient specific to the complaint of chest pain, the emergency nurse should ask about:
A. Any history of recent surgery or long-bone fractures
B. The date of the patient's last chest radiograph
C. The patient's previous occupation
D. History of hyperventilation

19. The patient states she recently had an abdominal hysterectomy. A fluid bolus of 500 ml normal saline brings the patient's blood pressure to 100/60. A lung scan is performed and demonstrates a pulmonary embolus. What medication should be started in the emergency department to treat this patient?
A. Heparin calcium
B. Dicumarol
C. Dipyridamole
D. Vitamin K

20. Based on the patient's initial blood pressure, which nursing diagnosis is appropriate?
A. Injury, high risk for, related to recent surgery
B. Tissue perfusion, altered cardiopulmonary, manifested by hypotension
C. Thought processes, altered, related to hypotension
D. Skin integrity, impaired, related to hypotension

21. The patient is given a bolus of 10,000 units of heparin, and a drip is begun at the rate of 1000 units/h. Potential complications of heparin administration include:
A. Intracerebral hemorrhage
B. Chills, fever, and urticaria
C. Oral and rectal bleeding
D. All of the above

A 17-year-old man comes to triage complaining of shortness of breath, severe chest pain, and difficulty swallowing. The triage nurse notes that the patient's voice is hoarse and he is sitting forward to help him breathe.

22. What important piece of history should the triage nurse obtain?
A. Date of the patient's last immunization
B. Recent use of illicit drugs
C. Presence of breath sounds bilaterally
D. Presence of ST elevation in lead II

23. The patient is taken emergently into the treatment area. A physical finding that may indicate a pneumomediastinum is:
A. Hamman's crunch
B. Kernig's sign
C. Kerr's sign
D. Homans' sign

24. A complication of pneumomediastinum includes:
A. Neck pain
B. Sore throat
C. Pneumothorax
D. Pericardial tamponade

The rescue squad brings a 53-year-old man to the emergency department. The patient was found camping outside and states he is from out of town and has yet to find a new home. He states that he has a history of alcohol abuse and has not eaten for 2 days. The patient is complaining of shortness of breath, a cough, and fatigue.

25. All of the following place this patient at risk for tuberculosis except:
A. Alcohol abuse
B. Homelessness
C. Proper diet
D. His age

26. A primary screening tool for tuberculosis is:
A. Chest radiograph
B. Sputum smears for acid-fast bacteria
C. Blood cultures
D. Purified protein derivative

Pediatric Respiratory Emergencies

27. A rare cause of chest pain in the pediatric patient is:
A. Asthma
B. Pneumonia
C. Kawasaki's disease
D. Rib fracture

28. A 5-year-old girl is brought to the emergency department by her family. The child and her parents are from Central America, and they report that she has never received immunizations. They also state through an interpreter that she has had a high fever, has been lethargic and unable to lie down, and has been drooling. During the initial assessment of this patient, the emergency nurse should do all of the following except:
A. Assess the child's level of consciousness
B. Look down the child's throat
C. Assess the child's respiratory status
D. Assess the child's circulatory status

29. Initial care for the child who is suffering respiratory distress from epiglottitis would include:
A. Administering cefuroxime intravenously
B. Administering racemic epinephrine through a nebulizer
C. Obtaining radiographs of the child's neck to diagnose her problem
D. Preparing for intubation of the child by skilled personnel

30. The most common cause of epiglottitis is:
A. *Streptococcus*
B. *Haemophilus influenzae*
C. *Staphylococcus*
D. *Pneumococcus*

31. A mother comes to the emergency department carrying her 18-month-old child, who has stridor and is cyanotic. The mother states that the child was eating a hot dog before her symptoms began. The emergency nurse's initial interventions should include:
A. Opening the child's mouth and trying to remove the food
B. Delivering four back blows and four chest thrusts
C. Grabbing the child by the legs and turning her upside down
D. Performing a cricothyrotomy with a 14-gauge needle

32. The emergency nurse performs the appropriate sequence of foreign body airway obstruction management for the conscious infant. An indication that the maneuvers are not being effective is:
A. Expulsion of the object
B. The child begins to cry
C. The child becomes unconscious
D. The child's color improves

33. The item most commonly aspirated by children younger than 3 years of age is:
A. A toy
B. A hot dog

C. A peanut
D. Hard candy

34. Foreign body aspiration should be suspected in the pediatric patient when:
A. The child does not respond to conventional management for respiratory distress
B. The child's chest radiograph does not show infiltrates or pneumothoraces
C. The child's respiratory rate returns to normal after conventional interventions
D. The child is afebrile after hydration in the emergency department

35. The initial treatment of the child experiencing an acute asthma attack is:
A. Administration of β-agonist bronchodilators
B. Hydration with 20 ml/kg of normal saline
C. Administration of high-flow oxygen by nasal cannula
D. Administration of prophylactic antibiotics

36. A 3-month-old infant is brought to the emergency department by his parents because of a "stuffy" nose and difficulty breathing. When teaching the parents how to care for the sick infant, the emergency nurse should be sure that the parents understand all of the following except:
A. Infants lose fluids through rapid breathing
B. Infants are obligate nose breathers
C. Infants cry when sick and may be impossible to console
D. Infants need to be kept warm but not made excessively warm

37. Respiratory syncytial virus is not transmitted by:
A. Large-droplet aerosols
B. Sneezing
C. Visitors
D. Hand washing

Pneumothorax

A 30-year-old man has attempted suicide by shooting himself in the left upper chest. On arrival in the emergency department, the patient is alert, complaining of shortness of breath, and is pale and diaphoretic. His vital signs are B/P 80 by palpation, P 140, and R 32.

38. The emergency nurse needs to assess quickly:
A. Breath sounds
B. Peripheral edema
C. Capillary refill
D. Altered mental status

39. No breath sounds are audible on the left side. The patient's respiratory distress increases and he becomes agitated. Until a physician is available, a critical intervention the emergency nurse may perform is:
A. Obtain central line access to begin fluid resuscitation
B. Perform needle thoracostomy on the patient's affected side
C. Connect the patient to a pulse oximeter to determine his oxygenation
D. Obtain a chest radiograph to rule out a tension pneumothorax

40. Based on the emergency nurse's initial assessment of this patient, the primary nursing diagnosis would be:
A. Injury, high risk for, related to the gunshot wound to the chest
B. Fluid volume deficit related to the gunshot wound to the chest
C. Activity intolerance related to the gunshot wound to the chest
D. Gas exchange, impaired, related to the gunshot wound to the chest

41. After the emergency nurse performs the needle thoracostomy, evaluation of the effectiveness of this procedure would include all of the following except:
A. A rush of air after insertion of the needle
B. Improvement in the patient's blood pressure
C. A dramatic increase in the patient's shortness of breath
D. Decrease in the patient's shortness of breath

42. The classic signs and symptoms of a tension pneumothorax include all of the following except:
A. Equal breath sounds bilaterally
B. Tracheal deviation away from the affected side
C. Distended neck veins
D. Cyanosis and diaphoresis

43. A flail segment may be stabilized by:
   A. Placing sandbags on the injured segment
   B. Strapping the patient to a backboard
   C. Positioning the patient on the injured side
   D. Applying skin traction to the injured chest wall

Myocardial Contusion

A 19-year-old man was riding his bicycle and hit a hole in the road at a high rate of speed. His chest struck the ground. On arrival in the emergency department, the patient is alert and complaining of chest pain. His vital signs are stable, but the rescue squad reports that the patient's pulse is irregular.

44. Because of the mechanism of injury, initial assessment of this patient should include inspection for:
   A. Chest wall ecchymosis
   B. Periorbital ecchymosis
   C. Scrotal ecchymosis
   D. Abdominal ecchymosis

45. An important intervention in the care of this patient would be:
   A. Monitoring and managing cardiac dysrhythmia
   B. Performing and documenting a Glasgow Coma Scale evaluation
   C. Preparing the patient for hospitalization
   D. Administering prescribed medications for pain

46. Because of the possibility of cardiac dysrhythmia in this patient, the nursing diagnosis the emergency nurse may base interventions on is:
   A. Fluid volume deficit, high risk for, related to the mechanism of injury
   B. Infection, high risk for, related to the skin abrasions on his chest
   C. Skin integrity, impaired, related to the skin abrasions on his chest
   D. Cardiac output, decreased, related to a myocardial contusion

47. The patient continues to have frequent premature ventricular contractions and is given lidocaine 50 mg as an IV bolus. A continuous infusion is maintained at 2 mg/min. The emergency nurse evaluates the patient for lidocaine toxicity by observing for:
   A. Onset of seizures
   B. Absence of ventricular dysrhythmia
   C. Redness at the IV site
   D. Chest pain

Pulmonary Contusion

An 18-year-old woman was an unrestrained passenger in the back seat of an automobile involved in a collision. The patient was thrown against the back of the front seat. On arrival in the emergency department, she is awake and complaining of chest pain. Her vital signs are B/P 110/70, P 90 and regular, and R 32.

48. All of the following signs and symptoms indicate a possible pulmonary contusion in this patient except:
   A. A sucking chest wound
   B. Shortness of breath
   C. Restlessness and agitation
   D. Presence of severe chest injuries

49. Because of the mechanism of injury and bruising on the patient's chest, a pulmonary contusion is suspected and confirmed with a chest radiograph. During the initial treatment of this patient, the emergency nurse should:
   A. Give the patient a fluid bolus to keep her blood pressure above 120/80
   B. Prepare the patient for elective intubation to maintain an oxygen saturation of 98%
   C. Limit fluids unless the patient develops hypovolemia from an associated injury
   D. Administer 3 L per minute of oxygen by a nonrebreather face mask

50. Based on the medical diagnosis given to this patient, the emergency nurse would base care on which of the following nursing diagnoses?
   A. Thought processes, altered, related to emergency department admission
   B. Gas exchange, impaired, related to the injury of the lung parenchyma from the pulmonary contusion
   C. Thermoregulation, ineffective, related to the patient's 30-minute entrapment
   D. Activity intolerance, related to the patient's chest injury

51. A 16-year-old male is brought to the emergency department after having been thrown 25 feet from his car. He is complaining of severe chest pain and shortness of breath. During the primary assessment, bowel sounds are heard over the right side of the chest. What injury is suspected?

A. Pneumothorax
B. Hemothorax
C. Aortic dissection
D. Ruptured diaphragm

52. A 3-year-old girl arrives in the emergency department in severe respiratory distress. The emergency physician has decided the child needs to be intubated. What size and type of tube should the emergency nurse prepare?

A. A 4.5 uncuffed endotracheal tube
B. A 4.5 cuffed endotracheal tube
C. A 3.0 uncuffed endotracheal tube
D. A 3.0 cuffed endotracheal tube

53. Which of the following is an advantage of a laryngeal tracheal mask in the emergency department?

A. It is available only in adult sizes, so it cannot be used in children
B. It requires direct laryngoscopy for correct insertion
C. It can be inserted successfully by emergency nurses
D. It can be inserted only in patients with normal upper airway anatomy

54. Emergency department preparation for patients who are infected with SARS virus should include:

A. A screening tool that evaluates only patients who come to the emergency department with symptoms
B. Preparation of private rooms so that patients can be comfortable while being treated in the emergency department
C. No additional training for equipment cleaning because the SARS virus does not remain viable outside of the patient's body
D. Instruction on the proper isolation equipment and clothing needed to protect patients and staff from infection

55. Which of the following statements is true about mechanical ventilation?

A. Increased intrathoracic pressure from mechanical ventilation increases venous return to the heart, which may result in hypotension
B. Whenever there is a complication with mechanical ventilation that causes patient compromise, the patient should be removed from the ventilator and manual ventilation performed until the problem is identified
C. Mechanical ventilation is never a cause of barotrauma and will never contribute to development of a pneumothorax
D. Every patient placed on a ventilator should receive neuromuscular blocking agents without sedation to prevent hypotension

ANSWERS

1. **B. Assessment.** Retractions of the sternocleidomastoid muscle usually indicate severe asthma. This occurs because of increased air trapping, which forces the patient to use accessory muscles to lift the rib cage in order to generate higher negative pleural pressures.[4,13]
2. **C. Assessment.** Obtaining a PEF from the patient having an asthma attack will provide the emergency nurse with important information about the patient's pulmonary status. A PEF of less than 100 L/min indicates severe obstruction, and a PEF of 100 to 200 L/min indicates moderate obstruction. The PEF can also be used to assess the effectiveness of the medical treatment the patient receives while in the emergency department. The PEF should improve more than 10% over baseline after treatment, or reach a minimum of 300 L/min.[5,15,16]
3. **C. Intervention.** A β-agonist, which will cause bronchodilation, is used as the initial treatment of the asthmatic patient.[4,5] Frequently used β-agonists include metaproterenol sulfate and albuterol.
4. **D. Analysis.** The inability to breathe, no matter what the cause, will generate anxiety. The emergency nurse will need to include interventions that will help decrease the patient's anxiety, as well as provide medication and physical comfort. A useful intervention would be structuring the environment so that the patient is not left alone. This can be done by placing the patient in an area of the department that allows continual observation.[15,17]
5. **A. Intervention.** Steroids have come into common use for acute asthma management in the emergency department. However, the method of administration remains controver-

sial. Research has demonstrated that intramuscular or intravenous administration is not more effective than oral administration. Inhaled steroids continue to be evaluated in the acute setting but currently are not recommended.[5,16,18]

6. **C. Evaluation.** All of the symptoms, except the blood gas results, would indicate that the asthmatic patient may need to be intubated. If the patient were unable to verbalize or cough, this would be an indication of severe distress that may need to be managed with intubation.[16]
7. **B. Assessment.** Of children who have asthma and who live in an urban environment, 23% to 60% have a sensitivity to cockroaches.[19]
8. **D. Assessment.** A "silent chest" in an asthmatic patient is an indication of marked airflow obstruction. Wheezes indicate that air is getting in and out even though there is obstruction. No sound means no air movement and is a premoribund sign that requires immediate intervention.[5,16,20]
9. **B. Intervention.** Continuous nebulization is most effective in the initial care of the patient with acute asthma.[5,16]
10. **A. Intervention.** The patient should remove the mouthpiece from the medication canister for cleaning. The mouthpiece should be cleaned daily with soap and water, and the medication canister should be cleaned twice a week. The MDI should be protected from freezing and overheating. The patient should use the MDI only as instructed and either contact his or her physician or return to the emergency department if the symptoms do not improve.[20]
11. **D. Assessment.** When evaluating the causes of wheezing, the following mnemonic may be of use:[16]

A	Asthma	Various precipitating events
S	Stasis	Pulmonary embolus
T	Toxins	Smoke inhalation Insecticides Chemical irritants
H	Heart	Congestive heart failure Noncardiogenic pulmonary edema
M	Mechanical	Foreign body aspiration
A	Allergy	Anaphylaxis Near drowning Aspiration of gastric contents
T	Trauma	Upper airway trauma
	Tumor	Endobronchial tumor
I	Infection	Bronchitis Pneumonia Bronchiolitis Croup
C	Chronic lung disease, Congenital lung disease	COPD Cystic fibrosis

12. **C. Assessment.** Bacteria that cause pneumonia include *Legionella, Mycoplasma,* and *Streptococcus pneumoniae.* HIV infection is a risk factor for pneumonia but does not cause it.[20-22]
13. **B. Intervention.** The patient with pneumonia is at risk of becoming dehydrated. Providing fluids for these patients is an important nursing intervention.[20]
14. **C. Evaluation.** The pulse oximeter does not provide information about the ventilatory status of the patient. In order to monitor the ventilatory status of this patient, the emergency nurse should connect the patient to a carbon dioxide monitor. Ventilatory status is measured by carbon dioxide tension and acid-base balance (pH).[21]
15. **B. Assessment.** Factors that limit the usefulness of pulse oximetry include carboxyhemoglobin, methemoglobin, hypovolemia, excess ambient light, patient motion, and nail polish.[21]
16. **D. Intervention.** Active tuberculosis provides a risk for transmission to other patients and to the people caring for the patient. The patient needs to be moved and admitted to a room with controlled airflow.[13,22]
17. **B. Intervention.** Guideline-recommended care of the patient who is to be discharged from the emergency department should include:
    - Assess level of oxygenation by pulse oximetry or arterial blood gas analysis before discharge
    - Administer first antibiotic dose before leaving the emergency department
    - Initiate appropriate empiric antibiotic regimen according to guidelines as to whether the patient does or does not reside in a nursing home[11]
18. **A. Assessment.** When obtaining a history from a patient who is experiencing chest pain, the emergency nurse obtains information about the possible causes of the chest pain. A part of this

history is identification of risk factors. Recent surgery, immobility, trauma, use of oral contraceptives, pregnancy, and obesity are risk factors for pulmonary embolus.[4]

19. **A. Intervention.** Because the patient has suffered an acute pulmonary embolus, initial treatment would include a direct-acting anticoagulant. Heparin calcium is a direct-acting anticoagulant, because it activates antithrombin III and factor Xa, which neutralize thrombin.[20,23]
20. **B. Analysis.** Tissue perfusion, altered cardiopulmonary, would be an appropriate nursing diagnosis. This condition is a result of pulmonary emboli. Included in the signs and symptoms of this nursing diagnosis is the patient's low blood pressure. Initial care of this patient by the emergency nurse will be based on interventions to improve tissue perfusion.[17]
21. **D. Evaluation.** Heparin can cause all of the complications listed, including, in rare instances, the actual formation of more clots, which may cause chest pain, neurological deficits, and diminished pulses in extremities.[23]
22. **B. Assessment.** When obtaining historical information from a patient with this type of symptomatology, the triage nurse should elicit whether the patient has been smoking crack or inhaling cocaine. Answers C and D are physical assessment parameters, not historical parameters.[23,24]
23. **A. Assessment.** Hamman's crunch, an indication of a pneumomediastinum, is a crunching sound heard during systole.[23,24]
24. **C. Evaluation.** Pneumomediastinum is air in the mediastinal tissues. This is the result of barotrauma (e.g., from smoking crack or inhaling cocaine), which causes increased pressure and alveoli rupture. Signs and symptoms include chest and neck pain, sore throat, difficulty swallowing, and subcutaneous emphysema. Complications of pneumomediastinum include pneumothorax.[23,24]
25. **C. Assessment.** Risk factors for tuberculosis include close contact with people with the disease, foreign-born people in countries with high incidence of tuberculosis, extremes of age, malnutrition, homeless people and migrants, alcohol and drug abuse, HIV, chronic renal failure, and certain malignancies.[13]
26. **D. Assessment.** In the emergency department, tuberculosis is generally a suspected diagnosis, because definitive diagnosis usually takes several days. Tuberculosis should be suspected if the patient complains of a constellation of signs and symptoms including fatigue, night sweats, cough, and low-grade fever. A chest radiograph may show cavitations or diffuse infiltrates. The primary screen for tuberculosis is the purified protein derivative. Results are obtained 2 to 3 days after it is administered.[13]
27. **C. Assessment.** Kawasaki's disease is a rare cause of chest pain in the pediatric patient. It causes cardiac ischemia.[7]
28. **B. Assessment.** The history and physical picture of this child are strongly suggestive of epiglottitis. Because of the possibility of obstruction, the child's throat should not be examined until she is in a safe environment that includes personnel capable of emergency airway management. The dangers of evaluating the child's throat include precipitating laryngospasm and complete obstruction, leading to respiratory arrest.[7,8]
29. **D. Intervention.** When the child is suffering acute respiratory distress from epiglottitis, the first intervention is to prepare the child for intubation. Administration of antibiotics would come after airway stabilization. Administration of racemic epinephrine is not recommended for the child with epiglottitis because of the potential for laryngospasm.[7,8]
30. **B. Assessment.** The most common cause of epiglottitis is *Haemophilus influenzae* infection.[7,8]
31. **B. Intervention.** According to the Basic Life Support Guidelines for infant foreign body airway obstruction management (conscious) of the American Heart Association, the emergency nurse should determine airway obstruction, place the infant face down and deliver four back blows, and then turn the infant on the back and deliver four thrusts in the midsternal region. This is repeated until the object is expelled or the infant becomes unconscious.[3]
32. **C. Evaluation.** As noted in the previous answer, an indication that these maneuvers are not effective would be the child's becoming unconscious.[3]
33. **B. Assessment.** The most common item aspirated by children younger than age 3 years is the hot dog.[3,7,8]
34. **A. Evaluation.** If the child does not respond to conventional therapy for respiratory distress, the emergency nurse should suspect foreign

body aspiration, particularly if the history is unclear.[3,7,8]

35. **A. Intervention.** Treatment of the child with asthma is based on bronchodilation. This can be done well with a β-agonist such as albuterol, terbutaline, or metaproterenol.[3,7,8]
36. **C. Evaluation.** An early indication of hypoxia in the infant is irritability. It is important for the emergency nurse to teach parents the signs and symptoms of early hypoxia so that there may be early intervention in the management of pediatric respiratory emergencies.[3,7,8]
37. **D. Assessment.** Respiratory syncytial virus is highly contagious. It is transmitted by direct contact from large-droplet aerosols, sneezing, and multiple visitors. The most effective way to decrease transmission is by hand washing and limiting visitors.[7,8]
38. **A. Assessment.** Following the formula of airway, breathing, and circulation, the emergency nurse would assess the patient's ability to maintain his airway. This patient is alert and able to speak but is complaining of shortness of breath. In assessing ventilation (breathing), the emergency nurse would auscultate for the presence or absence of breath sounds. Because one of the major interventions in the management of chest trauma is ensuring adequate ventilation, the absence of breath sounds and the complaint of shortness of breath indicate the need for interventions to reestablish adequate airflow.[6,9]
39. **B. Intervention.** Until a chest tube can be inserted to improve the patient's ventilation, the emergency nurse should prepare for and perform a needle thoracostomy. Two areas can be used for a needle thoracostomy: the second intercostal space in the midclavicular line or the fifth intercostal space in the midaxillary line. A large-bore needle is used (14-gauge), and the area should be prepared with antiseptic solution; the needle is inserted on the injured side.[24,25]
40. **D. Analysis.** Once again, based on the ABCs, the nursing diagnosis on which to establish initial nursing interventions would be impaired gas exchange. The emergency nurse's interventions would be directed toward managing the injuries that are impairing the patient's gas exchange.
41. **C. Evaluation.** The purpose of a needle thoracostomy is to improve the symptoms of tension pneumothorax, which include shortness of breath and hypotension. If there is no improvement or the patient's shortness of breath increases, another needle may need to be placed. The needle may not have completely entered the chest cavity, or it may have become kinked.
42. **A. Assessment.** Signs and symptoms of a tension pneumothorax include tracheal deviation, respiratory distress, unilateral absence of breath sounds, distended neck veins, and cyanosis.[24,25]
43. **C. Intervention.** Positioning the patient on the injured side is one method that may be used to stabilize a flail segment and improve oxygenation. However, the patient's cervical spine needs to be appropriately immobilized until cervical spine injury is ruled out.[6]
44. **A. Assessment.** Because the mechanism of injury involves the patient striking his chest and the patient is complaining of chest pain, the emergency nurse should assess the patient for chest wall injury, including abrasions or contusions on the chest wall.[24]
45. **A. Intervention.** Cardiac contusions leave the patient at risk for life-threatening injuries related to cardiac damage. The most important initial intervention based on an irregular pulse would be monitoring and management of cardiac dysrhythmia.
46. **D. Analysis.** The patient with myocardial contusion may suffer decreased cardiac output for several reasons. First, damage to the myocardium may result in pericardial tamponade, valvular disruption, and coronary artery occlusion. In addition, the patient may suffer cardiac dysrhythmia, such as premature ventricular contractions and tachycardia, and conduction abnormalities.[24,25]
47. **A. Evaluation.** There are many indications of lidocaine toxicity, including hypotension, bradycardia, drowsiness, dizziness, and seizures.[23]
48. **A. Assessment.** Signs and symptoms of pulmonary contusion include a high index of suspicion based on the mechanism of injury, dyspnea, ineffective cough, restlessness and agitation, and the presence of other severe chest injuries.[24,25]
49. **C. Intervention.** If the patient does not have hypotension from a related injury, such as an abdominal injury, fluids should be restricted for the patient with a pulmonary contusion. Because of the injury to the patient's lungs, the

patient is at risk for developing complications from fluid overload, such as acute respiratory distress syndrome and hypoxia. Diuretics and steroids may be considered for the treatment of these patients.[6]

50. **B. Analysis.** Because of the injury to the patient's lungs and the possibility of a pulmonary contusion, the patient's care should be based on keeping her oxygenated. Defining characteristics of this nursing diagnosis include confusion, somnolence, restlessness, irritability, inability to move secretions, hypoxia, and hypercapnia.[17]
51. **D. Assessment.** Based on the mechanism of injury and bowel sounds in the patient's chest cavity, a ruptured diaphragm would be suspected.[24,25]
52. **A. Intervention.** The formula for calculating the tube size is 16 plus the age of the child divided by 4. The approximate size is 4.5. The tube should be uncuffed for a 3-year-old child.[3]
53. **C. Intervention.** Advantages of the laryngeal mask in the emergency department include:[26]
    - No need for direct laryngoscopy
    - Ability to secure airway of patients with difficult upper airway anatomy
    - Can be used easily
54. **D. Intervention.** When caring for patients diagnosed with SARS in the emergency department, it is imperative that emergency department personnel have received and use appropriate isolation precautions. Personal protection equipment should be used per policy. Health care providers should be screened before providing patient care and quarantined, if warranted. The virus that causes SARS can survive on equipment for several hours, so equipment must be cleaned properly. Before patient resuscitation is performed, health care providers need to be sure that they are prepared. Patients should be placed in negative-pressure isolation rooms. The care of a patient with SARS or any potential communicable disease requires a plan and commitment from health care facilities. Guidelines may change frequently, so it is important that there is a system that can be quickly and safely initiated within each emergency department.[27,28]
55. **B. Intervention.** Whenever there is a problem with the ventilator that causes patient compromise, the patient should be removed from the ventilator and ventilated manually until the problem is found. Ventilators can cause barotrauma leading to pulmonary injury, including tension pneumothorax. Intrathoracic pressure is increased, which leads to hypotension, and patients should receive sedation when neuromuscular blocking agents are administered for ventilation management.[29]

References

1. Bates B: *Guide to physical examination and history taking,* Philadelphia, 1995, JB Lippincott.
2. Engel J: *Pediatric assessment,* St Louis, 1993, Mosby.
3. Hazinski F: *PALS provider manual,* Dallas, 2002, American Heart Association.
4. Mackey D: Pulmonary emergencies. In Kitt S, Selfridge-Thomas J, Proehl J et al, editors: *Emergency nursing: a physiologic perspective,* Philadelphia, 1995, WB Saunders.
5. National Heart Lung And Blood Institute: Update of selected topics 2002, National Institutes of Health Pub No 025074, Bethesda, MD, June 2003 Author.
6. Sherwood S, Hartsock R: Thoracic injuries. In McQuillan K, Von Rueden KT, Harstock RL, et al, editors: *Trauma nursing: from resuscitation through rehabilitation,* ed 3, Philadelphia, 2002, WB Saunders.
7. Phelan A: Respiratory emergencies. In Kelley S, editor: *Pediatric emergency nursing,* Norwalk, CT, 1994, Appleton & Lange.
8. Emergency Nurses Association: *Emergency pediatric core course,* Des Plaines, IL, 2004, Emergency Nurses Association.
9. James C: Respiratory emergencies. In Jordan KS, editor: *Emergency nursing core curriculum,* ed 5, Philadelphia, 2000, WB Saunders.
10. American Thoracic Society: Definition, diagnosis and staging of COPD, www.thoracic.org. Accessed May 31, 2004.
11. Yealy DM, Auble TE, Stone RA et al: The emergency department community-acquired pneumonia trial: methodology of a quality improvement intervention, *Ann Emerg Med* 43(6):770-782, 2004.
12. Varghese G, Crane L: Evaluation and treatment of HIV-related illnesses in the emergency department, *Ann Emerg Med* 24:503-511, 1994.
13. Curry J: Identifying the patient with tuberculosis and protecting the emergency department staff, *J Emerg Nurs* 20:293-304, 1994.

14. Brillman J et al: Hantavirus: emergency department response to a disaster from an emerging pathogen, *Ann Emerg Med* 24:429-436, 1994.
15. Candioty V: Shortness of breath. In Davis M, editor: *Signs and symptoms in emergency medicine,* St Louis, 1999, Mosby.
16. Hamilton G, Sanders A, Strange G et al: *Emergency medicine: an approach to clinical problem-solving,* Philadelphia, 2003, WB Saunders.
17. Kim MJ, McFarland GK, McLane AM: *Pocket guide to nursing diagnoses,* St Louis, 1993, Mosby.
18. Afilalo M, Guttman A, Colacone A et al: Efficiency of inhaled steroids (beclomethasone dipropionate) for treatment of mild to moderately severe asthma in the emergency department: a randomized clinical trial, *Ann Emerg Med* 33(3):304-309, 1999.
19. Mattera CJ: Crashing asthmatics, *J Emerg Med Serv* 24(10):30-33, 1999.
20. Koran Z, Howard PK: Respiratory emergencies. In Newberry L, editor: *Sheehy's emergency nursing: principles and practice,* ed 5, St Louis, 2003, Mosby.
21. Durren M: Getting the most from pulse oximetry, *J Emerg Nurs* 18:340-342, 1992.
22. Almeida S: Infectious and communicable diseases. In Newberry L, editor: *Sheehy's emergency nursing: principles and practice,* ed 5, St Louis, 2003, Mosby.
23. *Mosby's drug consult 2005,* St Louis, 2005, Mosby.
24. Peavey AA, Newberry L: Thoracic trauma. In Newberry L, editor: *Sheehy's emergency nursing: principles and practice,* ed 5, St Louis, 2003, Mosby.
25. Emergency Nurses Association: *Trauma nursing core course,* Des Plaines, IL, 2003, Emergency Nurses Association.
26. Danks R, Danks B: Laryngeal mask airway: review of indications and use, *J Emerg Nurs* 30(1):30-41, 2004.
27. Farquharson C, Baguley K: Responding to the severe acute respiratory syndrome (SARS) outbreak: lessons learned in a Toronto emergency department, *J Emerg Nurs* 29(3):222-228, 2003.
28. Centers for Disease Control: Severe acute respiratory syndrome. Supplement C: preparedness and response in health care facilities, www.cdc.org. Accessed January 8, 2004.
29. Proehl J, editor: *Emergency nursing procedures,* ed 3, Philadelphia, 2004, WB Saunders.

CHAPTER 18

Shock Emergencies

REVIEW OUTLINE

I. Definition of shock
   A. Shock is not a disease
   B. Clinical manifestation of inadequate tissue perfusion as the result of a clinical insult, such as excessive blood loss from a pelvic fracture
II. Causes of shock
   A. Alterations in circulating volume: loss of blood or other body fluids
   B. Alterations in cardiac pump function: heart is unable to function well enough to circulate blood to the body's tissues
   C. Alteration in peripheral vascular resistance: there is enough volume, but something has caused vasodilation or redistribution of blood in the periphery
III. Pathophysiology of shock[1]
   A. Amount of oxygen available for tissue consumption (DO_2)
   B. Amount of oxygen extracted from tissue ($\dot{V}O_2$)
   C. Oxygen consumption dependent upon
      1. Cardiac output
      2. Hemoglobin concentration
      3. Arterial oxygen saturation
      4. Venous oxygen saturation
   D. Oxygen debt is the difference between tissue oxygen demand and oxygen consumption
      1. Patient's preexisting condition will have an impact on how the body responds to a clinical insult that interferes with oxygen demand and consumption
         a. Chronic obstructive pulmonary disease
         b. Sickle cell anemia
         c. Cardiovascular disease
   E. Heat shock proteins
      1. Accumulate after a wide variety of clinical insults
      2. Associated with stress tolerance
      3. Potential biomarkers of early tissue injury
      4. Resistance to subsequent insult
   F. Apoptosis
      1. Physiological process of cell deletion that occurs during embryogenesis, metamorphosis, tissue atrophy, and tumor regression
      2. Active process
         a. Energy dependent
         b. Requires a cascade of signal-transducing events
         c. Programmed cell destruction
IV. The body's response
   A. Cellular response
      1. Cells shift from aerobic to anaerobic metabolism
         a. Cell destruction
         b. Cellular enzymes are released, which will damage and destroy other cells
   B. Immune system response
      1. Activation of complement cascade system
      2. Macrophage response
      3. Neutrophils
      4. Slow-reacting substance of anaphylaxis
      5. Platelet aggregation
   C. Neurological system response
      1. Alteration in cerebral perfusion pressure
      2. Seizures from hypoxia
      3. Coma
   D. Cardiac system response
      1. Decrease in cardiac output
      2. Development of dysrhythmia
      3. Myocardial depressant factor
   E. Pulmonary system response
      1. Acute lung injury
      2. Acute respiratory distress

F. Renal system response
   1. Decrease in urinary output
   2. Decrease in detoxification
G. Gastrointestinal system response
   1. Priming beds for circulating neutrophils
   2. Provokes multiple organ failure
H. Integumentary system response
   1. Pale, cooler, fragile skin
   2. Less protection
   3. Hypothermia

V. Compensatory mechanisms
A. Neural response
   1. Triggering of baroreceptors
   2. Release of catecholamines
   3. Vasoconstriction
B. Hormonal response
   1. Production of angiotensin II: vasoconstriction
   2. Aldosterone
   3. Pituitary gland
   4. Fall in thyroid hormone
   5. Increased insulin resistance
C. Fluid shifts
   1. Into the general circulation
   2. Fluid resuscitation: third spacing
D. Skeletal muscle
   1. Major reservoir of amino acids
   2. Proteolysis

VI. Classification of shock
A. Systemic inflammatory response syndrome[2]
   1. Body temperature higher than 38° C or lower than 36° C
   2. Heart rate higher than 90 beats per minute
   3. Hyperventilation evidenced by a respiratory rate higher than 20 breaths per minute or $PaCO_2$ lower than 32 mm Hg
   4. White blood cell count higher than 12,000 cells/µl or lower than 4000 cells/µl
B. PIRO system for staging sepsis
   1. Predisposition
   2. Insult
   3. Response
   4. Organ dysfunction
C. Multiple organ dysfunction syndrome
D. Pediatric multiple organ dysfunction
E. Compensated
F. Uncompensated
G. Irreversible

VII. Patient assessment
A. History of a clinical insult
   1. Trauma: blood and fluid loss
   2. Infection
      a. Sources
         (1) Indwelling urinary catheter
         (2) Indwelling intravenous access device
         (3) Feeding tube
   3. Myocardial infarction
   4. Tension pneumothorax
   5. Pericardial tamponade
   6. Allergic reaction
   7. Medical illness
      a. Gastrointestinal bleeding
      b. Hepatic disease
      c. Pancreatitis
   8. Vaginal bleeding
   9. Trauma in pregnancy, ruptured ectopic pregnancy
   10. Immunocompromised conditions
      a. Positive for human immunodeficiency virus
      b. Organ transplant
B. Source of clinical insult
C. Airway
D. Breathing
E. Circulation
   1. Skin color
   2. Skin temperature
   3. Level of consciousness
   4. Central and peripheral pulses
   5. Urinary output
F. Neurological
G. Diagnostic procedures
   1. Complete blood count with differential
   2. Serum electrolytes
   3. Liver function tests
   4. Lactate level
   5. Creatinine and blood urea nitrogen values
   6. Coagulation studies
   7. Arterial blood gas analysis
   8. Toxicological screen
   9. Cardiac enzyme values
   10. Cultures
   11. Type and crossmatch
   12. Electrocardiogram
H. Radiology
   1. Chest radiograph
   2. Pelvic radiograph
   3. Computed tomography

4. Magnetic resonance imaging
5. Angiography

I. FAST examination
1. Focused
2. Abdominal assessment
3. Sonography for
4. Trauma

VIII. Related nursing diagnosis
A. Impaired gas exchange
B. Fluid volume deficit
C. Decreased cardiac output
D. Altered tissue perfusion
E. Spiritual distress
F. Grieving, anticipatory

IX. Collaborative care of the patient in shock
A. Airway management
1. 100% oxygen by mask
2. Airway adjuncts
B. Ventilation management
1. Intubation for oxygenation
2. Neuromuscular blockade
3. Sedation and analgesia
C. Circulatory management
1. Fluid resuscitation
2. Vasoactive drugs
3. Other medications
a. Antibiotics
b. Antiviral agents
c. Steroids
4. Pneumatic antishock garments (PASG)
5. Operative management
D. Prevention
1. Vaccinations
2. Injury prevention
3. Age-related interventions

X. Age-related considerations
A. Pediatric patient[3]
1. Pediatric myocardial fibers are shorter and less compliant
a. To increase cardiac output, the child's heart rate will increase
2. Infants have a higher cardiac output and less oxygen reserve
3. Infant circulating blood volume 90 ml/kg and 80 ml/kg in the child
a. small blood loss can be significant
4. Hypotension is a late sign of circulatory compromise in the infant and child
5. Because a greater percentage of the child's body weight is water, children at greater risk of becoming dehydrated with fluid loss

B. Geriatric patient[4]
1. Preexisting cardiovascular disease may limit the geriatric patient's ability to respond to the initial clinical insult that causes systemic inflammatory response syndrome
2. Cardiac output and stroke volume decrease with aging, leaving the patient at risk of rapidly developing hypoxemia and hypoxia with blood and fluid loss
3. Decreased blood flow to the lungs and the possibility of preexisting lung disease place the elderly at greater risk of developing hypoxia
4. Renal changes due to aging affect the kidneys' abilities to reabsorb and to concentrate urine, which may result in fluid and electrolyte imbalances
5. Medications such as beta-blockers will alter normal compensatory mechanisms

---

Shock has been described as the "rude unhinging of the machinery of life." It is a syndrome that results from inadequate perfusion of tissues.[2] Shock was diagnosed initially using vital signs as a guide; for example, a systolic blood pressure of 90 mm Hg or lower or a heart rate of 100 beats per minute or more in the adult patient. Today, shock has been recognized as a systemic response to a clinical insult that results in inadequate tissue perfusion and decreased oxygen delivery to the cells.[3] The syndrome of shock has begun to be described as systemic inflammatory response syndrome to encompass all of the physiological responses that the body goes through.[5] Examples of clinical insults include trauma, infection, and an allergic reaction to a specific source such as an insect sting.

When the patient is in shock, all of the body systems will respond. Many of these responses produce familiar signs and symptoms such as altered mental status, skin pallor, diaphoresis, hypotension, and decreased urinary output.

Treatment of the patient in shock begins with recognition of its cause. If the patient has lost volume or is acutely infected, the source of the systemic response must be identified and dealt with. Airway, breathing, and circulation are ensured so that adequate oxygen is available to the cells.[5]

However, the most effective management for shock remains prevention. Ensuring that people are properly vaccinated, wear seat belts, understand fire safety, and stay healthy and injury-free are but a few examples of how to prevent shock and its devastating consequences.

REVIEW QUESTIONS

1. An 84-year-old male was brought to the emergency department by air medical transport. He was the unrestrained front-seat passenger involved in a head-on collision at a busy intersection. His 82-year-old wife was driving and was killed. The patient is awake and alert and asking about his wife. His blood pressure is 80 systolic by palpation only, and his heart rate is 80 beats per minute. His skin is cold and clammy. He has a history of congestive heart failure and takes numerous medications, but he does not remember the names. He has only one large-bore intravenous line and has received 1 liter of Ringer's lactate during transport. Based upon this initial assessment, which of the following critical interventions should be performed next?
   A. Insertion of another large-bore intravenous line and additional fluid resuscitation
   B. Preparation for emergency intubation due to hypotension and signs of shock
   C. Insertion of a urinary catheter for circulatory monitoring as soon as he is undressed
   D. Preparation for emergency computed tomography of the head, chest, and abdomen to discover active bleeding

2. The patient has received 3 liters of Ringer's lactate. Indications of adequate resuscitation would include:
   A. A decrease in the patient's peripheral pulses and level of consciousness
   B. A decrease in urinary output because of the poor renal function related to his age
   C. An increase in his systolic blood pressure and stronger peripheral pulses
   D. Bilateral basilar crackles and shortness of breath

3. The patient's history of congestive heart failure will affect:
   A. Oxygen delivery
   B. Oxygen use
   C. Oxygen demand
   D. Oxygen debt

4. Oxygen consumption is dependent upon all the following except:
   A. Cardiac output
   B. Hemoglobin concentration
   C. Arterial carbon dioxide
   D. Oxygen saturation

5. A unit of O-negative packed red blood cells is to be administered because of persistent hypotension. The emergency nurse administers the blood through a blood filter because:
   A. The filter will prevent the hypothermia that may develop with the administration of blood
   B. The filter will prevent debris found in banked blood from being infused and causing complications
   C. The filter will prevent clotting problems that are associated with the infusion of banked blood
   D. The filter will prevent hypokalemia that is associated with the infusion of banked blood

6. An example of a hormonal influence on blood flow and volume in shock is:
   A. Vasodilation to increase cardiac output and increase preload
   B. Production of angiotensin II to increase systolic blood pressure
   C. Proteolysis of muscle tissue to produce adenosine triphosphate
   D. Decrease in fluid reabsorption and sodium retention

7. A 56-year-old male was riding an all-terrain vehicle looking for loose cattle. When his tire hit a large hole, he was thrown off the vehicle. He now complains of "numbness all over." His vital signs are B/P 88/48, P 48 and regular, and R 12. He is probably in:
   A. Cardiogenic shock
   B. Neurogenic shock
   C. Hemorrhagic shock
   D. Anaphylactic shock

8. Once the primary interventions have been completed, which nursing diagnosis would be most appropriate on which to base the patient's care:
   A. Hyperthermia related to the patient's inability to maintain his body temperature
   B. Infection, high risk for, related to the abrasions he sustained in the fall
   C. Hypothermia related to his inability to maintain his body temperature
   D. Noncompliance related to his refusal to wear a helmet when riding his all-terrain vehicle

9. The neurosurgeon has ordered high-dose steroid administration. The patient weighs 155 pounds. His loading dose should be:
   A. 1500 mg of methylprednisolone over 15 minutes
   B. 1150 mg of methylprednisolone over 25 minutes
   C. 2325 mg of methylprednisolone over 15 minutes
   D. 4650 mg of methylprednisolone over 20 minutes

10. In anaphylaxis, chemical mediators target:
    A. Smooth muscle of the bronchopulmonary tree
    B. Smooth muscle of the abdominal cavity
    C. Striated muscles in the lower extremities
    D. Myocardial muscle to decrease cardiac output

11. An 18-month-old male child is brought to the emergency department with severe shortness of breath, wheezing, and facial edema. His mother states he was playing in the yard and may have been stung by a bee. The initial dose of epinephrine for this child is (he weighs 22 pounds):
    A. 0.10 ml epinephrine 1:1000 subcutaneous
    B. 0.10 ml epinephrine 1:10,000 subcutaneous
    C. 0.10 ml epinephrine 1:1000 PR
    D. 0.10 ml epinephrine 1:1000 IV

12. A 20-year-old male fell 20 feet from a tree, striking his chest. He is awake and alert, complaining of severe shortness of breath. No breath sounds are heard on the right side, and crepitus is palpable on the right side of his chest. His heart rate is 138 beats per minute, and there is no palpable blood pressure. He is experiencing:
    A. Hemorrhagic shock
    B. Distributive shock
    C. Obstructive shock
    D. Vasogenic shock

13. The initial critical intervention for this patient is:
    A. Insertion of a 14-gauge needle into his left second intercostal space, midclavicular line, followed by chest tube insertion
    B. Insertion of a 14-gauge needle into his right second intercostal space, midclavicular line, followed by chest tube insertion
    C. Administration of high-flow oxygen by a bag-valve-mask device in order to decrease his shortness of breath and improve his ventilation
    D. Turning the patient on his affected side or placing a pillow over the injured area in order to assist his ventilations

14. The mother of an 11-month-old infant carries her child into triage. The mother states that the child has been vomiting and has had diarrhea for the past 24 hours. The baby is lethargic, pale, cool, and clammy. No peripheral pulses can be palpated, and she has weak central pulses. Her capillary refill is longer than 6 seconds. This child is in:
    A. Compensated hypovolemic shock
    B. Compensated septic shock
    C. Decompensated hypovolemic shock
    D. Cardiopulmonary failure from fluid loss

15. A high-flow oxygen mask is placed on the child, and an intraosseous needle is inserted in her right tibia. An initial fluid bolus is ordered. The child weighs 22 pounds. How much fluid should be administered to this child?
    A. 200 ml of normal saline
    B. 220 ml of normal saline
    C. 200 ml of dextrose in water
    D. 100 ml of normal saline

16. An indication that the child is improving is:
    A. A decrease in her level of consciousness
    B. A palpable radial pulse or pedal pulse
    C. A decrease in her body temperature
    D. A capillary refill time of longer than 5 seconds

17. The parents of a 15-month-old male bring him to the emergency department. They state that he has had a high fever and vomiting and is now very irritable. His mother states that he has "bruises" on his leg but has no history of recent trauma. The child's vital signs are P 160 and regular, R 38, and Temp 103° F rectal. There is purpura on both lower extremities. The most probable cause of this child's illness is:
    A. *Neisseria meningitidis*
    B. *Haemophilus influenzae*
    C. *Streptococcus pneumoniae*
    D. Any of the above

18. The initial systemic response that occurs in septic shock is caused by:
A. Loss of volume that occurs in sepsis due to fever
B. Endotoxins of the infecting bacteria, virus, or fungus
C. Immune system response to the invading organism
D. Cardiovascular system response to the invading organism

19. A 62-year-old patient in septic shock has been started on a norepinephrine (Levophed) infusion at 2 mcg/min. Norepinephrine will cause:
A. A significant decrease in this patient's cardiac output
B. A significant decrease in this patient's urinary output
C. A significant increase in this patient's mean arterial pressure
D. No significant change in this patient's serum lactate level

20. An example of a preventive strategy that may be used in the emergency department to decrease the risk of sepsis in the elderly population is:
A. Administration of the pneumococcal vaccine to patients over 65 years of age
B. Provision of information related to recognition of the signs and symptoms of sepsis
C. Referral of elderly patients to a health care provider to ensure that all their vaccinations are up to date
D. Provision of written material that outlines when all vaccinations should be obtained

21. A 23-year-old Hispanic patient is brought to triage by her husband. She is complaining of severe abdominal pain. Her skin is cool and clammy. Initial B/P is 78/40, P 150, R 30, and Temp 104° F. She states that her last menstrual period was 12 weeks ago and she has been bleeding for the past 3 days. Which of the following interventions should the emergency nurse initiate?
A. Administer 650 mg of acetaminophen orally to manage the patient's fever
B. Place the patient on 100% oxygen with a nonrebreather mask
C. Obtain large-bore intravenous access for administration of normal saline
D. Draw blood cultures from two separate sites to identify the source of her fever

22. PASG in an injured patient is indicated to:
A. Provide protection of a gravid abdomen in an injured female patient
B. Control internal bleeding for the patient who has suffered a traumatic arrest
C. Stabilize an isolated lower extremity fracture in an injured patient
D. Support a suspected pelvic fracture in an injured hypotensive patient

23. Complications of massive fluid resuscitation include:
A. Increased tissue perfusion to injured cells
B. Decreased risk of developing metabolic derangements
C. Decreased length of stay in the critical care unit
D. Increased risk of developing hypothermia

24. A 52-year-old male is brought to the emergency department complaining of 10/10 chest pain for the past 3 days. His vitals signs are B/P 90/50, P 110, R 24. He is pale and diaphoretic. His electrocardiogram demonstrates an acute anterior myocardial infarction. Which of the following interventions should this patient be prepared for?
A. Administration of fibrinolytic therapy
B. Transfer to a cardiac catheterization lab for angioplasty
C. Insertion of an intraaortic balloon pump
D. Administration of an antiarrhythmic medication

25. A 41-year-old male is brought to the emergency department after he collided with another skier. He is complaining of severe left-sided chest pain (10/10) and shortness of breath. His B/P is 90/58, P 120, and R 28. He is pale and cold. He asks the emergency nurse for something for pain. Which of the following is true?
A. The patient who is hypotensive should never receive medication for pain, because it further decreases the blood pressure
B. A patient with rib fractures should not receive any analgesia, because it will interfere with his breathing and may cause pneumonia
C. Appropriate use of analgesia and sedation can only serve to support the patient in

shock, by decreasing the effects of the stress response on the body

D. Analgesic agents should not be administered to a patient who may be hypothermic, because they may interfere with the patient's compensatory mechanisms

ANSWERS

1. **A. Intervention.** The patient is currently awake and alert and appropriately asking about his wife. However, because he has only had 1 liter of fluid, the most appropriate intervention would be to insert another parenteral line and continue his fluid resuscitation.[4,7,8]
2. **C. Evaluation.** Fluid resuscitation end points include maintaining the patient's level of consciousness; maintaining an adequate blood pressure, generally a systolic pressure between 90 and 100 mm Hg, or even lower with uncontrolled hemorrhage; and maintaining the patient's peripheral perfusion.[7]
3. **D. Assessment.** Oxygen debt is the difference between tissue oxygen demand and oxygen consumption. The effects of the patient's injury and current health status will affect the oxygen debt.[9]
4. **C. Assessment.** Oxygen consumption is dependent upon the patient's cardiac output, hemoglobin concentration, and the oxygen saturation.[7]
5. **B. Intervention.** Debris in banked blood may cause additional injury to the patient. Blood should always be administered with a filter to prevent this complication.[3,5]
6. **B. Assessment.** The body's hormonal compensatory mechanisms to maintain blood flow and volume include triggering the renin-angiotensin system. Once released, renin allows the conversion of angiotensinogen to angiotensin I, which is converted to angiotensin II. Angiotensin II is a potent vasoconstrictor, which also stimulates aldosterone release and causes the kidneys to retain sodium and water.[8]
7. **B. Assessment.** Injuries to the spinal cord and brain will block the outflow of the sympathetic nervous system. This results in hypotension and bradycardia.[1]
8. **C. Analysis.** The loss of vasomotor tone leaves the patient at great risk of becoming hypothermic, because he is unable to maintain his body temperature through vasoconstriction (poikilothermia).[8,10]
9. **C. Intervention.** The patient weighs approximately 136 lb, which is 62 kg. The loading dose of methylprednisolone is 30 mg/kg over 15 minutes.[3]
10. **A. Assessment.** The slow-reacting substance of anaphylaxis targets specific organs, including the smooth muscle of the bronchopulmonary tree and tissue in the upper airway. This leads to bronchospasm and airway edema, compromising the patient's airway and ability to ventilate effectively.[1,8]
11. **A. Intervention.** The correct calculation is 0.01 ml/kg epinephrine 1:1000 subcutaneous. The child weighs 22 lb, or 10 kg; therefore, the dose is 0.10 ml of epinephrine 1:1000 subcutaneous. The epinephrine may be given IV if the child's condition dictates; however, it would be 0.10 ml 1:10,000.[9-13]
12. **C. Assessment.** The patient is experiencing obstructive or mechanical shock. Causes of obstructive shock include tension pneumothorax, pericardial tamponade, and myocardial contusion. The injury causes obstruction of venous return and lowers cardiac output.[6]
13. **B. Intervention.** A 14-gauge needle should be inserted in this patient's chest in the second intercostal space, at the midclavicular line. Because his breath sounds are decreased on the right side, that is where the needle should be inserted. Chest tube insertion should follow.[2,6]
14. **C. Assessment.** This child is in decompensated hypovolemic shock. Her level of consciousness, skin color and temperature, capillary refill longer than 5 seconds, and the absence of peripheral pulses indicate uncompensated shock.[13]
15. **A. Intervention.** The initial fluid bolus for this baby is 200 ml of normal saline. The baby weighs 22 lb (10 kg). 10 kg × 20 ml = 200 ml.[13]
16. **B. Evaluation.** Return of peripheral pulses would be an indication that the fluid resuscitation is effective.[9]
17. **D. Assessment.** All of the above. The child has significant signs and symptoms of meningitis or meningococcemia. Any of these bacteria can cause these signs and symptoms, and it may be difficult to differentiate the cause in the emergency department. History of recent exposure to any of these diseases would assist in differentiation, but management should not be

delayed. A key piece of history is whether the child has been exposed to an infected child or the presence of meningococcemia cases in the community.[3,6,11]

18. **B. Assessment.** The initial response of the body to the invading organism's endotoxins initiates a systemic response. For example, the immune system responds by releasing interleukins, tissue necrosis factor, and slow-reacting substance of anaphylaxis.[1-10]
19. **C. Evaluation.** Norepinephrine is a potent α-agonist. It will significantly increase the patient's mean arterial pressure, with little change in heart rate or cardiac output. It is more potent than dopamine in reversing hypotension in patients with septic shock. Even though norepinephrine can cause vasoconstriction that may cause renal injury in other shock states, by improving the mean arterial pressure in the hyperdynamic state of sepsis, it will also improve glomerular filtration.[15]
20. **A. Intervention.** Written information and referral does not ensure follow-up. Actual administration of vaccines in the emergency department provides the first step in preventive health care.[14,16]
21. **B. Intervention.** The initial intervention for the patient in shock is airway management to improve oxygenation. Because there is no indication for endotracheal intubation, administration of 100% oxygen by mask would be the first intervention.[4]
22. **D. Intervention.** Indications for the use of PASG in the treatment of a patient in shock include suspected pelvic fracture with hypotension, profound hypotension (less than 60 mm Hg), and suspected intraperitoneal or retroperitoneal hemorrhage. Contraindications for PASG use include penetrating thoracic trauma, stabilization of an isolated extremity fracture, evisceration of abdominal organs, objects impaled in the abdomen, pregnant abdomen, and traumatic arrest.[17]
23. **D. Analysis.** Complications of massive fluid resuscitation include decreased perfusion to injured cells, increased risk of metabolic derangements such as hypokalemia and coagulopathy, and increased length of stay in the critical care unit.[18]
24. **B. Intervention.** Based on the American Heart Association recommendations for the management of acute coronary syndrome, the best treatment for this patient is reperfusion. Because it has been longer than 12 hours since the start of his chest pain, fibrinolytic therapy would not be beneficial.[19]
25. **C. Intervention.** Although the patient is hypotensive, pain management can be beneficial. Pain causes triggering of the stress response, which can cause further injury to the patient.[20]

REFERENCES

1. McCance KL, Huether SE: *Pathophysiology: the biologic basis for disease in adults and children,* ed 4, St Louis, 2002, Mosby.
2. Levy MM, Fink M, Marshall J et al: 2001 SCCM/ESICM/ACCP/ATS/SIS International Sepsis Definitions Conference, *Intensive Care Med* 29:530-538, 2003.
3. Emergency Nurses Association: *Emergency nursing pediatric course,* ed 3, Des Plaines, 2004, Emergency Nurses Association.
4. Emergency Nurses Association: *Trauma nursing core course,* ed 5, Des Plaines, 2000, Emergency Nurses Association.
5. Shoemaker WC: Diagnosis and treatment of shock and circulatory dysfunction. In Grenvik A, editor: *Textbook of critical care,* ed 4, Philadelphia, 2000, WB Saunders.
6. Bone R: Sepsis, sepsis syndrome, and the systemic inflammatory response syndrome (SIRS). Gulliver in Laputa, *JAMA* 273:155-156, 1995.
7. Chapman C: Shock emergencies. In Newberry L, editor: *Sheehy's emergency nursing: principles and practice,* ed 5, St Louis, 2003, Mosby.
8. Emergency Nurses Association: *Course in advanced trauma nursing-II: a conceptual approach to injury and illness,* Des Plaines, IL, 2003, Emergency Nurses Association.
9. Selfridge-Thomas J: Shock. In Kitt S, Selfridge-Thomas J, Proehl J et al, editors: *Emergency nursing: a physiologic and clinical perspective,* Philadelphia, 1995, WB Saunders.
10. Fowler R, Pepe P, Lewis R: Shock evaluation and management. In Campbell JE, editor: *Basic trauma life support,* ed 4, Upper Saddle River, NJ, 2000, Brady/Prentice Hall Health.
11. Horvath C: Shock emergencies. In Jordan KS, editor: *Emergency nursing core curriculum,* ed 5, Philadelphia, 2000, WB Saunders.
12. www.mosbysdrugconsult.com. Accessed October 4, 2004.

13. Chameides L, Hazinski MF: *Pediatric advanced life support,* Dallas, 2002, American Heart Association.
14. Task Force on Community Preventative Services: Reviews of evidence regarding interventions to improve vaccination coverage in children, adolescents, and adults, *Am J Prev Med* 18(1S):97-140, 2000.
15. Society of Critical Care Medicine: Practice parameters for hemodynamic support of sepsis in adult patients, *Crit Care Med* 27(3):639-660, 1999.
16. Steffen S, Herringshaw M: Fulminate pneumococcal septicemia in the asplenic patient: a case study with urgent implications for recognition and prevention, *J Emerg Nurs* 25(2):102-106, 1999.
17. McSwain NE, Frame S, Salomone JP: *PHTLS: basic and advanced trauma life support,* St Louis, 2003, Mosby.
18. Rueden K, Dunham CM: Sequelae of massive fluid resuscitation in trauma patients, *Crit Care Nurs Clin North Am* 6:463-472, 1994.
19. Cummins RO: *ACLS provider manual,* Dallas, 2001, American Heart Association.
20. Semonin Holleran R: The problem of pain in emergency care, *Nurs Clin North Am* 37(1):67-78, 2002.

CHAPTER 19

TOXICOLOGICAL EMERGENCIES

REVIEW OUTLINE

I. General treatment of the patient with a toxicological emergency
    A. Ensure safety of the health care providers
    B. Environment in which the patient was found
    C. Remove patient from the toxic environment
    D. Assess and maintain the patient's airway, breathing, circulation, and disability
II. History related to amount of toxin exposed to
    A. Was it an intentional or unintentional exposure?
    B. How was the patient exposed?
        1. Ingestion
        2. Dermal
        3. Inhalation
        4. Ocular
        5. Bite or sting
        6. Parenteral
        7. Aspiration
    C. When did it occur?
    D. What has been done since the exposure?
    E. Medical history
        1. Allergies
        2. Medications
        3. History of mental health problems
            a. Suicide attempts
            b. Depression
        4. History of recent loss
        5. History of substance abuse
III. Objective data
    A. Level of consciousness
    B. Vitals signs
    C. Seizure activity
    D. Skin assessment
        1. Color
        2. Rashes
        3. Debris
        4. Needle marks, tracks
        5. Bruising
    E. Pupils
    F. Nystagmus
    G. Gait
    H. Cardiac rhythm
IV. Identification of the toxin
    A. Presence of burns around or in the mouth
    B. Odor of the patient's breath
        1. Alcohol
        2. Garlic
        3. Oil of wintergreen
        4. Bitter almond
    C. Eyes
        1. Pinpoint pupils: narcotics, chloral hydrate, phenothiazines, insecticides
        2. Dilated pupils: alcohol, amphetamines, cocaine, tricyclic antidepressants
        3. Nystagmus: vertical, horizontal
    D. Vital signs
        1. Bradycardia: beta-blockers, digitalis toxicity, organophosphate poisoning
        2. Tachycardia: tricyclic antidepressants, cocaine and crack, amphetamines, hallucinogens
    E. Neurological assessment
        1. Mental depression
        2. Excitability
        3. Pupillary changes
        4. Extraocular eye movements
    F. Changes in respiratory patterns
        1. Tachypnea
            a. Amphetamines
            b. Alcohols
            c. Salicylates
            d. Cocaine
            e. Cyclic antidepressants
        2. Bradypnea
            a. Barbituates
            b. Cyclic antidepressants
            c. Narcotics
            d. Alcohol

G. Changes in body temperature
   1. Hypothermia
      a. Ethanol
      b. Carbon monoxide
      c. Barbiturates
   2. Hyperthermia
      a. Salicylates
      b. Cyclic antidepressants
H. Excessive salivation and lacrimation
   1. Organophosphates
I. Carbamates

V. Collaborative care of the patient with a toxicological emergency
   A. ABCs, the primary interventions
      1. Ensure a patent airway
      2. Adequate ventilation
      3. Cardiac monitor
      4. Large-bore intravenous line
      5. Specific antidote when available
      6. Neurological assessment
      7. Terminate toxic exposure
      8. Identify nature of the toxin
         a. Poison information center
         b. Internet
         c. Toxicologist
         d. Federal agencies
         e. Local experts

VI. Decontamination
   A. Ipecac
   B. Charcoal
   C. Gastric lavage
   D. Whole bowel irrigation
   E. Cathartics
   F. Hemodialysis
   G. Charcoal hemoperfusion
   H. Alkaline diuresis
   I. Ocular decontamination
   J. Dermal decontamination

VII. Antidotes
   A. Oxygen
   B. Naloxone
   C. Atropine
   D. N-acetylcysteine
   E. Glucagon
   F. Calcium
   G. Nitrites, sodium thiosulfate
   H. Digoxin fab antibodies
   I. Protamine
   J. Deferoxamine
   K. Pyridoxine
   L. Dimercaprol (BAL), ethylenediamine tetraacetic acid (EDTA), dimercaptosuccinic acid (DMSA)
   M. Methylene blue
   N. Ethanol
   O. Sodium bicarbonate
   P. Vitamin K

VIII. Diagnostic testing
   A. Laboratory
      1. Whole blood glucose
      2. Serum drug screen
      3. Arterial blood gas analysis
      4. Carbon monoxide level
      5. Liver function tests
      6. Renal profile
      7. Coagulation studies
      8. Toxicology screen
      9. Specific toxin levels: aspirin, acetaminophen
   B. Radiographs
      1. Chest
      2. Flat plate of the abdomen
      3. Computed tomography
   C. Electrocardiogram (ECG)

IX. Related nursing diagnoses
   A. Airway clearance, ineffective, related to toxic exposure
   B. Aspiration, high risk for
   C. Breathing pattern, ineffective, related to toxic exposure
   D. Cardiac output, decreased, related to toxic exposure
   E. Coping, ineffective, related to a drug overdose
   F. Fluid volume deficit related to toxic exposure
   G. Gas exchange, impaired, related to toxic exposure
   H. Hyperthermia related to toxic exposure
   I. Injury, high risk for, related to toxic exposure
   J. Interrupted family processes
   K. Knowledge deficit
   L. Poisoning, high risk for
   M. Sensory or perceptual alterations related to toxic exposure
   N. Skin integrity, impaired, potential, related to toxic exposure
   O. Violence, high risk for: self-directed or directed toward others, related to toxic exposure

X. Age-related differences
   A. Pediatric
      1. Curious children may ingest things not normally ingested

2. Brightly colored packages and pills that look like candy can be tempting
3. Oral gratification important in infants and young children
4. Physiological differences in the pediatric digestive system influence the toxicity of substances
5. Increased metabolism can affect absorption of poisons

B. Geriatric
1. Patients may take multiple medications and unintentionally become poisoned
2. Slower metabolic rate will affect the absorption of toxic substances
3. Physiological changes in the neurological, pulmonary, and cardiovascular systems will effect the absorption of toxins and the body's response to them

XI. Specific toxicological emergencies
A. Acetaminophen poisoning
B. Salicylate poisoning
C. Alcohol poisoning
1. Ethanol
2. Methanol
3. Ethylene glycol
D. Sedative-hypnotic poisoning
E. Household products poisoning
1. Hydrocarbons and petroleum distillates
2. Caustic agents
F. Cyanide
G. Heavy metals
1. Iron
2. Lead
H. Cyclic antidepressants
I. Toxic inhalants
J. Cardiovascular medications
1. Beta-blockers
2. Calcium channel blockers
3. Digitalis
K. Food poisonings
L. Herbal toxicity
M. Plant poisoning
N. Organophosphates
O. Carbon monoxide
P. Substance abuse
1. Methamphetamine
2. Cocaine
3. Heroin
4. Hallucinogens
5. Drugs of the day

A person who has been "poisoned" has suffered a chemical injury to one or more body systems. Each year millions of patients are cared for in the emergency department after being intentionally or unintentionally poisoned. Although most continue to be unintentional, intentional poisonings still account for a significant number of deaths in the United States each year. Many times patients are poisoned by medications that were prescribed to help, not hurt, them. Most poisonings still occur in children younger than the age of 6 years.[1,2] However, most substance abuse or intentional exposure to poisons occurs in the 18- to 34-year-old age group.[3]

There are literally thousands of medications, plants, and chemicals that can poison patients. Very few antidotes are available, although research continues to be directed toward affecting the most toxic substances.[4,5] The American Heart Association has issued specific guidelines for the resuscitation of a patient who has suffered a toxic exposure.[6]

The review questions presented in this chapter offer examples of some of the most frequent types of poisonings seen by the emergency department nurse. The assessment, analysis, intervention, and evaluation components in the care of the poisoned patient are addressed.

Treatment of the Poisoned Patient

Supportive care is the key to treatment of the poisoned patient. Airway, ventilation, and circulatory maintenance are the mainstays of care. Unfortunately, compared with the number of poisons contained in the human environment, there are few known antidotes.

In addition to meeting the physical and physiological needs of the poisoned patient, the emergency nurse needs to provide emotional care. Particular attention needs to be given to why or how the patient was poisoned. Was it an environmental problem, an unintentional poisoning, or an intentional poisoning? It is important to assess whether the poisoning may have been a form of abuse, particularly if a child or elderly adult is involved.

Acetaminophen Poisoning

Acetaminophen is contained in many over-the-counter drugs. Its most popular name is Tylenol. Poisoning by acetaminophen can be lethal. The drug, if not properly eliminated, can cause hepatic, renal, and cardiac failure. Ingestions of 7.5 g or 150 mg/kg are potentially toxic.[7]

Salicylate Poisoning

Aspirin is the most common type of salicylate. It is one of the oldest nonprescription drugs used by humankind. As with acetaminophen, many over-the-counter drugs contain salicylates. There are three types of salicylate toxicity. Mild toxicity occurs with ingestions of less than 150 mg/kg, moderate toxicity with ingestions of 150 to 300 mg/kg, and severe toxicity with ingestions of 300 to 500 mg/kg.[8]

Cyclic Antidepressant Poisoning

Antidepressant medications are used to manage depression in adults, nocturnal enuresis, and painful neuropathies in diabetic patients, as well as chronic pain. In addition to tricyclic antidepressants, there are bicyclic and tetracyclic antidepressants. However, the most frequently prescribed antidepressants are tricyclic.[4]

The exact toxic level of poisoning cannot always be determined, because the drug accumulates in body tissues. The patient is treated according to symptoms. Tricyclic antidepressants in toxic amounts induce the release of norepinephrine and then inhibit its reuptake, directly block alpha action, exert a quinidine-like effect on myocardial tissue, and cause atropine-like anticholinergic effects.[2] The most common cause of death in cyclic poisoning is related to cardiac toxicity. Signs and symptoms of cardiac toxicity include depression of myocardial contractility, prolongation of the QT interval, heart block, atrial and ventricular dysrhythmias, and sudden cardiac death.[9-10] It is very important to remember that these drugs can be very toxic to the pediatric patient in what would appear to be small amounts to the adult patient.

Hydrocarbon Poisoning

Hydrocarbons are contained in many substances that may be ingested, inhaled, or spilled directly onto the skin. Examples of hydrocarbons include gasoline, kerosene, turpentine, and camphor. The most common types of hydrocarbon poisoning seen by the emergency department nurse include ingestion of gasoline and kerosene, and dermal exposure to these same substances.[4]

Hydrocarbon poisoning may cause pulmonary and cutaneous injuries. The major effects of hydrocarbon ingestion are on the lungs, gastrointestinal tract, and central nervous system.[3]

Organophosphate Poisoning

Organophosphates are contained in many commercial insecticides. Their mechanism of action is achieved by their ability to combine with acetylcholinesterase. This causes increased salivation, vomiting, bronchospasm, bradycardia, muscle fasciculations, paralysis, ataxia, confusion, seizures, and coma.[11]

REVIEW QUESTIONS

A 20-year-old woman is brought to the emergency department by the rescue squad. Her mother states that the patient has been anxious about her new job and has been taking alprazolam (4 mg daily), which was prescribed by the family physician. An empty pill bottle, along with a bottle of wine, was found by her bed. Currently the patient is responding only to deep, painful stimuli and she has vomited.

1. Initial assessment of this patient would include which of the following?
   A. Consult the poison information center to determine what is a lethal dose of alprazolam
   B. Evaluate the patient's ability to protect her airway from aspiration
   C. Evaluate the effect of the toxic ingestion on the patient's heart by ordering an ECG
   D. Identify the reason why the patient may have taken an overdose of her medication

2. What would be the most appropriate intervention in the initial treatment of this patient?
   A. Prepare the patient for intubation to protect her airway
   B. Obtain intravenous access to administer flumazenil
   C. Connect the patient to a cardiac monitor to assess her rhythm
   D. Administer ipecac as soon as possible to empty her stomach

3. The emergency physician has decided to administer flumazenil to confirm the diagnosis of suspected benzodiazepine poisoning. Flumazenil should be administered:
   A. Slowly over 5 minutes
   B. Rapidly over 15 to 30 seconds
   C. Mixed with sodium bicarbonate
   D. Through a small vein

4. A life-threatening side effect to flumazenil administration is:
   A. Agitation
   B. Sweating
   C. Seizures
   D. Dizziness

5. What would be an appropriate nursing diagnosis for this patient?
   A. Coping, ineffective individual, related to use of drugs and alcohol to manage her anxiety
   B. Poisoning, potential for, related to ingestion of an unknown amount of alprazolam and alcohol
   C. Family processes, altered, related to attempted suicide by a family member who is having work problems
   D. Infection, potential for, related to poisoning and being immobile for several hours of treatment in the emergency department

6. One of the parameters that must be monitored to evaluate the effectiveness of flumazenil is:
   A. The patient's level of consciousness
   B. The patient's urinary output
   C. The patient's peripheral pulses
   D. The patient's drug screen results

7. Benzodiazepines potentiate the activity of:
   A. Epinephrine
   B. Gamma-aminobutyric acid
   C. Acetylcholine
   D. Dopamine

8. The purpose of charcoal in the care of the poisoned patient is to:
   A. Absorb toxins from the gastrointestinal tract
   B. Induce vomiting and remove all the remaining toxins
   C. Prevent cardiac dysrhythmias that may result from absorbed toxins
   D. Decrease the possibility of bleeding from absorbed toxins

9. Charcoal administration is contraindicated when:
   A. The patient has ingested a toxic amount of salicylate
   B. The patient has ingested a toxic amount of a tricyclic antidepressant
   C. The pediatric patient is younger than 5 years of age
   D. The patient has ingested a toxic amount of alcohol

10. What is an important assessment parameter in the care of the patient who has ingested a toxic amount of acetaminophen?
    A. The serum acetaminophen level immediately following ingestion
    B. The serum acetaminophen level 24 hours after ingestion
    C. The serum acetaminophen level 4 hours after ingestion
    D. The serum acetaminophen level 48 hours after ingestion

11. A 23-year-old female is brought to the emergency department by her family after having taken 30 extra-strength acetaminophen tablets. She states that she has had a severe headache and "just wants the pain to go away." She states she took the pills about 12 hours before arriving in the emergency department. She decided to come in because she cannot stop vomiting. Which of the following treatments should be considered to manage this patient's toxicity?
    A. Administration of 50 g of activated charcoal through a gastric tube
    B. Administration of a normal saline solution with sodium bicarbonate
    C. Administration of 15 ml of ipecac in a glass of orange juice
    D. Administration of N-acetylcysteine 150 mg/kg over 1 hr intravenously

12. N-acetylcysteine counteracts the effect of acetaminophen by:
    A. Stimulating the production of vitamin K to prevent bleeding
    B. Increasing hepatic production of glutathione, protecting the liver
    C. Stimulating the production of glucagon and absorbing the acetaminophen
    D. Decreasing the effects of liver enzymes stimulated by the acetaminophen

13. Which of the following assessment parameters may be used by the emergency department nurse to evaluate the toxicity of an acetaminophen poisoning?
    A. Liver function studies
    B. Serial arterial blood gases

C. Coagulation studies
D. Electrolyte values

A 15-year-old girl comes to the emergency department complaining of abdominal pain. She states that she took a bottle of aspirin after having a fight with her boyfriend. She is currently alert, and her skin is hot and dry. Her vital signs are B/P 90/50, P 130, and R 32. A set of blood gases is drawn, and the results are pH 7.37, Po_2 100, Pco_2 20, and HCO_3 18.

14. These blood gas results reflect the patient's:
A. Metabolic acidosis
B. Respiratory alkalosis
C. Respiratory acidosis
D. Metabolic alkalosis

15. In addition to gastric emptying and charcoal administration for the patient who has suffered salicylate poisoning, which of the following interventions may be useful?
A. Administering a salicylate antidote
B. Administering fresh frozen plasma
C. Initiating forced diuresis and alkalinization
D. Administering N-acetylcysteine intravenously

16. What nursing diagnosis would pertain to the patient who has a toxic level of salicylates?
A. Swallowing, impaired, related to mental status changes caused by salicylates
B. Fluid volume deficit, high risk for, related to fluid loss from nausea and vomiting
C. Family processes, altered, related to the patient taking an intentional overdose
D. Infection, high risk for, related to the skin injury that may occur with bleeding

17. Because of the bleeding complications that may occur with salicylate poisoning, what laboratory value should the emergency department nurse evaluate?
A. Platelet count
B. Creatinine level
C. Prothrombin time
D. Arterial blood gases

18. An 18-month-old boy has ingested an unknown amount of his mother's amitriptyline. His sister gave the pills to him, believing they were candy. He is brought to the emergency department protecting his airway but responding only to deep, painful stimuli. His mother reports that it could not have been longer than 45 minutes since the ingestion. Signs and symptoms of tricyclic antidepressant toxicity include:
A. Hypothermia
B. Constricted pupils
C. Urinary incontinence
D. Sinus tachycardia

19. The first step in the treatment of this child is:
A. Insert a gastric tube and begin lavage with room temperature water
B. Insert a gastric tube and instill 50 g of charcoal along with a cathartic
C. Secure the child's airway by intubation with a cuffed endotracheal tube
D. Secure the child's airway by intubation with an uncuffed endotracheal tube

20. Which of the following is the recommended method of decontamination for this child?
A. Insertion of a gastric tube for lavage with measured amounts of saline
B. Administration of 30 ml of syrup of ipecac and saline through a gastric tube
C. Administration of activated charcoal mixed in 500 ml of orange juice given orally
D. Administration of syrup of ipecac orally, followed by eight glasses of warm distilled water

21. A pertinent nursing diagnosis for the patient who has been poisoned by cyclic antidepressants would be:
A. Noncompliance related to excessive ingestion of prescribed medications despite appropriate instructions
B. Social isolation related to depression and inability to express their need for counseling
C. Cardiac output, decreased, related to the quinidine-like effects of cyclic antidepressant toxicity
D. Injury, high risk for, related to the effects of cyclic antidepressant poisoning on the neurological and cardiovascular systems

22. Because of the capability of tricyclic antidepressants to block the reuptake of norepinephrine, what assessment parameter should be evaluated constantly by the emergency department nurse?
A. Temperature
B. Capillary refill

C. Blood pressure
D. Urinary output

23. A gastric tube is to be inserted for gastric lavage. The optimal patient position for this procedure would be:
A. Side-lying right lateral decubitus position
B. Side-lying left lateral decubitus position
C. Prone with the head of the bed lowered
D. Supine with pillow under the shoulders

24. Tricyclic antidepressant toxicity is very difficult to manage because the medications bind to:
A. Hemoglobin
B. Plasma proteins
C. White blood cells
D. Muscle cells

A 1-year-old child has ingested an unknown amount of gasoline from an open container. He is awake, alert, and crying appropriately, with a respiratory rate of 40. He smells like gasoline.

25. Because the patient has ingested a hydrocarbon, the initial assessment of this patient will be focused on his:
A. Cardiac rhythm
B. Respiratory system
C. Gastrointestinal system
D. Central nervous system

26. Initial interventions for the treatment of this child should include:
A. Placement of a temperature probe
B. Supplemental oxygen as tolerated
C. Placement in an isolation room
D. Placement in a protective crib

27. The patient is given 100% oxygen by mask. His respiratory rate has decreased to 28 breaths per minute. However, he continues to smell of gasoline. In order to prevent any further injury to this child, the emergency nurse should:
A. Prepare the child for endotracheal intubation to secure his airway as a precaution related to gasoline ingestion
B. Wash the child's skin with soap and water to prevent further absorption of the gasoline and the possibility of burns
C. Administer 50 g of charcoal to prevent further absorption of the gasoline internally and prevent the possibility of aspiration
D. Administer 15 ml of ipecac to prevent further absorption of the gasoline and the possibility of aspiration pneumonia

28. A relevant nursing diagnosis in the care of this child would be:
A. Injury, high risk for, related to his age and curiosity
B. Gas exchange, impaired, related to pulmonary injury
C. Cardiac output, decreased, related to hydrocarbon ingestion
D. Aspiration, high risk for, related to hydrocarbon ingestion

29. What additional information should be obtained by the emergency department nurse to evaluate the child's home environment?
A. The number of siblings in the house in which the child lives
B. The location of the gasoline and other possible toxins in the home
C. Who is responsible for the child's care on a day-to-day basis
D. The distance from the child's home to the emergency department

An elderly man attempted to commit suicide by locking himself in a closet and spraying himself with insecticide. On arrival in the emergency department, the patient is comatose, and his ECG shows sinus bradycardia.

30. In addition to the initial assessment of the patient's ABC status, the emergency nurse should consider:
A. How the patient was exposed to the toxin
B. The age of the patient and the effects of the toxin
C. Whether the patient is depressed or has attempted suicide in the past
D. Whether the patient has any other medical or psychological problems

31. In addition to stabilizing this patient's ABCs, the emergency nurse should prepare to:
A. Administer epinephrine 1:1000 intravenously
B. Administer 50 g of charcoal through a gastric tube
C. Decontaminate the patient with soap and water
D. Connect the patient to a pulse oximeter

32. The initial drug of choice to reverse the toxic effects of organophosphate poisoning is:
A. Lidocaine 1 mg/kg
B. Sodium bicarbonate 1 mEq/kg
C. Atropine 2 mg IM or IV
D. Calcium chloride 10 mg

33. Pralidoxime is used in the management of organophosphate poisoning because it:
A. Blocks acetylcholinesterase
B. Regenerates acetylcholinesterase
C. Regenerates acetylcholine
D. Blocks epinephrine

34. An appropriate nursing diagnosis for this patient would be:
A. Knowledge deficit related to the inappropriate use of an insecticide
B. Coping, ineffective individual, related to depression
C. Thought processes, altered, related to organophosphate poisoning
D. Family processes, altered, related to age

35. What outcome in this patient would indicate the effectiveness of atropine in the management of organophosphate poisoning?
A. Decreased salivation
B. Increased bradycardia
C. Increased ataxia
D. Cardiopulmonary arrest

36. The antidote administered for iron toxicity is:
A. N-acetylcysteine
B. Vitamin K
C. Deferoxamine
D. There is no antidote

A 2-year-old child is brought to the emergency department by her mother. The mother states that the child has chickenpox, has become confused and hyperactive, and is having difficulty walking. She does not have a fever, and her other vital signs are also within normal range. The only medication the mother has been using is Caladryl lotion to decrease the child's itching.

37. What type of toxicity is this child suffering from?
A. Acetaminophen
B. Diphenhydramine
C. Salicylate
D. Calcium chloride

38. A 40-year-old woman has taken an overdose of atenolol. She arrives in the emergency department awake, with B/P of 80/56 and P 38. Which of the following medications will be administered to manage this patient's toxicity?
A. Atropine sulfate
B. Epinephrine 1:1000
C. Calcium chloride
D. Glucagon hydrochloride

39. A 4-year-old boy took 10 tablets of his grandmother's Calan SR (verapamil). He comes to the emergency department with B/P 86/48, P 32, and R 30. The drug of choice to reverse the effects of the verapamil is:
A. Calcium chloride
B. Digitalis
C. Adenosine
D. Epinephrine

40. Gamma hydroxybutyrate (GHB) toxicity is managed by:
A. Administration of syrup of ipecac and water
B. Administration of flumazenil intravenously
C. Supporting the patient's ventilations
D. Gastric lavage 4 hours after ingestion

ANSWERS

1. **B. Assessment.** The most important component of the initial assessment of the poisoned patient is the ability to use his or her airway. Many poisons alter the patient's mental status, and the patient could quickly be at risk for aspiration, hypoventilation, and apnea.[4,12]
2. **A. Intervention.** Initial treatment of the poisoned patient is based on supportive management of ABCs. Because this patient has an altered level of consciousness and has vomited, intubation is indicated. Ipecac should not be given to a patient who is not capable of protecting the airway.[4,12]
3. **B. Intervention.** Flumazenil should be administered rapidly over 15 to 30 seconds through a large vein. The drug should not be mixed with any other medications.[9]
4. **C. Assessment.** A serious and life-threatening side effect of flumazenil administration is seizures. Patients with a history of seizures and those with mixed overdoses, particularly tricyclic antidepressants, should not be given this drug.[9]
5. **B. Analysis.** The most appropriate nursing diagnosis, and one on which the emergency nurse could develop this patient's plan of care,

would be poisoning, potential for, related to ingestion of an unknown amount of alprazolam and alcohol. Because of the possible life-threatening complications that may occur with poisoning, and the nature of the episodic care provided by the emergency department nurse, this particular diagnosis would encompass many of the relevant nursing actions that would be required by this patient.[13]

6. **A. Evaluation.** The patient's level of consciousness should be monitored closely. One potential problem with flumazenil administration in the patient with benzodiazepine overdose is resedation.[10]
7. **B. Intervention.** Benzodiazepines potentiate the affects of γ-aminobutyric acid, which is an inhibitory neurotransmitter. A positive side effect is a decrease in anxiety and, in some cases, amnesia. However, an overdose of the drug can cause sedation and a depressed mental status.[13]
8. **A. Intervention.** Charcoal is a finely divided black powder with an extensive internal network of pores that absorb substances. For charcoal to be effective, it needs to be given as quickly as possible after ingestion of the toxic substance.[13] In certain poisonings, charcoal alone, rather than combined with the use of ipecac, may be useful in the initial treatment of the alert poisoned patient. Many patients are unable to keep charcoal down until several hours after ipecac has been administered, thus being deprived of the charcoal's ability to absorb the poison.[11]
9. **D. Intervention.** Charcoal is contraindicated when the patient has ingested alcohol, a caustic or corrosive substance, hydrocarbons, and heavy metals such as iron, lead, mercury, lithium, and arsenic. When administering charcoal to children, the age, weight, and method of delivery need to be considered in order to administer an effective dose.[4]
10. **C. Assessment.** All patients should have a serum acetaminophen level drawn 4 hours after ingestion. The serum level immediately following ingestion will offer little information about the potential toxic level.[7]
11. **D. Intervention.** N-acetylcysteine is indicated when the serum acetaminophen level remains at a toxic level after 4 hours or if an acetaminophen level cannot be obtained before 10 hours after ingestion. N-acetylcysteine can be given orally or by intravenous infusion (Acetadote). When the patient has uncontrolled vomiting, the drug may be administered through a gastric tube. However, N-acetylcysteine has been administered intravenously in Australia and in other countries for many years. Recent research in the United States in toxicology centers has demonstrated that intravenous administration is more effective, and the drug can be given safely by this route. If it is used within 48 hours, the chances of hepatotoxicity are greatly reduced. The recommended dosage is 150 mg/kg over 1 hour as a loading dose and an infusion of 15 mg/kg per hour for 4 hours. Administration is continued at 7.5 mg/kg per hour for 16 hours, if needed. The infusion may be stopped for the following reasons: the patient is asymptomatic or is improving clinically, transaminase levels are decreasing or are normal, and serum acetaminophen level is undetectable.[7,8,14]
12. **B. Intervention.** N-acetylcysteine stimulates an increase in the production of glutathione, which preferentially conjugates with the injested dose of acetaminophen to form a nontoxic substance that is secreted by the kidneys.[2,8,13,14]
13. **A. Evaluation.** Because acetaminophen is particularly toxic to the liver, blood should be drawn for baseline hepatic studies. Peak hepatotoxicity occurs 72 to 96 hours after ingestion.[7,8,14]
14. **B. Assessment.** Salicylate poisoning initially will stimulate the respiratory center of the central nervous system. This manifests itself in an increased respiratory rate and causes respiratory alkalosis.[15]
15. **C. Intervention.** Salicylate poisoning is managed with gastric emptying, charcoal administration, and alkaline diuresis. Alkaline diuresis will increase the pH of the patient's urine and improve free salicylate excretion.[8,12]
16. **B. Analysis.** Salicylate poisoning may cause excessive fluid loss from nausea, vomiting, sweating, and hyperventilation, all of which can lead to dehydration.[15]
17. **C. Evaluation.** Bleeding problems may develop in severe salicylate poisoning. This occurs because of impaired platelet aggregation and decreased circulating thrombin.[8,12]
18. **D. Assessment.** Because tricyclic toxicity stimulates anticholinergic activity and has quinidine-like effects on the cardiovascular system, the signs and symptoms of tricyclic toxicity include altered level of consciousness,

decreased respirations, seizures, urinary retention, sinus tachycardia with widened QRS complexes, hyperpyrexia, and hypotension.[4,12,16]

19. **D. Intervention.** Because the child already has an altered mental status, his airway should be protected. The age of the child requires that the child be intubated with an uncuffed endotracheal tube.[4]
20. **A. Intervention.** Because this child is responsive only to painful stimuli, will be intubated, and ingested the pills less than an hour ago, gastric lavage may be of some benefit. It is important to closely monitor a patient who is being lavaged to prevent complications such as aspiration and hypoxia.[4,16]
21. **C. Analysis.** The most appropriate nursing diagnosis would be C, because the toxic cardiac and neurological effects of cyclic antidepressants are lethal.[10]
22. **C. Evaluation.** Because the supply of norepinephrine is depleted by the body, and the tricyclic antidepressant is blocking the reuptake of norepinephrine, hypotension will result. It is important to recognize this toxic effect early so that appropriate intervention can be initiated.[4,10]
23. **B. Intervention.** The patient should be placed in the side-lying left lateral decubitus position to protect his airway, particularly if he is not intubated, and to facilitate drainage of the lavage fluid.[13]
24. **B. Assessment.** Tricyclic antidepressants bind to the plasma proteins, which makes them very difficult to remove from the body.[9,10]
25. **B. Assessment.** Because hydrocarbon ingestion initially affects the respiratory system, the patient's respiratory status will need to be assessed. Included should be the patient's normal respiratory rate and any indications of respiratory distress, including dyspnea, wheezes, stridor, hemoptysis, and cyanosis.[4,16]
26. **B. Intervention.** If the child has suffered pulmonary injury, supplemental oxygen will be needed.[4]
27. **B. Intervention.** Because some hydrocarbons, particularly gasoline, can be absorbed through the skin, and the emergency nurse is unsure of the amount of gasoline ingested, the child's skin should be decontaminated by washing it with soap and water. External gasoline can cause burns.[4,16]
28. **D. Analysis.** One of the major complications with hydrocarbon ingestion is the potential for aspiration because of vomiting. The emergency nurse's plan of care needs to include interventions that will prevent further injury to the pulmonary system from aspiration.[4,10]
29. **B. Evaluation.** An important role for the emergency nurse is teaching prevention. Obtaining information about the location of possible poisons, and then teaching the child's parents how to prevent further accidents, could prevent a tragedy.[4]
30. **A. Assessment.** The method of exposure needs to be considered, particularly in relation to insecticide poisoning. As noted in the history, the patient sprayed the insecticide all over himself in an enclosed place.[4,11,12]
31. **C. Intervention.** He suffered not only inhalation exposure but also dermal exposure. Therefore, he will need to have his clothes removed and his skin cleansed with soap and water to remove any remaining insecticide.[4,11,12]
32. **C. Intervention.** Atropine is administered in doses of 2 mg IM or IV until symptoms disappear and repeated every 15 minutes.[4,11,12]
33. **B. Intervention.** Pralidoxime is an additional antidote for organophosphate poisoning. It works by regenerating acetylcholinesterase.[15]
34. **B. Analysis.** A suicidal patient is displaying ineffective coping. The patient has chosen behavior that is detrimental, and suicide precautions will need to be instituted while he is in the emergency department.[17]
35. **A. Evaluation.** Atropine will reverse the muscarinic effects of organophosphate poisoning, which include salivation, lacrimation, urinary and fecal incontinence, vomiting, miosis, bronchospasm, and bradycardia.[4,11,12]
36. **C. Intervention.** Deferoxamine is the antidote for iron toxicity. This medication will turn the urine a *vin rosé* color, which indicates that the iron is binding with the drug.[4]
37. **B. Assessment.** Caladryl lotion contains diphenhydramine to help decrease the amount of itching that accompanies some skin lesions, such as those of chicken pox. If the lotion is applied in large amounts, to large areas of skin, or to broken skin, it can be absorbed and cause toxic side effects. Diphenhydramine toxicity causes anticholinergic effects, including confusion, paradoxical hyperactivity, disorientation, and ataxia. The lotion needs to be removed to prevent further absorption.[18]
38. **D. Intervention.** Glucagon hydrochloride is effective in the management of propranolol tox-

icity. Glucagon may increase the intracellular level of calcium within the myocardium.[4]

39. **A. Intervention.** Calcium chloride is the drug used to manage the toxic side effects of calcium channel blocker intoxication. Unlike verapamil toxicity, which causes hypotension and bradycardia, nifedipine toxicity causes hypotension and tachycardia.[4]
40. **C. Intervention.** GHB toxicity can cause respiratory depression, so supporting the patient's ventilation is the best answer. Flumazenil and naloxone have no therapeutic effect on GHB toxicity, and lavage and ipecac have limited use because the drug is rapidly absorbed. Vomiting should not be induced because of the potential for respiratory depression.[19,20]

REFERENCES

1. Watson W, Litovitz T, Rodgers G et al: 2002 annual report of the American Association of Poison Control Centers toxic surveillance system, *Am J Emerg Med* 21(5):353-421, 2003.
2. McCaig LF, Burt CW: Poisoning-related visits to emergency departments in the United States, 1993-1996, *J Toxicol Clin Toxicol* 77(7):817-826, 1999.
3. Department of Health and Human Services: *Mid-year 1998 preliminary emergency department data from the drug abuse warning network,* Rockville, MD, July, 1999, SAMHSA.
4. Emergency Nurses Association: *Emergency nursing pediatric course,* ed 3, Des Plaines, IL, 2004, Emergency Nurses Association.
5. Zimmerman HE, Burkhart KK, Donovan JW: Ethylene glycol and methanol poisoning: diagnosis and treatment, *J Emerg Nurs* 25(2):116-120, 1999.
6. International Liaison Committee on Resuscitation: *ILCOR advisory statements: special resuscitation situations,* Dallas, 1999, American Heart Association.
7. Perry H, Shannon M: Acetaminophen. In Haddad L, Shannon M, Winchester J, editors: *Poisoning and drug overdose,* ed 3, Philadelphia, 1998, WB Saunders.
8. Kao L, Kirk M, Furbee R et al: What is the rate of adverse events after oral N-acetylcysteine administered by the intravenous route to patients with suspected acetaminophen poisoning? *Ann Emerg Med* 42(6):741-750, 2003.
9. Pentel P, Keyler D, Haddad L: Tricyclic antidepressants and selective serotonin reuptake inhibitors. In Haddad L, Shannon M, Winchester J, editors: *Poisoning and drug overdose,* ed 3, Philadelphia, 1998, WB Saunders.
10. McKinney PE, Rasmussen R: Reversal of severe tricyclic antidepressant-induced cardiotoxicity with intravenous hypertonic solution, *Ann Emerg Med* 42(1):20-24, 2003.
11. Diaz J, Lopez A: Voluntary ingestion of organophosphate insecticide by a young farmer, *J Emerg Nurs* 25(4):266-268, 1999.
12. McDeed-Breault C: Toxicological emergencies. In Jordan KS, editor: *Emergency nursing core curriculum,* ed 5, Philadelphia, 2000, WB Saunders.
13. Proehl J, editor: *Emergency nursing procedures,* ed 3, Philadelphia, 2004, WB Saunders.
14. Dribben WH, Porto SM, Jeffords BK: Stability and microbiology of inhalant N-acetylcysteine used as an intravenous solution for the treatment of acetaminophen poisoning, *Ann Emerg Med* 42(1):9-13, 2003.
15. Krenzelok E, Kerr F, Proudfoot AT: Salicylate toxicity. In Haddad L, Shannon M, Winchester J, editors: *Poisoning and drug overdose,* ed 3, Philadelphia, 1998, WB Saunders.
16. Eddleston M, Juszcazk, Buckley N: Does gastric lavage really push poisons beyond the pylorus? A systemic review of the evidence, *Ann Emerg Med* 42(3):359-364, 2003.
17. Kim MJ, McFarland GK, McLane AM: *Pocket guide to nursing diagnoses,* St Louis, 1993, Mosby.
18. *Mosby's drug consult 2005,* St Louis, 2005, Mosby.
19. Albertson TE, Derlet RW, Foulke GE: Superiority of activated charcoal in the treatment of acute toxic ingestions, *Ann Emerg Med* 18:56, 1989.
20. Criddle LM: Toxicologic emergencies. In Newberry L, editor: *Sheehy's emergency nursing: principles and practice,* ed 5, St Louis, 2003, Mosby.

CHAPTER **20**

WOUND MANAGEMENT EMERGENCIES

REVIEW OUTLINE

I. Anatomy of the integumentary system[1]
   A. Largest organ system
   B. Epidermis
      1. Avascular
      2. Composed primarily of epithelial cells
      3. Responsible for regeneration of skin
   C. Dermis
      1. Composed of connective tissue, fibroblasts, microphages, and fat cells
      2. Vascular
      3. Has lymph channels and nerves
   D. Hypodermis
      1. Contains subcutaneous tissues
      2. Contains smooth muscle, the areolar bed, blood vessels, and nerves

II. Function of the skin
   A. Protection
   B. Temperature regulation
   C. Excretion of salt and water
   D. Preservation of body fluids
   E. Production of vitamin D

III. Resolution and repair[2]
   A. Methods of wound healing
      1. Primary intention
      2. Secondary intention
      3. Tertiary intention
   B. Acute inflammation: occurs after tissue injury
      1. Inflammatory exudates: neutrophils, macrophages, bacteria, erythrocytes, and dead cells
      2. Macrophages release angiogenesis factor to attract epithelial factors and vascular endothelial cells
      3. Macrophages also release fibroblast-activating factor to attract fibroblasts
   C. Reconstructive phase, begins 3 to 4 days after injury, may last up to 2 weeks
      1. Granulation: growth of granulation tissue inward from surrounding healthy connective tissue
      2. Epithelialization: growth of epithelial cells into the wound from surrounding healthy tissue
      3. Cellular differentiation
         a. Fibroblasts
         b. Procollagen
         c. Myofibroblasts
      4. Contraction
   D. Maturation phase, about 2 weeks after injury
      1. Remodeling of scar tissue
      2. Development of an avascular scar

IV. Assessment of the integumentary system[1]
   A. History
      1. Mechanism of injury
         a. Direction and amount of force
         b. Associated injuries
         c. What may have been responsible for the injury: weapon, fall, animals, insects, and so on
      2. Time when injury occurred
      3. Risk for contamination
      4. Amount and type of bleeding
      5. Level of pain
      6. Amount of disability
      7. Numbness or tingling distal to the injury
      8. Interventions prior to arrival in the emergency department
   B. Medical history
      1. Chronic illness
         a. Diabetes
         b. Cancer
         c. Peripheral vascular disease
         d. Osteoporosis
         e. Arthritis
         f. Sickle cell anemia
         g. Immunosuppressive diseases
         h. Transplant
      2. History of recent surgery
      3. Medications
         a. Aspirin

b. Immunosuppressants
c. Steroids
d. Anticoagulants

C. Tetanus immunological status
D. Psychosocial history
1. Intentional versus unintentional injury
E. Age-related characteristics[1,3]
1. Pediatric
a. Growth and development
(1) Younger children have thinner skin, more easily injured
(2) Skin changes occur with adolescence
(3) Immunization status
(4) Intentional versus unintentional injury
2. Geriatric
a. Changes in skin texture and turgor, wrinkling, fragility
b. Less skin elasticity
c. Diminished temperature sensation
d. Skin becomes dry, flaky
e. Skin discoloration
(1) Liver spots
(2) Seborrheic keratosis
(3) Cherry angiomas
F. Inspection
1. General appearance of the patient
2. Edema
3. Redness
4. Foreign bodies
5. Extent of damage to the skin
6. Bite or fang marks
G. Neurovascular assessment
1. Flexion
2. Extension
3. Palpation of distal pulses
4. Palpation of skin temperature
5. Capillary refill
6. Sensation
7. Two-point discrimination
8. Neurological function
9. Vascular status

V. Collaborative care of the patient with surface trauma[4-7]
A. Airway, breathing, circulation, disability
B. Control of bleeding
C. Assess for other life-threatening injuries
D. Assess and manage patient's pain
E. Goals of wound care
1. Prevention of infection
2. Promotion of rapid healing
3. Prevention of scarring
F. Forensic considerations
1. Always keep in mind that the wound may be evidence or contain evidence
2. Describe or draw wound in documentation
3. Preserve evidence in appropriate containers
4. Label containers with patient's identification, location where evidence was obtained, and date and time
5. Maintain chain of evidence
G. Wound care
1. Assessment of the wound
2. Assessment of neurovascular status
3. Cleansing of the wound
4. Irrigation of the wound
5. Anesthesia
6. Hair removal: never shave eyebrows
7. Closure
a. Sutures
b. Staples
c. Adhesive tape
d. Tissue adhesives
8. Suture, staple, adhesive tape removal
9. Dressing application
a. Dry dressings
b. Occlusive dressings
c. Semi-occlusive dressings
10. Discharge instructions
H. Medications
1. Tetanus or tetanus immune globulin
2. Anesthesia
3. Sedation and pain management
4. Antibiotics
5. Rabies prophylaxis

VI. Related nursing diagnoses
A. Anxiety
B. Infection, high risk for
C. Fluid volume deficit
D. Knowledge deficit
E. Pain
F. Skin integrity, impaired

VII. Selected wounds
A. Abrasion
B. Abscess
C. Avulsion
D. Amputation
E. Bites
F. Contusion
G. Combination wounds
H. Crush wounds

I. Lacerations
J. Puncture wounds
K. Wound-related infections

The skin, or integumentary system, is the largest organ system of the body. Its functions are protection, regulation of body temperature, primary sensation, excretion of water and salt, preservation of body fluids, and production of vitamin D. Injuries to the skin, or integumentary system, are a common reason for patients to come to the emergency department. There are many sources of these injuries, including thermal or chemical sources, punctures (or penetrating trauma), lacerations, and abrasions.[4] This chapter focuses on some of the most common types of surface trauma seen in the emergency department.

Collaborative care of the patient who has suffered an injury to the integumentary system includes prevention of infection, promotion of rapid healing, and prevention of scarring.[5] Proper cleansing of the wound is important in the prevention of infection.[5] Many types of solutions can be used to cleanse a wound. It is important to be familiar with the solution being used to prevent further injury to the wound. Many solutions should be diluted.[6] In addition, irrigation of the wound with sterile water or normal saline helps to remove debris and contaminants.[6]

Whenever the skin has been penetrated, disrupted, or abraded, the tetanus status of the patient should be evaluated. Recommendations for tetanus prophylaxis are provided by the Centers for Disease Control and Prevention.[7]

The type of wound determines interventions, such as suturing, stapling, or the use of tissue adhesives. The time when the wound occurred and the extent of injury also influence care. Surface injuries older than 6 hours are generally considered contaminated and may not be closed in the same manner as wounds that occurred closer to the time of intervention.

Wounds may result from either intentional or unintentional injury. Observing the pattern of injury will provide the emergency nurse with important information. Wound patterns may indicate the presence of other injuries, and signs of defense or intentional injury may indicate that the patient needs to be protected from himself or others. Finally, wounds may be evidence of a crime.[8] If photographs cannot be obtained, the wound should either be drawn or described on the patient's chart. Any evidence that is collected should be labeled and placed in a paper bag to prevent degradation.

Integumentary injuries are some of the most common problems seen in the emergency department. Early recognition of potential complications and high-quality wound management will prevent further injury to the patient.[9]

REVIEW QUESTIONS

1. Which of the following wounds has the greatest potential for becoming infected?
   A. Eyebrow laceration sustained by a 3-year-old child who fell
   B. Facial abrasion sustained by an 18-year-old bicycle rider who was not wearing a helmet
   C. Avulsion injury from a skin tear sustained by a 30-year-old person
   D. A crushed foot injury sustained by a 25-year-old factory worker

2. Wounds to which area of the body are at greatest risk for infection?
   A. The forearm
   B. The scalp
   C. The digits
   D. The face

3. The most common skin pathogen is:
   A. *Pasteurella multocida*
   B. *Staphylococcus aureus*
   C. *Vibrio vulnificus*
   D. *Pseudomonas aeruginosa*

4. An 81-year-old male cut his finger on a car door. He states that he has not been injured since he was in the military in WW-II. He is unsure as to whether he has ever had a tetanus shot. The wound is jagged but not deep. What type of immunizations would he require?
   A. Human tetanus immune globulin and tetanus toxoid
   B. A tetanus immune globulin vaccination
   C. A diphtheria, tetanus, and pertussis vaccination
   D. No vaccination is necessary at this time

5. Which of the following is an indication for antibiotic therapy in wound management?
   A. A wound that is repaired within 2 hours of injury
   B. An uncomplicated wound without any drainage

C. An open wound over a prosthetic joint
D. A superficial abrasion to the scalp

6. An 18-year-old man comes to the emergency department and states that he was riding his motorcycle and lost control, scraping his legs on the road. Physical examination reveals large abrasions on the tops of both thighs. A wound complication common to abrasions is:
A. A large loss of fluids from the skin
B. Contamination of the wound by debris
C. Wounds open to the bone
D. Loss of sensation to the injured area

7. Contamination of an abrasion by asphalt may leave a patient at risk for:
A. A third-degree burn from the asphalt
B. An anaphylactic reaction to the asphalt
C. Tattooing from retained asphalt
D. Tetanus from the asphalt

8. A 20-year-old woman comes to the triage nurse with a severe laceration on her right wrist. The patient states that she tripped and put her hand through a plate-glass door. The patient has a towel wrapped around the extremity. She is pale and diaphoretic. Her B/P is 90/60, P 120. Initial care of this patient should be based on which of the following nursing diagnoses?
A. Fluid volume deficit related to blood loss from the wrist laceration
B. Skin integrity, impaired, related to the wrist laceration
C. Pain related to the wrist laceration
D. Anxiety related to the potential for disfigurement from the wrist laceration

A 32-year-old male painter comes to the emergency department complaining of pain in his left hand. The patient states that earlier that day he injected his left index finger with his paint gun. Upon evaluation, his left index finger is found to be swollen, pale, and tender to the touch.

9. The extent of this type of high-pressure injection injury depends on all of the following except the:
A. Age of the patient who has been injured
B. Site of the injury
C. Characteristics of the substance injected
D. Amount of the substance injected

10. The emergency nurse should prepare this patient for:
A. Immediate débridement of the injured left finger to determine the extent of damage
B. Immediate infiltration of the injured finger to manage the patient's pain during evaluation
C. Immediate administration of the antidote to the paint substance that has been injected
D. Immediate evaluation and admission to the operating room for surgical evaluation of the wound

11. Which of the following will delay wound healing?
A. Optimal nutrition
B. Adequate hydration
C. Corticosteriods
D. Adequate circulation

12. An injury in which skin is peeled away from an extremity is:
A. Contusion
B. Laceration
C. Abscess
D. Avulsion

13. A 23-year-old male suffered a 1.5-cm–deep laceration to his left forearm when a chunk of rock struck it while he was digging a ditch. The bleeding has been stopped. The initial nursing diagnosis upon which to base this patient's care would be:
A. High risk for infection related to the size and depth of his left forearm laceration
B. Knowledge deficit related to the safety regulations that prevent work injuries
C. Risk for impaired skin integrity related to his left forearm laceration
D. Impaired physical mobility related to his left forearm laceration

14. An example of a vegetative foreign body is:
A. Metal splinter
B. Straight pin
C. Glass shard
D. Wood splinter

15. A method that is effective in decreasing the pain of infiltration when administering a local anesthetic is:
A. Injecting the local anesthetic directly into the wound

B. Cooling the local anesthetic before injection
C. Injecting the local anesthetic into the wound edges
D. Buffering the anesthetic agent with epinephrine

16. A 2-year-old child suffered a 2.5-cm laceration to his head above his right eyebrow after tripping on a rug and striking his head on a coffee table. There was no loss of consciousness. Preparation of this child's wound for closure should include:
A. Shaving his eyebrow to remove hair and decrease the risk of infection
B. Scrubbing the wound with a hard sterile brush and undiluted povidone-iodine
C. Allowing devitalized tissue to remain in the wound to enhance healing
D. Irrigating the wound with normal saline, using a protective shield to decrease splattering

17. The parents have chosen to have the child's wound closed with a tissue adhesive. An advantage of using a tissue adhesive is:
A. Tissue adhesive application causes significantly more pain than suturing
B. A tissue adhesive costs more than suturing a facial wound
C. Use of a tissue adhesive instead of suturing decreases the risk of wound infection
D. Use of tissue adhesives increases the risk of foreign body reactions

18. Tissue adhesives can be used for wound closure for all of the following except:
A. Neck laceration
B. Forehead lacerations
C. Knee laceration
D. Eyebrow laceration

19. Discharge instructions for the patient whose wound has been closed with a tissue adhesive should include:
A. The tissue adhesive should be peeled off in 2 weeks
B. The patient may shower but should not soak the wound
C. No explanation of signs and symptoms of infection
D. Application of a moisturizing cream will enhance healing

20. Sutures placed over a finger joint should be removed:
A. In 3 to 5 days
B. In 4 to 6 days
C. In 10 to 14 days
D. In 7 to 10 days

21. Which of the following used for wound cleansing provides the most effective antimicrobial activity?
A. Baby shampoo
B. Hydrogen peroxide
C. Povidone-iodine
D. Pluronic F-68

22. Fibroblasts secrete:
A. Fibrin
B. Collagen
C. Lymphocytes
D. Giant cells

23. Which of the following topical agents may be used to anesthetize a laceration on the dorsal surface of a finger?
A. Lidocaine, epinephrine, and tetracaine (LET)
B. Tetracaine-adrenaline-cocaine (TAC)
C. Lidocaine (Xylocaine)
D. Lidocaine-prilocaine (EMLA) cream

24. Which of the following is an indication to use surgical tape closures to manage a wound?
A. A laceration over a finger joint
B. A wound too old to be sutured
C. A wound surrounded by hair
D. A wound with irregular edges

25. A 15-year-old male was shot in the arm, suffering a minor wound. When removing the patient's clothes, the emergency nurse should:
A. Cut around the area where the bullet wound is located
B. Cut through the area where the bullet wound is located
C. Allow the patient to throw his bloody clothes away
D. Place the bloody shirt in a plastic patient belongings bag

ANSWERS

1. **D. Assessment.** Crush injuries have the greatest potential to become infected because of the extent of injury and vascular compromise.[9]

2. **C. Assessment.** The digits are most likely to become infected because of decreased blood flow to the peripheral areas of the body. Both the face and scalp are very vascular areas.[9]
3. **B. Assessment.** *Staphylococcus aureus* and streptococci are the most common pathogens on skin.[9]
4. **A. Intervention.** Because the patient is unsure of whether he had a tetanus shot, and it has been longer than 10 years, the patient should receive human tetanus immune globulin 250 to 500 units and tetanus toxoid 0.5 ml; with these, his immunization should be complete.[8]
5. **C. Intervention.** Indications for antibiotic therapy for wound management include delay in wound closure of longer than 3 hours; pus in the wound; wounds contaminated with feces, saliva, or vaginal secretions; prevention of endocarditis; wounds over prosthetic joints; and bites to the hand.[9]
6. **B. Assessment.** Abrasions result from the skin being forced against a hard surface, such as a road. Injury can occur to both the epidermis and the dermis. The resultant injury is similar to a burn. Often, because of the mechanism of injury, these wounds are contaminated.[6]
7. **C. Assessment.** Asphalt is one of the most common contaminants found in an abrasion. If the abrasion is not properly cleansed and débrided, tattooing can occur because of the dark color of the asphalt. This can be especially disfiguring when the abrasion is on the patient's face.[5]
8. **A. Analysis.** Based on the initial assessment of this patient, the triage nurse's care would be based on the nursing diagnosis of fluid volume deficit related to blood loss from the wrist laceration.
9. **A. Assessment.** The extent and the potential complications that may result from a high-pressure injury depend on the site of the injury (usually the nondominant hand), characteristics and amount of the substance injected (accidental epinephrine for a health care provider, paint and paint solvents in industrial settings are very toxic), and the underlying anatomy that will be affected.[10]
10. **D. Intervention.** Management of this type of injury requires immediate recognition of the type of injury it is (high-pressure injection injury) and preparation for further evaluation in the operating room. The wound should not be infiltrated or débrided in the emergency department. Occasionally, the patient may have a toxic reaction to the substance injected, requiring supportive care.[10]
11. **C. Assessment.** Risk factors that will contribute to delayed wound healing include inadequate blood supply, corticosteriod therapy, obesity, diabetes mellitus, poor general health, and anemia.[6,8]
12. **D. Avulsion.** Skin that has been peeled away from an extremity has suffered a severe form of an avulsion known as a *degloving injury.*[6]
13. **A. Analysis.** Initial care of this patient should be based on decreasing the risk for infection. The patient's skin is already impaired.[11,12]
14. **D. Assessment.** Examples of vegetative foreign bodies include thorns or wood. These foreign bodies are highly reactive and sometimes difficult to see.[11,12]
15. **C. Intervention.** Methods to decrease the pain of administering local anesthetic include injecting the local anesthetic into the wound edges, warming the local anesthetic, buffering it with sodium bicarbonate at a 1:10 ratio, slow injection, and pretreatment with a topical anesthetic.[8]
16. **D. Intervention.** Wound preparation includes removing hair to decrease the risk of infection. However, eyebrows should not be shaved, because they may not grow back and they may also be used for exact approximation of wound edges. Wounds should not be scrubbed with a hard brush or an undiluted solution, because additional injury may be caused. Wounds should be irrigated with normal saline. A splashguard should be applied to decrease splattering.[8]
17. **C. Analysis.** Tissue adhesives are associated with a low rate of infection. When compared with suturing, other advantages include decreased pain with application, decreased foreign body reaction, and lower cost.[13]
18. **C. Assessment.** Tissue adhesives are associated with early bond weakness and are not recommended for use over joints or areas with high mobility. Tissue adhesives can become ineffective in moist or wet environments.[13]
19. **B. Intervention.** Discharge instructions after application of tissue adhesives should include:
    - Avoid getting the area wet for a prolonged period, or applying creams or ointments that may loosen the adhesive
    - The patient may shower

- Signs and symptoms of wound infection
- Leave the tissue adhesive alone, because it will fall off naturally within 2 weeks of application[13,14]

20. **D. Intervention.** Sutures placed over a joint should be removed 7 to 10 days after placement.[14]
21. **C. Intervention.** Hydrogen peroxide is a weak disinfectant and ineffective against anaerobic organisms. Baby shampoo can be used to cleanse a wound, but it has no antimicrobial activity. Pluronic F-68 (Shur Clens) has no antimicrobial activity but can be used to cleanse open wounds and eyes. Povidone-iodine provides antimicrobial activity against gram-positive and gram-negative organisms, fungi, and viruses.[14]
22. **B. Assessment.** Fibroblasts secrete and synthesize collagen, which is the material of tissue repair.[2]
23. **C. Intervention.** LET, TAC and EMLA are topical anesthetics. LET should not be used on digits because of the epinephrine, TAC is not recommended for use any more, and EMLA cream should not be applied to open skin. The most commonly used anesthetic is lidocaine.[14]
24. **B. Assessment.** Some of the indications for surgical tape closures include:[14]
    - To provide additional support to a sutured wound or one from which sutures have been removed
    - To approximate wound edges on a wound too old to suture
    - To hold skin flaps and grafts in place
    - To approximate wounds in patients on long-term steroid use whose skin is compromised
25. **A. Intervention.** To preserve evidence, the emergency nurse should cut around the area where the bullet entered the patient. Clothing should be collected in a paper bag.[14]

REFERENCES

1. Bickley L: *Bates guide to physical examination and history taking,* ed 8, Philadelphia, 2002, Lippincott.
2. McCance KL, Huether S: *Pathophysiology: the biologic basis for disease in adults and children,* St Louis, 2002, Mosby.
3. Engel J: *Pediatric assessment,* St Louis, 1993, Mosby.
4. Daly W, Munier-Sham J: Burns. In Kelley S, editor: *Pediatric emergency nursing,* Norwalk, 1994, Appleton & Lange.
5. Hackley L: Surface trauma. In Kitt S, Selfridge-Thomas J, Proehl J et al, editors: *Emergency nursing: a physiologic and clinical perspective,* Philadelphia, 1995, WB Saunders.
6. Trott A: *Wounds and lacerations: emergency care and closure,* ed 2, St Louis, 1998, Mosby.
7. Centers for Disease Control and Prevention: Tetanus surveillance-United States 1995-1997, *MMWR* 47:1-13, 1998.
8. Herman M, Newberry L: Wound management. In Newberry L, editor: *Sheehy's emergency nursing: principles and practice,* ed 5, St Louis, 2003, Mosby.
9. Harrahill M: Patterns of sharp force injury, *J Emerg Nurs* 18:355-356, 1992.
10. Stiles N: High-pressure injection injury of the hand: a surgical emergency, *J Emerg Nurs* 20:351-354, 1994.
11. Eron L: Antimicrobial wound management in the emergency department: an educational supplement, *J Emerg Nurs* 17(1):189-195, 1999.
12. Mitchell B: Wound management emergencies. In Jordan KS, editor: *Emergency nursing core curriculum,* ed 5, Philadelphia, 2000, WB Saunders.
13. King M, Kinney A: Tissue adhesives: a new method of wound repair, *Nurs Pract* 24(10):66-74, 1999.
14. Proehl J, editor: *Emergency nursing procedures,* Philadelphia, 2004, WB Saunders.

CHAPTER 21

Disaster Preparedness and Management

REVIEW OUTLINE

I. General overview
   A. Disaster: any situation that overwhelms the existing resources of an institution, community, state, or nation[1]
   B. Types of disaster
      1. Internal: institutional structure impaired; loss of electrical power as the result of a storm, floods, fire, terrorist activity; may require outside responders to assist
      2. External: takes place outside of the hospital, but has an impact on the hospital's operations; earthquake, flood, tornado, terrorist activity
   C. Emergency operations planning[1,2]
      1. Organized disaster committee
      2. Organized plan
         a. Authority: who or what activates the disaster plan
         b. Preestablished hospital operations centers
         c. Communication plan
         d. Coordination of patient care
         e. Security
         f. Deactivation
         g. Debriefing
   D. Effects of disasters
      1. Loss of life
      2. Physical injuries
      3. Psychological trauma
      4. Property damage
      5. Environmental destruction
   E. National-level and state-level interfaces
      1. Federal Emergency Management Agency: the central point of contact in the federal government for a variety of emergency management activities with which hospitals may need to interact
      2. National Disaster Medical System: federal-level system functioning to respond to major catastrophic disasters
      3. Joint Commission on the Accreditation of Healthcare Organizations (JCAHO) requirements: hospitals must devise, implement, and practice a hospital-wide disaster plan
   F. Key components of emergency preparedness and emergency operations
      1. Command center
      2. Administrative operations center
      3. Medical operations center
      4. Nursing operations center
      5. Operating room operations center
      6. Personnel operations center
      7. Security operations center
      8. Emergency department operations center
      9. Public relations operations center
   G. Emergency disaster response
      1. Patient care
         a. Personal protective equipment (PPE)
            (1) Level A: self-contained breathing apparatus (SCBA) and vapor protective, fully encapsulated chemical-resistant suit
            (2) Level B: SCBA or positive pressure–supplied air respirator; hooded, splash-protective chemical-resistant suit
            (3) Level C: air-purifying respirator and hooded, splash-protective chemical-resistant suit
            (4) Level D: No respiratory equipment or protective equipment
         b. Receiving, triaging, distributing
         c. Proper use of resources and facility
         d. Documenting care
         e. Evaluating care

2. Communication
   a. Internal
   b. External
   c. Media
   d. Emergency operations center
3. Resources
   a. Personnel
   b. Supplies
   c. Security
   d. Coordination
   e. Hospital resources
   f. Community resources
4. Security, safety
   a. Traffic control
   b. Controlled access to department
5. Coordination
   a. Local, state, federal
   b. Intradepartmental
   c. Interdepartmental
   d. Emergency medical services community
   e. Health care community
6. Documentation
   a. Medical record
   b. Disaster tags: METTAG, the universal triage tag
   c. Paper flow

H. Deactivation
1. Communication
2. Dispersal of additional resources
3. Community notification

I. Critical incident stress management (CISM)
1. Immediate reactions
2. Delayed reactions
3. Effect on care providers and community

II. Causes of disasters

A. Weapons of mass destruction and effect: nuclear, biological, chemical
1. Radiation
2. Routine industrial chemicals
3. Vesicants
4. Riot control agents
5. Nerve agents
   a. Cyanide
6. Biological agents
   a. Botulin
   b. Ricin
   c. Staphylococcal enterotoxin B
7. Viral agents
   a. Smallpox
8. Toxins

B. Terrorist activities

C. Nature: earthquakes, tornado, flood, and so on

III. Disaster preparedness

A. Philosophy related to disaster preparation and response

B. Disaster drills and exercises

C. Critique and education

IV. Postdisaster care

A. Acute stressors
1. Noise
2. Decreased oxygen
3. Malnutrition
4. Prolonged exertion
5. Fear

B. Physiological responses
1. Fight-or-flight syndrome
2. Increased catabolism of proteins
3. Gluconeogenesis leading to hyperglycemia
4. Decreased lymphocytes and immune response
5. Increased heart rate and blood pressure

C. Posttraumatic stress response
1. Causes
   a. Involvement in a disaster of human origin
   b. Severe motor vehicle crash
   c. Diagnosed with a life-threatening illness
   d. Victim of a violent crime
   e. Torture
2. Symptoms
   a. Reexperiencing
      (1) Nightmares
      (2) Flashbacks
      (3) Muscle tremors
   b. Avoidance numbing
      (1) Isolation
      (2) Moodiness
      (3) Depression
   c. Increased arousal
      (1) Anxiety
      (2) Restlessness
      (3) Sleep disturbances
3. Treatment
   a. Education
   b. Prevention
   c. CISM
   d. Therapy
   e. Medication

A disaster has been defined as any situation, natural or of human origin, that overwhelms an institution, community, state, or even a nation, so that it is incapable of responding with existing resources.[1,2] Over the years, we have witnessed a variety of disasters, ranging from earthquakes and floods to terrorist attacks that include bombings and biological weapons. The terrorist acts of 2001 have prompted all state, local, and community agencies to evaluate their disaster plans. In many cases, the emergency department is the initial place where victims will be transported. Emergency operations planning and disaster preparedness are integral pieces of emergency care.

The influx of casualties from a disaster can greatly tax or overwhelm the emergency department. To prevent overpowering the system, a plan is necessary to deal with the resultant increase in patient volume, increased workload, and the increased need for supplies and other resources. An emergency operations plan is an obligatory component of emergency department clinical operations and management.[2,4]

Hospitals are required by the JCAHO to prepare for disaster situations. The JCAHO requires hospitals to have a documented plan for the environment of care that (1) addresses emergency preparedness, (2) has an orientation and education component, (3) establishes performance standards to measure its effectiveness on the environment of care, and (4) ensures the organization conducts emergency drills to test the responsiveness to emergency situations[3] (see Environment of Care and Human Resource Standards in JCAHO Manual).[4]

The emergency department disaster preparedness plan must include detailed guidelines that collaborate with both the hospital and the community plans. Key components of the disaster plan include patient care, communication, resources, safety or security, coordination, and documentation. Recent attention has also been focused on both national and international response to disasters, particularly those caused by chemical or biological weapons.[5]

Because of an increase in terrorist activities, greater risks for disaster situations exist in the world today. Emergency department personnel must be familiar with the disaster plan and know their role in executing the plan, when needed. They also need to understand the stages of a disaster so they can better understand what has happened to patients before their arrival in the emergency department and what they will likely experience after treatment and admission to the hospital or discharge from the hospital. They need to be able to assess the impact of a disaster upon themselves, their co-workers, and the rescue personnel and assist them in coping with the effects of the disaster experience.

The role of the emergency department nurse in disaster preparedness and management involves the following areas: (1) development and practice of the plan, (2) implementation of the plan, (3) development of an emergency operations center to serve as a communications link with the hospital and external environment, (4) triage activities, (5) secondary triage, (6) stabilization, and (7) CISM. Emergency nurses are well equipped for disaster preparedness and management because of their rapid assessment and triage skills, crisis management abilities, and links with community resource persons.

Of specific concern is knowing how to handle the effects of weapons of mass destruction that include chemical, biological, and radiation hazards. Donning and removing PPE, using proper decontamination procedures, and evaluating the disaster drills in which one participates are all important to the efficient functioning of the staff during a real situation. Practice helps keep the staff and patients safe and makes for a smoother operation when a real disaster occurs.

The emergency department plan must provide for the efficient management of incoming casualties and must include charge nurse responsibilities, disposition of patients currently in the department, preparation of triage site, patient flow, extent of initial and ongoing treatment, alternative patient care areas, and staffing and supply needs.

Sanford describes the eight principles of disaster management as follows: (1) preventing the occurrence of a disaster, (2) minimizing the number of casualties, (3) rescuing, (4) providing first aid, (5) evacuating the injured, (6) providing definitive care, (7) facilitating reconstruction, and (8) recovery.[6] Whether in the prehospital care arena or in the emergency department, the emergency nurse is one of the best prepared to handle disaster situations. It is important, however, for the nurse to be aware of the differences in triage priorities "in the field" versus in the emergency department.

Comprehensive disaster preparedness incorporates the community, the hospital, the emergency department, and the local, state, and federal domains. Disaster preparedness and management requires careful planning, frequent practice, critiques, and ongoing improvement and revisions. The emergency nurse must be knowledgeable about these disaster systems and be in a constant state of readiness to quickly implement and execute the plan.

REVIEW QUESTIONS

There has been an explosion at a chemical plant in an inner city area. Employees, people passing by in cars, and people in nearby houses and buildings have been injured. The number of injured is unknown. The emergency nurse has been called to assist with field triage and, on arrival, finds the following victims:

- Patient #1: 28-year-old man in acute respiratory distress who is cyanotic and diaphoretic. Vital signs are B/P 70/40, P 140, and R 40 and labored. There is bruising on the left side of his chest.
- Patient #2: 64-year-old man in cardiac arrest with dilated and fixed pupils. There is no pulse or respiration. There are no physical signs of injury.
- Patient #3: 30-year-old pregnant woman who is full term and in active labor, with contractions every 5 minutes. This is her fourth child. She is upset and crying. There are no physical signs of injury.
- Patient #4: 35-year-old woman with head, face, and leg lacerations with bleeding. She is incoherent. Her vital signs are B/P 96/60, P 110, and R 30.
- Patient #5: 60-year-old man with a head laceration who is unresponsive to verbal or painful stimuli. Vital signs are B/P 100/70, P 96, R 24.

1. Which patient should be cared for first?
A. Patient #1
B. Patient #2
C. Patient #3
D. Patient #4

2. The most obvious nursing diagnosis for patient #1 in this scenario is:
A. Airway clearance, ineffective
B. Tissue perfusion, altered
C. Gas exchange, impaired
D. Cardiac output, decreased

3. Which patient in this scenario should receive last priority for treatment?
A. Patient #2
B. Patient #3
C. Patient #4
D. Patient #5

4. Disaster management principles include:
A. Maximize the number of casualties
B. Prevent occurrence of a disaster
C. Treating all injured at the scene
D. Only one form of communication

5. The nurse who enters an internal disaster scene begins an evaluation to control the disaster. The first and foremost step for the emergency nurse to take is to:
A. Take photographs of the situation so that mechanism of injury can be identified
B. Tell everyone else to stand back while the nurse cares for the victims
C. Ensure that the area where the disaster occurred is safe before entering
D. Notify the National Disaster Management Services before entering

6. The emergency nurse receives a patient who has been exposed to radiation and admits him in the decontamination room. The largest part of the decontamination procedure is accomplished by:
A. Removing the patient's clothing and placing it in a sealed container
B. Washing the patient with soap and water before removing clothing
C. Washing the patient with water only after removing the clothes
D. Using a specific antidote for decontaminating radiation materials

7. The initial care of the patient who has suffered a radiation exposure includes:
A. Preventing further exposure to the radiation
B. Management of life-threatening emergencies
C. Notifying the patient's family about the exposure
D. Calling the state health and safety regulatory agency immediately

8. Which of the following PPE should a health care provider wear when exposed to a Level A toxic substance?
A. A cloth shirt and pants and no respiratory protection
B. A work uniform and no respiratory protection until the substance has been identified

C. Chemical-resistant clothing and full-face air-purifying canister
D. Fully encapsulating suit and an SCBA

9. The primary method of decontamination for most chemical exposures is:
A. Application of a specific antidote to the affected area
B. Placement in a hyperbaric chamber for oxygenation
C. Administration of an aerosolized specific antidote
D. Showering with large quantities of water to dilute the agent

10. A 23-year-old patient arrives from a construction site cave-in in critical condition. Which triage tag would indicate his condition to the triage nurse?
A. Yellow tag
B. Red tag
C. Green tag
D. Black tag

11. Which of the following bacterial agents has been used in military and civilian populations?
A. Smallpox
B. Sarin
C. Cyanide
D. Anthrax

12. The critique following a disaster exercise should include:
A. Patient triage and tracking
B. Security operations
C. Deactivation of the disaster
D. All of the above

13. Following a disaster, the staff may need to deal with their feelings about the situation and the patients they cared for. This could best be accomplished by:
A. Calling the chaplain to come to the emergency department and conduct a debriefing
B. Asking the staff to talk openly in a group session with the nurse manager
C. Calling the CISM team to conduct a defusing
D. Asking a physician to prescribe sleeping medication for all personnel who request it

14. The most important tool to have in the emergency department to serve as a first line of defense for disasters is:
A. A well-organized disaster plan, which has been rehearsed
B. A medical director who has disaster medicine experience
C. Red Cross nurse on staff who works with the medical assistance team
D. Alarm system that connects to the local fire department

15. JCAHO requires:
A. All hospitals experience one real disaster a year in order to be accredited
B. All hospitals schedule a disaster drill each year in order to remain accredited
C. All hospitals experience two drills (one with patients) or actual events each year
D. That hospitals do not have to have any drills if they feel qualified to handle them

16. A 16-year-old female was involved in a motor vehicle collision that killed several of her friends. Her mother notices that she will not talk about the event, which occurred about 3 months ago, and she spends a great deal of time in her room. The daughter is exhibiting signs of:
A. Chronic posttraumatic stress response
B. An acute stress response
C. Acute posttraumatic stress response
D. Normal behavior after the loss of a friend

17. What other conditions may be associated with posttraumatic stress disorder?
A. Depression
B. Panic disorder
C. Substance abuse
D. All of the above

18. Which of the following steps should be followed in order to ensure appropriate use of PPE?
A. Universal sizes should be stored in the emergency department, because everyone can use the same size in an emergency
B. All equipment should be inspected for holes or other defects before being used by emergency department personnel
C. Orientation to each piece of equipment is not necessary, because its use is self-

explanatory and easy to use no matter what the level of training

D. Only tight-fitting masks should be used as respirators in order to protect emergency department personnel in an emergency

19. Standard hospital-approved disinfectants are effective for decontaminating patients exposed to which of the following biological agents?

A. Q-fever
B. Glanders
C. Cholera
D. All of the above

20. When using a color-coded triage system, a minimally injured patient may be classified as which color?

A. Black
B. Green
C. Yellow
D. Red

ANSWERS

1. **A. Assessment.** Always remember the airway, breathing, circulation rule and that field triage is geared toward saving the greatest number of lives using the simplest measures possible. Triage in the emergency department is focused on doing the greatest good for the greatest number. For patient #1, an airway needs to be established or cleared; the patient then needs to be transported to the emergency department.[1,2,7]
2. **A. Analysis.** The patient's airway is not patent. The airway must be opened so that breathing and circulation can be assessed further.[1]
3. **A. Assessment.** The life of this patient could not be saved "simply" or in a short time. Other patients whose lives might be saved would have to wait if this patient were dealt with first.[2,4-6]
4. **B. Assessment.** The principles of disaster management include prevent disasters, minimize casualties, prevent further casualties, rescue the injured, provide first aid, evacuate the injured, provide definitive care, and facilitate recovery.[2]
5. **C. Intervention.** The nurse who goes to a disaster situation should do a three-step evaluation of (1) the safety of the area, (2) the organization of the disaster system, and (3) the provision of the most appropriate patient care.[1]
6. **A. Intervention.** Ninety to ninety-five percent of the decontamination procedure is accomplished by removing the patient's clothing. The clothing is placed in bags, tagged, and removed to a remote section of the contaminated area, to be disposed of later by qualified personnel. The remaining decontamination is accomplished by washing the patient with soap and water.[1,8]
7. **B. Intervention.** Initial treatment of the patient who has been exposed to radiation is the management of any life-threatening emergencies, management of the patient's ABCs, and decontamination.[1]
8. **D. Intervention.** PPE for a Level A toxic exposure should include an SCBA and a fully encapsulating chemical-resistant suit.[9]
9. **D. Intervention.** An effective method of decontamination for most chemical exposures consists of showering with large quantities of water.[1]
10. **B. Assessment.** A colored tag system should be used to identify patient priority. One of the most common is based on red: critical condition, yellow: serious condition, green: stable condition, and black: dead.[5]
11. **D. Assessment.** Anthrax, or *Bacillus anthracis,* is a bacterial agent that has been used against both military and civilian populations.[6]
12. **D. Evaluation.** Critique of a disaster exercise should include emergency department operations, emergency department staff, communications, security operations, patient management and tracking, and deactivation.[1]
13. **C. Intervention.** The debriefing team is best prepared to handle this situation. Team members remain objective and are most helpful to the staff, enabling them to discuss their feelings and providing a tool to prevent and alleviate symptoms caused by the event. This offers immediate crisis intervention, helping the staff to return to their previous level of functioning.[1,2,6]
14. **A. Evaluation.** A well-defined disaster plan that has been practiced and critiqued will provide emergency nurses with guidelines for dealing with real disaster situations.[6]
15. **C. Intervention.** The JCAHO requires that hospitals have two drills (one with patients) or actual events each year.[1]
16. **C. Assessment.** The child is experiencing signs of acute posttraumatic stress response. Symptoms that occur within 3 months of the incident are considered acute. These include isolation and depression. Symptoms that persist longer than 3 months are considered chronic, and over 6 months, delayed.[10]

17. **D. Assessment.** Posttraumatic stress disorder may be associated with major depression, panic disorder, substance abuse, and generalized anxiety disorder.[10]
18. **B. Intervention.** All equipment should be inspected for holes or other defects on a routine basis. All staff should be trained about how to use the equipment and what chemicals that they might have to protect against. Hoods may be used instead of tight-fitting respirators. A tank may be too large for an employee of small stature. Hoods may be more popular and more comfortable.[9]
19. **D. Intervention.** Standard hospital-approved disinfectants are effective when treating patients contaminated by any of these biological agents.[2]
20. **B. Assessment.** Generally green indicates a minimally injured patient or "walking wounded."[2]

REFERENCES

1. Klein J: Disaster preparedness/disaster management. In Jordan KS, editor: *Emergency nursing core curriculum,* ed 5, Philadelphia, 2000, WB Saunders.
2. O'Shields M: Emergency operations preparedness. In Newberry L, editor: *Emergency nursing principles and practice,* ed 5, St Louis, 2003, Mosby.
3. Newberry L: *Practical suggestions for helping nurses handle mass casualties,* Disaster Management and Response, September 2002.
4. Joint Commission on Accreditation of Healthcare Organizations: *Accreditation manual,* Oakwood, IL, 2000, Joint Commission on Accreditation of Healthcare Organizations.
5. Institute of Medicine and Board on Environmental Studies and Toxicology: National Research Council: *Chemical and biological terrorism. Research and development to improve civilian medical response,* Washington, DC, 1999, National Academy Press.
6. Elliot D, Cushing B: Mass casualty incidents. In Maull K, Rodriguez A, Wiles C, editors: *Complications in trauma and critical care,* Philadelphia, 1996, WB Saunders.
7. Moatman D, Alson R, Baldwin J et al: Multicasualty incidents and triage. In Campbell J, editor: *Basic trauma life support,* ed 5, Upper Saddle River, NJ, 2004, Brady Prentice Hall Health.
8. Proper C, Solotkin K: One urban hospital's experience with false anthrax exposure disaster response, *J Emerg Nurs* 25(6):501-504, 1999.
9. Lehmann J: *Considerations for selecting personal protective equipment for hazardous materials decontamination,* Disaster Management and Response, September, 2002.
10. Mitchell A, Sakraida T, Karneg K: *Overview of post-traumatic stress,* Disaster Management and Response, September 2002.

ADDITIONAL READINGS

Lanros N: *Assessment and intervention in emergency nursing,* ed 2, Bowie, MD, 1983, Robert J. Brady.

National Council on Radiation Protection and Measurements: Management of persons accidentally contaminated with radionuclides, Rep No 65, Bethesda, MD, 1985, US Government Printing Office.

Wash M: *Accident and emergency nursing: a new approach,* ed 2, Oxford, 1990, Honeymoon Medical.

CHAPTER 22

BIOLOGICAL AND HAZMAT RESPONSE

REVIEW OUTLINE

I. Sources of biological and hazmat emergencies
   A. Biological weapons[1]
      1. One of the first reported uses of biological warfare was sixth century BC when a well was poisoned with rye ergot
      2. Corpses infected with plague were used as weapons during the fourteenth century in Crimea, which may have been the seed of the Black Death in Europe
      3. Fifteenth- and eighteenth-century European explorers spread smallpox to native populations in North and South America
      4. Twentieth-century use of biological warfare in both the first and second world wars using plague and anthrax bacteria
      5. Other twentieth-century use includes ricin assassination, "yellow rain" in Southeast Asia and Iraq
   B. World infections
      1. Human immunodeficiency virus
      2. Severe acute respiratory syndrome
      3. Flu viruses
      4. Ebola virus
      5. Others still unknown
   C. Bacterial agents
      1. Anthrax
      2. Brucellosis
      3. Glanders and melioidosis
      4. Plague
      5. Q-fever
      6. Tularemia
   D. Viral agents
      1. Smallpox
      2. Venezuelan equine encephalitis
      3. Viral hemorrhagic fevers
   E. Biological toxins
      1. Botulin
      2. Ricin
      3. Staphylococcal enterotoxin B
      4. T-2 mycotoxins
   F. Chemical agents
      1. Blistering agents
         a. Sulfur mustard
      2. Nerve agent
         a. Sarin
         b. Tabun
         c. VX
      3. Phosgene
      4. Cyanide
   G. Hazmat: a material is categorized as hazardous if it poses a risk to people, property, or the environment when it is not properly controlled
      1. Explosives
      2. Gases
         a. Flammable gases
         b. Nonflammable gases
         c. Gases toxic by inhalation
         d. Corrosive gases
      3. Flammable liquids
      4. Flammable solids
         a. Spontaneously combustible solids
         b. Materials that are dangerous when wet
      5. Oxidizers and organic peroxides
      6. Toxic substances and infectious substances
      7. Radioactive materials
      8. Corrosive materials
         a. Sulfuric acid
         b. Nitric acid
         c. Hydrochloric acid
         d. Phosphoric acid
         e. Perchloric acid
         f. Hydrofluoric acid
         g. Caustic soda
      9. Miscellaneous dangerous goods

II. Providers[2]
   A. Awareness
      1. Recognition
      2. Initial scene safety
      3. Notification of appropriate responders

- B. Operations
  1. Identification of the problem
  2. Isolation
  3. Prevention of individual contamination
- C. Technician
  1. Required to wear personal protective equipment (PPE)
  2. Works directly with the contaminated patients
- D. Specialist: thoroughly familiar with the toxin or hazardous material, may or may not be trained to care for victims
- E. Advanced hazmat life support level
  1. Nurses, paramedics, physicians, other health care professionals
  2. Trained in the recognition of signs and symptoms of exposure
  3. Protection of hazmat team members primary responsibility
- F. Medical control
- G. Incident command system

III. Recognition[1,2]

- A. Hazmat
  1. Crash of a vehicle carrying a hazardous substance
  2. Location of the incident, such as a chemical plant
  3. Unexplained multiple casualties
- B. Distinguishing between natural and intentional disease outbreaks[1]
  1. Epidemiological investigation
     - a. Affected population
     - b. Possible routes of exposure
     - c. Signs and symptoms of the disease
     - d. Laboratory studies
     - e. Identification of causative agents
  2. Biological or terrorist attack clues
     - a. Large similar population affected
     - b. More severe cases than usually expected from a particular bacteria or virus
     - c. Unusual route of exposure
     - d. Disease unusual for a given geographical area
     - e. Disease unusual for a specific age group
     - f. Higher concentration of a disease in specific areas, such as in an office building
     - g. Disease outbreaks occurring in noncontiguous areas
     - h. Intelligence about an impending attack

IV. Zones

- A. Hot zone
  1. Exclusion or restricted zone
  2. Red zone
- B. Warm zone
  1. Decontamination or contamination reduction zone
  2. Yellow zone
- C. Cold zone
  1. Support zone
  2. Green zone

V. Decontamination[3]

- A. PPE
  1. Level A: Completely encapsulating chemical-resistant suit and self-contained breathing apparatus (SCBA)
  2. Level B: Encapsulating suit with SCBA
  3. Level C: Splash suit and air-purifying respirator
  4. Level D: Work clothes including standard precautions
- B. Scene safety for prehospital care providers
  1. Aircraft land upwind from scene
  2. Follow direction of scene commander
  3. Patient decontamination
- C. Decontamination
  1. Decontamination rooms
  2. Portable decontamination systems
- D. Decontamination procedures
  1. Removal of contaminated clothing
  2. Showering or hosing off with water
  3. Disposal of wastewater
  4. Management for specific chemicals or agents
  5. Notification of appropriate agencies
- E. Poisoning management paradigm[2]
  1. A: alter absorption, administer antidote
  2. B: basic patient assessment and critical interventions
  3. C: change catabolism
  4. D: distributing them differently
  5. E: enhance elimination

REVIEW QUESTIONS

1. The first step in the treatment of a patient who has been exposed to a hazardous substance is:

A. Assess the patient's airway and breathing and perform any required critical interventions

B. Decontaminate the patient by placement either in a negative-pressure room or in a decontamination shower

C. Establish a diagnosis so that appropriate toxins can be obtained from the government with which to treat the patient
D. Ensure that staff who will be caring for the patient are wearing the appropriate PPE

2. An exposure to a corrosive toxin will cause:
A. Sleepiness to the point of stupor when inhaled
B. Stimulation of excessive acetylcholine accumulation
C. Chemical burns of any exposed area such as the skin
D. Displacement of oxygen from the ambient atmosphere

3. Which of the following biological agents may not be transmitted from one human to another?
A. Brucellosis
B. Smallpox
C. Plague
D. Botulism

4. Which of the following may be an indication that a disease outbreak may be related to a terrorist attack?
A. A disease that fails to respond to standard therapy such as antibiotics
B. An outbreak of the same disease at a college or office building
C. Disease transmitted by a vector not native to the affected area
D. A usual route of exposure for a pathogen such as droplet contact

5. Two students come to the triage area stating that they have been exposed to an acid in their chemistry class. They have burns on both upper extremities and obvious pitted areas on their pants. The triage nurse should:
A. Tell the students to return to their classroom until the type of acid has been identified
B. Call the local authorities and wait for directions in order to provide the appropriate decontamination
C. Have the students remove their clothes and shower in the decontamination room
D. Have the students remove their clothes and manage their burns with antibiotic ointment

6. A disadvantage of Level D PPE is:
A. It is expensive and requires training for proper use
B. Its dependence on an air line or limited air supply
C. It offers no protection against chemical or other agents
D. It can cause heat or other physical stresses when worn

7. First responders to the scene of an incident must have all of the following except:
A. Knowledge about basic hazards and risk assessment techniques
B. Ability to make all operational decisions related to the incident
C. Knowledge about how to implement basic decontamination procedures
D. Proper PPE and knowledge of its use

8. Which of the following biological agents requires the patient to be placed in a negative-pressure room during treatment in the emergency department?
A. Anthrax
B. Smallpox
C. Plague
D. Q-fever

9. Decontamination of patients should take place in the:
A. Hot zone
B. Cold zone
C. Support zone
D. Warm zone

10. Which of the following antibiotics is recommended as part of the management regimen for anthrax?
A. Ciprofloxacin 400 mg IV every 12 hours
B. Penicillin 2 million units every 2 hours
C. Erythromycin 500 mg orally every 12 hours
D. Gentamicin 120 mg orally every 12 hours

ANSWERS

1. **D. Intervention.** The first step in the treatment of a patient who is contaminated is for health care providers to protect themselves by applying the appropriate PPE.[1-3]
2. **C. Assessment.** Exposure to a corrosive agent will cause chemical burns to the exposed parts of the body. When hydrocarbons are inhaled, they will cause sleepiness to the point of stupor and coma; excessive acetylcholine accumulation occurs with exposure to organophosphate pesticides or nerve agents; and displacement of

ambient oxygen will occur with inhalation of an asphyxiant such as carbon monoxide, methane, or propane.[2]

3. **D. Assessment.** Human-to-human transmission does not occur with botulism. Brucellosis has been transmitted by exposure to infected tissue or sexual contact but not through routine patient care. Smallpox is spread through respiratory droplets or direct contact with contaminated clothing. Plague is spread through droplet contamination.[3]
4. **A. Assessment.** Epidemiological clues that may indicate a biological or terrorist attack include:
   - More severe disease than is usually expected for a specific pathogen, or a pathogen that does not respond to usual therapies such as antibiotics
   - A large epidemic with a similar disease or syndrome
   - Many cases of unexplained diseases or deaths
   - A single case of a disease caused by an uncommon agent such as smallpox
   - A disease outbreak occurring in multiple and different places[1]
5. **C. Intervention.** The students should remove all clothing and shower in the decontamination room or area, so that the wastewater can be contained appropriately. Even though the exact substance is not known, decontamination usually can be accomplished with water.[3]
6. **C. Assessment.** Level D PPE consists of work clothes and the use of standard precautions, which will allow for increased mobility and decreased physical stresses and is less expensive, but offers no protection against chemical or other agents.[4]
7. **B. Analysis.** The person responsible for decision making is the scene incident commander. Many health care facilities refer to this person as the *decontamination officer.* This leader will oversee the entire operation, including selecting the appropriate PPE for the particular incident.[4]
8. **B. Analysis.** Most biological agents that have been used in terrorist attacks require standard precautions or droplet precautions. However, smallpox requires that the patient be placed in a negative-pressure room. All linen should be autoclaved. Infectious waste should be placed in biohazard bags and autoclaved before incineration.[3]
9. **D. Intervention.** Patient decontamination should take place within the warm zone. There are several names for these zones, including the hot zone or red zone. The hot zone is where there is imminent danger of exposure, and only appropriately trained and equipped personnel should be in this zone. The warm zone or yellow zone, decontamination zone, or contamination reduction zone is where decontamination takes place. In the warm zone, contaminated personal and equipment must remain. Finally, the cold zone, green or support zone, is where personnel ready to receive the patients are staged.[2]
10. **A. Intervention.** Even though anthrax has been managed successfully with intravenous penicillin, the military currently recommends ciprofloxacin until the strain of anthrax that has infected the patient demonstrates sensitivity to penicillin.[1] The Centers for Disease Control and Prevention recommends ciprofloxacin or doxycycline and one or two additional antibiotics. Current recommendations from the CDC can be found at www.cdc.gov.

REFERENCES

1. Kortepeter M, editor: *USAMRIID's medical management of biological casualties handbook,* Fort Detrick, MD, 2001, Operational Medicine Division.
2. Association of Air Medical Services: *Guidelines for air medical crew education,* Dubuque, IA, 2004, Kendall/Hunt.
3. Newberry L, editor: *Sheehy's emergency nursing,* ed 5, St Louis, 2003, Mosby.
4. Hick J, Hanfling D, Burstein J et al: Protective equipment for health care facility decontamination personnel: regulations, risks, and recommendations, *Ann Emerg Med* 42(3):370-380, 2003.

CHAPTER **23**

Legal and Ethical Issues in Emergency and Transport Nursing

REVIEW OUTLINE

I. Legal issues in emergency and transport nursing
  A. General overview
    1. Hospital's duty to provide care[1]
      a. *Wilmington General Hospital v Manlove* (1961): the hospital's duty to provide care outweighs the hospital's internal policies
      b. Hill-Burton Act (1946): if the hospital receives federal funds under this act, it must provide care regardless of the patient's ability to pay or the nature of the initial complaint
    2. Nurse's duty to provide care
      a. State nurse practice act: duty, responsibility, and scope of practice defined
      b. Hospital employment policies: obligation to follow directions and fulfill duties
    3. Sources of law[2]
      a. Constitutional: determines the validity of both the statutory decision and the case law within the provisions of the fourth, fifth, and fourteenth constitutional amendments
      b. Statutory: law enacted by a legislative body
      c. Regulatory: regulations developed by an official under empowerment by statutory law
      d. Case, common: interpretation by the courts on statutes, administrative rules, and common law
      e. Contract: written, oral, or implied agreement between parties
      f. Administrative: laws created by administrative agencies through power delegated to them by state or federal legislature
    4. Types of law
      a. Civil law: addresses injury to an individual or the individual's property
      b. Criminal law: addresses injury to society
    5. General legal terms, concepts
      a. Standards of care
        (1) Provide guidelines
        (2) Ordinary, reasonable, prudent person with like or similar training in like or similar circumstances
      b. Negligence: omission or commission of an act that should or should not have been performed coupled with unreasonableness or imprudence on the part of the doer
        (1) Standard
        (2) Deviation from standard
        (3) Elements of negligence (nonintentional tort)
      c. Malpractice: negligence on the part of a professional when his or her misconduct, lack of skill, omission, or misjudgment in the commission of duty causes harm to the person or property of the recipient of services
      d. Tort: unintentional negligent act on the person of another that results in injury to that person
    6. Assault: threat to do harm to another without the actual performance of that threatened harm
    7. Battery: actual touching of another person without the person's consent
    8. False imprisonment: restriction of a person's right to freedom of movement

9. Good Samaritan law: law passed to encourage assistance to be rendered in emergency conditions without fear of liability for the assistance provided
10. Respondent superior: liability that employers have for the negligent acts of their employees who act within the scope of their employment

B. Consent issues
   1. Types of consent
      a. Expressed consent: voluntary consent of an individual seeking medical treatment; patient must be competent to provide consent
      b. Implied consent: individual is in life-threatening or limb-threatening situation and is unable, because of unconsciousness or incompetence, to provide express consent
      c. Involuntary consent: individual refuses to consent to needed medical treatment, yet another individual (physician or police) can ensure that the individual receives treatment
      d. Informed consent: three components must be presented to the patient by the physician prior to the procedure
         (1) Must describe the procedure to be performed
         (2) Must explain the alternative available
         (3) Must detail the risks of the procedure
   2. Consent-related issues
      a. Minors
      b. Religious implications
      c. Against medical advice (AMA)
      d. Withholding or withdrawing life support
      e. Living wills
      f. Patient Self-Determination Act: a December 1991 federal law that provides hospitalized patients with the authority to make decisions regarding termination or continuation of life support
      g. Durable power of attorney for health care decision or living will: allows individuals to select someone to act for them in the area of health care decisions should they become unable to make their own decisions

C. Reporting requirements
   1. Medical record documentation
   2. Discharge instructions
   3. Handling information and confidentiality
   4. Reportable events and situations
      a. Local, state, and federal regulations
      b. Hospital policies and procedures

D. Emergency department record
   1. JCAHO requirements
   2. Hospital documentation requirements
   3. Confidentiality
   4. Health Insurance Portability and Accountability Act of 1996 (HIPAA)
      a. Signed into law in August 1996
      b. HIPAA administrative simplification regulations include:
         (1) Electronic health care transaction and code sets
         (2) Health information privacy
         (3) Unique identifier for employers
         (4) Security requirements
         (5) Unique identifier for providers
         (6) Unique identifier for health plans
         (7) Enforcement procedures
   5. Patient transfers: Consolidated Omnibus Budget Reconciliation Act (COBRA) and Omnibus Budget Reconciliation Act (OBRA)[3]
      a. OBRA: Part of the Medicare law preventing inappropriate transfers of individuals who seek emergency department care (antidumping law)[4]
      b. Emergency Medical Transport and Active Labor Act (EMTALA; Update 2004)[5]
         (1) Provide appropriate medical screening within the capability of the hospital's emergency department
         (2) If an emergency condition is determined to exist, provide any necessary stabilizing management and appropriate transfer
         (3) Definition of "comes to the emergency department" which assists in clarification

of emergency department diversion
(4) Definition of an emergency medical condition
(5) Definition of a patient
(6) Refusal of consent for treatment
(7) Clarification of delay in examination related to insurance information
(8) Recipient hospital responsibilities related to specialization such as shock-trauma units, burn centers
(9) Appropriate transport teams
(10) Landing of helicopters on hospital property for patient transport
6. Patient discharge and instructions: oral and written
7. Chain of evidence collection
E. Specific emergency situations
1. Triage guidelines
a. Hospital policy: triage guidelines
b. State law
c. Nurse practice act
2. Telephone advice
a. Hospital policy and procedure
b. Documentation
3. Restraining of patients
a. Out-of-control behavior
b. Danger to self or others
c. Nursing considerations
d. Documentation
(1) Less restrictive interventions were not effective
(2) Order for the restraints from a physician
(3) Ongoing patient evaluation including need for patient to remain restrained
(4) Assessments should include
(a) Neurovascular status
(b) Activities of daily living
(c) Nutrition
4. Psychiatric patients
a. Assess danger to self or others
b. Knowledgeable of policies, procedures, and laws regarding "holds"
5. Blood alcohol and drug screening
a. Hospital policy
b. State law
c. Medical purposes versus police request
6. Assault and abuse situations
a. Sexual assault
(1) Policies and procedures
(2) Documentation
(3) Collaboration with team members
(4) Preserving evidence and chain of evidence collection
(5) Referring of evidence collection for appropriate follow-up
b. Abuse and neglect
(1) Child
(2) Elderly

II. Going to court[6]
A. Expert witness
1. Practicing clinician
2. Experience relevant to the case
3. Communication skills
4. Experience with testifying in court
5. Certification in specialty
B. Patient-related issues
1. Sexual assault nurse examiner testimony
2. Evidence
C. Components of a lawsuit
1. Complaint
2. Discovery
3. Trial

III. Transport law[5,7]
A. EMTALA
1. Appropriate medical screening must occur before transport
2. Written consent should be obtained from patient or person acting for the patient for the transfer
3. Agreement for the receiving facility to accept the patient
4. Transfer in the most appropriate transport vehicle
5. Qualified transport crews
6. Copies of documentation
B. Responsibility for medical direction during transport
C. Whose patient is it during transport?

IV. Ethical issues
A. Sources of issues
1. Patients
2. Families
3. Institutions

4. Communities
5. Co-workers

B. Ethical decision-making model
1. Problem identification
2. List alternatives
3. List ethical values related to the problem
   a. Beneficence
   b. Fairness
   c. Patient self-determination
   d. Reparation
   e. Alternative
4. Frame an ethical statement
5. List consequences of actions
6. Examine personal values
7. Compare consequences to values
8. Are the consequences consistent or inconsistent with values?
9. Make a decision
10. Act on the decision

C. End-of-life issues
1. Cultural issues
2. Religious beliefs
3. Advance directives
4. Euthanasia
5. Family presence

D. Resuscitation
1. Advance directives
2. Do-not-resuscitate (DNR) orders
3. Transporting under full cardiopulmonary arrest
4. Pronouncing patients dead in the field
5. Pronouncing patients dead in other institutions

E. Resources
1. Hospital ethics committee
2. Case presentations
3. Professional associations
4. American Nurses Association Code of Ethics
5. Personal philosophy, spirituality, religion

The legal and ethical issues encountered by emergency and transport nurses are many and varied. Nursing practice is governed by state nursing practice acts and guided by standards of care from professional nursing associations, court opinions, administrative regulations, authoritative nursing texts and journals, and other associations such as JCAHO.[7] Nurses need to be aware of the legal issues that influence their practice and be prepared to be held accountable for their actions.

Legal issues faced by both emergency and transport nurses include consent, confidentiality, and evidence collection. Consent can be particularly challenging, because in emergency situations the patient may be unable to give consent, and family or legal guardians may not be available. There are three types of consent: expressed consent, implied consent, and informed consent. Many emergency and transport care circumstances involve implied consent; if the patient were able, he would consent to the care that is being rendered to him.

The prehospital care environment and the emergency department frequently are in the public spotlight because of both the nature of the incidents that occur and simple human curiosity. Nurses need to ensure that the patient is afforded as much privacy as possible. Federal, state, and local laws require that certain situations have to be reported. Suspicion of child maltreatment, attempted suicide or homicide, and sexual assault are some examples of such situations.

Nurses who practice in the emergency department and prehospital care environment will become involved in evidence collection. Evidence that may be collected by nurses includes clothing, weapons, and body fluids. Photographs of injuries are also examples of evidence.

Clothing and some body fluids should be air dried, labeled, and stored in paper bags. All evidence needs to be labeled with its source, date and time of collection, name of the patient, and place of storage in order to maintain a chain of custody.

Emergency and transport nurses' practice is based on and evaluated by standards set by their professional associations. Emergency Nurses Standards of Care, Standards for Critical Care and Specialty Rotor Wing Transport, and Standards for Critical Care and Specialty Ground Transport are generally evidence based and reflect the current practice environments. Standards undergo revision, and it is important to keep abreast of the most current ones.

In 1950, the American Nurses Association adopted a code of ethical nursing practice that offered a description and guidelines for the ethical practice of nursing.[8] Ethical decision making in nursing practice is influenced by several entities, including the nurse's obligation to care, standards of care, legal direction, and the nurse's life experiences.[8]

Ethical decisions may be based on four principles. These are beneficence (i.e., does the care or procedure benefit the patient), nonmaleficence (i.e., will the care or procedure harm the patient), autonomy (i.e., the patient's ability to participate in the decision making), and fidelity.[8]

Common ethical dilemmas encountered by emergency and transport nurses include refusal of treatment or transport, resuscitation issues, and transport of patients undergoing cardiopulmonary resuscitation.

One of the primary roles of nursing practice today is as a patient advocate, to ensure that patients receive competent and safe care.[9] Many patients come to the health care system with limited knowledge about their rights and the type of care they are about to receive. Emergency and transport nurses meet patients in crisis situations. The volatility of these situations requires that both emergency and transport nurses be prepared to assist families, as well as become a part of ethical decision making.

The practice of emergency and transport nursing continues to provide both legal and ethical challenges that we must be prepared to deal with effectively. Our patients and their families depend on us to be their voices and guides through very difficult and challenging life predicaments.

REVIEW QUESTIONS

A 75-year-old man with a history of intermittent confusion and disorientation is brought to the emergency department. The nursing home record confirms the report given by emergency medical services personnel that the patient has wandered about the nursing home during periods of confusion and disorientation and fallen without injury on more than one occasion. On admission, the patient is alert, oriented, and joking with the nurse about how young he feels. Fifteen minutes later, he becomes confused and disoriented, trying to get out of bed to turn on the radio. However, when instructed to remain in the bed, the patient is cooperative.

1. The nursing diagnosis for this patient that calls for immediate nursing intervention is:
   A. Thought processes, altered, related to his confusion
   B. Injury, high risk for, physical, related to his confusion
   C. Mobility, impaired physical, related to his confusion
   D. Infection, high risk for, related to his confusion

2. Nursing interventions for this patient should include:
   A. Placing the patient in four-point soft restraints and raising all of the bed's side rails
   B. Administering sedation, applying soft restraints, and raising all of the bed's side rails
   C. Administering sedation and placing the patient in four-point leather restraints
   D. Placing the patient in an area or room where he can be monitored closely

3. The nurse caring for this patient fails to put up one of the side rails and appropriately monitor this patient. The patient falls out of bed. Radiographs reveal a fractured hip and wrist. The patient's family files a lawsuit. The lawsuit would most likely accuse the emergency nurse of:
   A. Negligence
   B. Malpractice
   C. Battery
   D. Felony

4. In order to claim negligence, which of the following must be proved?
   A. The emergency nurse did not have a duty to care for this patient
   B. The emergency nurse did follow current standards or hospital policy
   C. The emergency nurse's action did cause the patient's injuries
   D. The damage the patient suffered was not related to his fall in the emergency department

5. An emergency or transport nurse who is notified by a lawyer that she is going to be sued should first:
   A. Contact her own legal counsel
   B. Obtain additional malpractice insurance
   C. Talk with co-workers about the case
   D. Contact her employer's risk manager

6. One of the best ways to prevent misinterpretation of a patient care situation is:
   A. Document what happened clearly and concisely

B. Call the supervisor to witness any unusual events
C. Ask the physician to add information to the dictation
D. Complete an exception report as a routine part of the chart

7. On entering the trauma room, the emergency nurse finds the surgical resident beginning to administer a research protocol drug to a patient who has just arrived. The patient is alert and oriented. What should the emergency nurse's first reaction be?
A. Ask the resident if the patient has been informed about the study and has signed a consent form
B. Not worry about bothering the patient with paperwork, because he is a trauma patient
C. Ask the patient if he knows whether the resident is allowed to perform the research study he is about to be involved in
D. Notify the resident's superior as soon as the research protocol has been initiated in the emergency department

8. A 15-year-old boy is brought to the emergency department by his 18-year-old sister. He is complaining of flulike symptoms. Permission to treat should be received from the:
A. Patient's parents
B. Patient's sister
C. Hospital administrator
D. Local court system

9. A 46-year-old woman is brought into the emergency department. She has the odor of alcohol on her breath. On transfer to the treatment stretcher, she becomes violent, cursing at the staff and attempting to hit anyone nearby. The first priority of the emergency department nurse would be to:
A. Call security and have the patient taken to jail
B. Try to calm the patient by establishing rapport
C. Protect the patient, family, and staff from physical harm
D. Prepare the patient for transfer to a psychiatric facility

10. A 24-year-old woman known to have diabetes passes out at work and hits her head. She is incoherent for a few seconds after she awakens and is brought to the emergency department. After the nurse and physician see the patient, blood is drawn for laboratory studies and computed tomography (CT) of the head is ordered. After waiting an hour, the patient tells the nurse that she is leaving before the CT is completed. What is the first and most important step for the nurse to take in this situation in which a patient wishes to act AMA?
A. Determine the patient's competence to decide refusal
B. Assist the patient in understanding the risks involved in leaving
C. Have the patient sign the AMA form on her way out of the department
D. Try to convince the patient to stay by offering her food and drink

11. A 21-year-old uninsured paranoid schizophrenic patient who has been deeply depressed has attempted suicide. She is brought to the community hospital emergency department with a large laceration on the right side of her neck and one on her left upper arm. She has some active bleeding from the arm, which is controlled with a pressure bandage. The emergency department physician asks the nurse to arrange a transfer to the county hospital, because that facility offers emergency psychiatric services. Before transport, the most important thing the nurse should ensure is that the:
A. Patient consents to the transfer to another facility and is not concerned that she is being transferred to a psychiatric facility
B. Receiving hospital agrees to the transfer of this patient and has a bed available in an appropriate unit
C. Reason for the transfer is clear and justifiable on the transport document when presented to the transport team and the receiving facility
D. Patient is stabilized prior to the transfer and deemed safe for transport to another facility willing to accept her

12. A 28-day-old infant is brought to the emergency department by his parents. They are concerned because he has been lethargic and feeding poorly for the last 24 hours. The infant is lethargic and pale. He has weak peripheral pulses. Oxygen by mask is applied, an intraosseous needle is inserted, and the patient is given multiple fluid boluses based on Pediatric Advanced Life Support guidelines. His condition shows little improvement, and the emergency physician contacts the pediatric center 50 miles away. The receiving physician recommends that the referring physician wait for the pediatric transport team to transfer the patient. The referring physician sends the infant with a basic life support service that is readily available. Which component of EMTALA has this physician violated?

A. The hospital must examine all patients who come to the emergency department, no matter what their insurance status
B. The transport vehicle should be equipped with appropriate personnel and equipment to transfer the patient safely and provide life support measures
C. All patients who come to the emergency department must be stabilized within the capabilities of the department before transfer to another facility
D. The receiving facility should agree to accept and have a bed available for the type of patient that is being transferred

13. During the transport, the infant suffers a respiratory arrest. The emergency medical technician initiates bag-valve-mask ventilation, but the child arrives at the receiving facility in full cardiopulmonary arrest . Who is responsible for any further injury that may have occurred to the infant during transport?

A. The medical technician who initiated resuscitation
B. The receiving emergency department
C. The referring emergency physician
D. The infant's parents or caregivers

14. A dedicated emergency department is:

A. A health care facility that provides care that requires an appointment for service and is located on the hospital campus
B. A health care facility that advertises that it provides care for emergency medical conditions and is located off the hospital campus
C. A health care facility that provides care that requires an appointment for service and is located off the hospital campus
D. A health care facility that advertises that it provides care only for a specific medical condition which requires an appointment for service

15. A 32-year-old man is transferred from the emergency department to the preanesthesia care unit to await an emergency appendectomy. The surgeon explains the procedure to the patient, as well as the risks. Which type of consent is the patient giving for this procedure?

A. Informed authorization
B. Implied consent
C. Expressed consent
D. Informed consent

16. When cutting clothes off a victim who has sustained a gunshot wound to the chest, the nurse should:

A. Cut through the clothing in the area of the gunshot wound and place the clothes in an unlabeled plastic bag
B. Leave the patient's clothes on the patient until the police arrive to remove them and label them as evidence
C. Cut around the gunshot wound and place the clothes in a labeled plastic bag until the police arrive
D. Cut around the area of the wound and place the patient's clothes in a labeled paper bag

17. When testifying in court related to a case in which the flight nurse provided patient care, the flight nurse should:

A. Not read the patient care record or any related documents before appearing in court
B. Provide an elaborate description of the incident, including current medical definitions
C. Answer only the questions that are asked and not offer additional information
D. Answer only the questions that the flight nurse believes that the hospital would like to have answered

18. Cardiopulmonary resuscitation should not be performed if the patient:

A. Is incompetent
B. Has written DNR orders
C. Has verbal DNR orders
D. Has not suffered a decapitation

19. The ethical principle that applies to the patient's ability to make his own decisions is:

A. Beneficence
B. Fidelity

C. Autonomy
D. Nonmaleficence

20. The air transport team has been called to a referring facility to transport a 73-year-old female in congestive heart failure and chronic renal failure. Upon arrival, they find a patient in severe respiratory distress with no palpable blood pressure. The transport team elects to intubate the patient before placing her in the aircraft. The referring emergency department physician states that the patient has a written DNR order. What should the transport team do?
A. Ask the patient if she understands that in order to be safely transported, she must be intubated
B. Attempt to contact the patient's family to determine what their wishes are regarding the care of this patient
C. Explain to the referring physician that the patient must be intubated in order to transport her safely, no matter what her wishes are
D. Intubate the patient because transport team members do not have to honor DNR orders outside of their own hospital

21. When deciding to physically or chemically restrain a patient in the emergency department, the emergency nurse should:
A. Ask the emergency physician to write an order stating that the patient can be restrained as needed, so that he will not have to be bothered about writing additional orders
B. Use the most restrictive means to restrain the patient, such as four-point leather restraints or neuromuscular blocking agents
C. Determine whether alternative methods many be used to treat the patient, such as asking a family member to stay with the patient in a monitored area
D. Give nothing by mouth to a nonsedated patient while restrained, so that there is little chance of the patient vomiting and aspirating

22. Which of the following statements is true?
A. A prudent lay person cannot determine if a patient needs an emergency examination or treatment based on appearance or behavior
B. An ambulance must always transport a patient to the facility that owns it, no matter what the patient's condition
C. Patient stabilization requires that when emergency treatment has been provided, there is no chance that the patient's condition may deteriorate during transport and transfer
D. A hospital may direct an air or ground ambulance to another facility if it is on diversionary status because it does not have staff or facility to accept additional emergency patients

23. HIPAA privacy standards:
A. Direct that patients may not have access to their medical records without a physician's order
B. Dictate that all emergency departments provide information to anyone who calls about the patient
C. Establish safeguards for the use of patient information by public health and law enforcement
D. Dictate full disclosure of a patient's medical records to appropriate research centers

24. A 25-year-old male has sustained a gunshot wound to the head. His friends state that it was self-inflicted. In order to preserve evidence, the emergency nurse should:
A. Remove all of the patient's clothes and place them in a plastic bag for storage
B. Place paper bags over both of the patient's hands and tape the bags in place
C. Use the same pair of gloves when collecting evidence from the patient
D. Seal all of the evidence envelopes by licking them

25. When collecting bite-mark evidence, the emergency nurse should:
A. Take photographs only of identifiable bite marks
B. Take photographs only after the wounds have been cleaned
C. Collect a saliva sample from the patient
D. Not draw any blood from the patient to monitor for blood-borne pathogens

ANSWERS

1. **B. Analysis.** Based on the patient's history and assessment, he is at great risk for falling and suffering physical injury.[7,8]
2. **D. Intervention.** It is important to determine that "less restrictive" methods have failed before restraining a patient. Placing the patient

in a room or area where he may be closely monitored, especially because he does follow commands, should be the first step in his treatment. In addition to a physical assessment, blood should be drawn to measure a glucose level to rule out hypoglycemia as a cause of his confusion.[10]

3. **A. Analysis.** Negligence, to be alleged and proved in court, must consist of the following four elements: (1) duty: accepting responsibility for care and then being obligated to provide acceptable care, (2) breach of duty: not providing care according to accepted standards, (3) damage or injury: damage must have occurred, and (4) proximate cause: a cause-and-effect relationship between damage and breach of duty must exist. In this case the nurse had a duty to protect this patient with an altered mental status from harm and injury. She neither put up the side rail nor restrained the patient. The damage, fractured hip and wrist, resulted from this negligence, although it was unintentional on the part of the nurse.[5,7]
4. **C. Intervention.** See discussion in question 3.
5. **D. Intervention.** When a nurse is informed that she is to be involved in a legal matter related to her work, she should immediately contact her institution's risk manager. It is a good idea to have malpractice insurance before an incident occurs.[5,7]
6. **A. Intervention.** Documenting what happened, clearly and concisely, is the best way to prevent misinterpretation of what happened.[7,11]
7. **A. Intervention.** The rights of human subjects must be a priority in research endeavors. If the research protocol has outlined that consent is to be signed, that policy must be adhered to. The role of the emergency department nurse in conjunction with research endeavors is often one of ensuring patient safety.[6,9]
8. **A. Intervention.** If a minor is brought to the emergency department by anyone other than the parents, all attempts must be made to contact the parents before treatment is rendered unless a life-threatening situation exists.[6,8]
9. **C. Intervention.** The first priority should be safety for all parties involved in providing emergency care.[6,8-10]
10. **A. Intervention.** The patient's competence to leave AMA must be determined. A competent, conscious patient has the right to refuse treatment after demonstrating understanding of the consequences of refusal. This should be confirmed by a signature on the AMA form. The patient's chart should include documentation that the risks or consequences of leaving AMA were explained.[6,8-10,12-14]
11. **D. Intervention.** Although all of these steps must be taken, the most important is the safety of the patient. The COBRA law requires that any hospital receiving Medicare funds must evaluate all emergency patients to determine whether an emergency condition exists. If it does, the hospital must provide immediate and stabilizing care before a transfer is considered.[1-5]
12. **B. Intervention.** When a patient is to be transferred to another facility, the level of care and equipment needed for safe transport should be available and provided. A pediatric patient, particularly an infant, requires educated and trained individuals who can provide safe care.[1-5,15]
13. **C. Intervention.** The referring emergency physician would be responsible for any injury that occurred to the infant during the transport. However, the emergency nurse at the referring facility should have documented any objections to this patient's care and attempted to stop it by notification of the appropriate authorities.[1-5]
14. **B. Assessment.** According to the most recent clarification of EMTALA, a dedicated emergency department means any department or facility of a hospital, regardless whether it is located on or off the main hospital campus, that meets the following requirements: (1) it is licensed as an emergency room or department by the state in which it is located, (2) the facility holds itself out to the public as a place that provides emergency care without an appointment, and (3) within the previous calendar year at least one third of all of the outpatient visits were for management of emergency medical conditions on an urgent basis without requiring a previously scheduled appointment.[5]
15. **D. Intervention.** The patient is giving informed consent, which consists of providing a description of the procedure, a discussion of alternative treatments, and a discussion of the risks of the procedure.[2]
16. **D. Intervention.** The nurse should cut around any bullet or knife wound holes in clothing. All clothing should be labeled as to its source, the patient's name and age, date and time collected, and placed in a paper bag to preserve evidence.[16]

17. **C. Intervention.** When testifying, the transport nurse should review the chart and any related materials before appearing in court, answer the questions (keeping the terminology simple and direct), answer only the questions, and always tell the truth.[17]
18. **B. Intervention.** Cardiopulmonary resuscitation should not be performed if the patient is competent and refuses it, has written DNR orders, is decapitated, or has rigor mortis or tissue decomposition.[11]
19. **C. Autonomy.**[8]
20. **A. Assessment.** Speak with the patient to be sure that she understands that she must be intubated to transport her safely. If the patient were unconscious or unable to understand, even though her wishes would be legally honored in most states, it would be wise to contact the patient's family and explain the situation. Discussing the case with the medical director would also be of assistance in this difficult situation.[18]
21. **C. Intervention.** When deciding whether to restrain a patient, the emergency nurse should attempt to use other methods first if safety is not an issue. For example, asking a family member to stay with the patient would be appropriate. Orders for restraint cannot be given on an as-needed basis. A patient's needs, such as food and hydration, must be met while in restraints. Finally, documentation of why the patient has been restrained and frequent monitoring are imperative.[10]
22. **D. Intervention.** If it is on diversionary status and does not have the facilities or staff to care for the patient, a hospital may divert an air or ground ambulance. However, if the transport ream disregards hospital diversion and comes to the hospital, the patient must be cared for by the receiving facility.[7]
23. **C. Assessment.** HIPAA gives patients the right to access their medical records, restricts disclosure of health information to the minimum needed for the intended purpose, and establishes safeguards and restrictions regarding the use and disclosure of records for public health, research, and law enforcement.
24. **B. Intervention.** To preserve evidence, the emergency nurse should place paper bags over the patient's hands, change gloves frequently to prevent cross contamination, not lick the envelope because that will leave the nurse's DNA, and never store evidence in plastic because it may damage the evidence.[19]
25. **C. Intervention.** When collecting bite-mark evidence, the emergency nurse should collect a saliva sample from the patient that can be used as a control. Blood should be drawn for a baseline for blood-borne pathogens which can be transmitted by biting, and even suspected areas where a bite mark may be should be photographed. When possible, a professional forensic photographer should be used.[19]

REFERENCES

1. *Wilmington General Hospital v Manlove,* 194 A 2d 135, State Court, Delaware, 1961.
2. Lee G: Legal issues. In Jordan KS, editor: *Emergency nursing core curriculum,* ed 5, Philadelphia, 2000, WB Saunders.
3. Consolidated Omnibus Budget Reconciliation Act (COBRA) of 1985 (42 USCA Section 1395 dd) as amended by the Omnibus Budget Reconciliation Act (OBRA) of 1987, 1989, and 1990, Washington, DC, US Government Printing Office.
4. Omnibus Budget Reconciliation Act of 1989, pub L, No 101-239, Washington, DC, US Government Printing Office.
5. Health Law Resource Center: Compiled EMTALA Regulations, www.medlaw.com. Accessed October 6, 2004.
6. Sheehy S: Understanding the legal process: your best defense, *J Emerg Nurs* 25(6):492-495, 1999.
7. Niersbach C: EMTALA, *J Emerg Nurs* 25(6):541-543, 1999.
8. Showers JL: What you need to know about negligence lawsuits, *Nursing 2000* 30(2):45-48, 2000.
9. Pryor-McCann JM: Ethics in trauma nursing. In McQuillan, Van Rueden KT, Harstock RL et al, editors: *Trauma nursing: from resuscitation to rehabilitation,* ed 3, Philadelphia, 2002, WB Saunders.
10. Lee G, Gurney D: The legal use of restraints, *J Emerg Nurse* 28(4):335-337, 2002.
11. Denke N: End of life in the emergency department. In Newberry L, editor: *Sheehy's emergency nursing: principles and practice,* ed 5, St Louis, 2003, Mosby.
12. Sheehy S: A duty to follow-up on laboratory reports, *J Emerg Nurs* 26(1):56-57, 2000.
13. George J, Quattrone M, Goldstone M: Nursing judgment—is it alive? *J Emerg Nurs* 25(1):43-44, 1999.

14. Cole F: Research. In Jordan KS, editor: *Emergency nursing core curriculum,* ed 5, Philadelphia, 2000, WB Saunders.
15. Akoi B, McCloskey K: *Evaluation, stabilization, and transport of the critically ill child,* St Louis, 1992, Mosby.
16. Southard P: Legal and legislative considerations in emergency practice. In Kitt S, Selfridge-Thomas J, Proehl J et al, editors: *Emergency nursing: a physiologic and clinical perspective,* ed 2, Philadelphia, 1995, WB Saunders.
17. Task Force on Interhospital Transport American Academy of Pediatrics: *Guidelines for air and ground transport of neonatal and pediatric patients,* Elk Grove Village, IL, 1999, American Academy of Pediatrics.
18. Air and Surface Transport Nurses Association: *Transport nurse advanced trauma course,* Denver, CO, 2002, Air and Surface Transport Nurses Association.
19. Proehl J, editor: *Emergency nursing procedures,* ed 3, Philadelphia, 2004, WB Saunders.

CHAPTER 24

RESEARCH

REVIEW OUTLINE

I. Purpose of research
   A. Describes the characteristics of a particular problem
   B. Explains phenomena
   C. Predicts outcome
   D. Controls occurrences of undesired outcomes
II. Purpose of emergency and transport nursing research
   A. Identifies and describes nursing knowledge
   B. Discovers whether nursing care does make a difference
   C. Provides scientific explanations for emergency nursing actions
   D. Discovers emergency and transport nursing professional identity
III. Two approaches to research in emergency and transport nursing
   A. Quantitative: used to examine the relationship between and among variables and determine cause and effect
      1. Explores causes and makes predictions
      2. Objective perspective
      3. Requires large sample sizes
      4. Data collection based on some objective instrument
      5. Data analysis is statistical
   B. Qualitative: a research method that investigates a research question or a phenomenon in an in-depth holistic manner
      1. Phenomenology
      2. Grounded theory
      3. Ethnography
      4. Historical
IV. Research process
   A. Identification of the research question or problem
      1. From clinical practice
      2. Duplication of previous study
      3. Current controversies in the literature
      4. Case study
      5. Quality management issues
   B. Review of the literature
   C. Implementation of a new procedure
   D. Need for change
   E. Theories
      1. Theory-practice-theory
      2. Practice-theory
      3. Research-theory
      4. Theory-research-theory
      5. Modified-practice-theory
   F. Conceptual models
      1. Johnson's behavioral systems model
      2. Leninger's sunrise model: transcultural nursing
      3. Watson's caring constructs
      4. King's open systems model
      5. Levine's conservation model
      6. Orem's self-care model
      7. Neuman's health care systems model
      8. Roger's science of unitary human beings
      9. Roy's adaptation model
      10. Parse's theory of human becoming
   G. Review of the current literature
   H. Research terms[1-4]
      1. Subject
      2. Population
      3. Sampling
      4. Consent
      5. Subject protection
      6. Dependent variable
      7. Independent variable
      8. Extraneous variable
   I. Hypothesis or research question
   J. Research design
      1. Experimental
      2. Quasi-experimental
      3. Descriptive
      4. Exploratory

5. Methodological
6. Historical

K. Methods of data collection
   1. Identification of the research population
      a. Consent issues
      b. Protection of subjects
      c. HIPAA
   2. Methods
      a. Observation
      b. Self-report methods
      c. Physiological measurements
      d. Scales
      e. Video- or audiotaping
      f. Chart reviews
   3. Reliability and validity issues
   4. Data entry

L. Analysis of the data
   1. Descriptive statistics
   2. Inferential statistics
   3. Multivariate statistical analysis

M. Interpretation of the results

N. Communication of the results
   1. Introduction
   2. Methods
   3. Results
   4. Discussion
   5. Implications to nursing practice

O. Critiquing research
   1. Research question, hypothesis, problem
   2. Methods used to collect data
   3. Ethical issues
   4. Interpretation of the results
   5. Presentation of the results
   6. Conclusions drawn from the study

P. Applying research to practice
   1. Identification of sources of research
   2. Evaluating research findings in practice
   3. Ethical issues

Q. Evidence-based research[4]
   1. Agency for Healthcare Research and Quality
   2. Bandolier evidence-based health care
   3. Centre for Evidence Based Medicine (Oxford, England)

Research always begins with a question or a problem to be solved, and research in nursing practice begins with questions or problems encountered or described in nursing practice.[1,2] Research provides a means of discovering and evaluating old and new ideas (knowledge) in emergency and transport nursing, which offers multiple opportunities for research. Evidence-based research has emerged as an important method of validating what emergency nursing practice is and does.[3] Research studies also provide a framework to discover new methods of providing patient care and enhancing clinical practice. Research helps us discover who we are and what difference we make in patient care.

There are two general approaches to research, quantitative and qualitative. Quantitative research explores causes in order to make predictions. It depends on control, reproducibility, and generalizability. The qualitative approach to research is perceptual and exploratory and produces themes that may or may not be generalizable. It is fluid and many times is better at describing what nursing is all about.[1-4]

There are myriad ways to discover knowledge in clinical practice, including observing, measuring, and describing phenomena. Equipment that emergency and transport nurses use on a daily basis, such as monitors, or the procedures that are employed to care for patients offer rich sources of data. However, the emergency or transport nurse must always put the rights of the patient before the need of the study. Patients and staff may refuse to participate in research projects. This can lead to difficult situations, especially in emergency situations when the research protocol cannot be explained to the patient, nor can consent be obtained (i.e., cardiopulmonary arrest), but could be beneficial to the patient. Both emergency and transport nurses need to be aware of patients' rights when they cannot protect themselves or no one is available to speak for them.[5-7]

The research process is composed of multiple steps, including identification of the problem, review of the literature, development of a theoretical framework, definition of research variables, hypothesis formation or formation of research questions, selection of a research design, sample selection, measurement of variables, collection of the data, data analysis, interpretation of the results, and communication of the research findings.[1-4]

It is important for emergency and transport nurses to read and evaluate research. Because of the multiple sources of knowledge needed to practice emergency and transport nursing, research studies in medicine, psychology, and sociology, for example, should be reviewed. Learning to apply research findings to emergency and transport nursing practice will serve to expand not only nursing knowledge, but that of other disciplines that collaborate with nursing, as well.[1-10]

REVIEW QUESTIONS

1. The primary purpose of nursing research is:
   A. To discover what care activities patients do not require while in the emergency department
   B. To discover which team, nurse-nurse or nurse-paramedic, provides the best care during air or ground transport of the critically ill or injured patient
   C. To develop a collaborative framework to describe patient care in the emergency and transport nursing environments
   D. To describe and validate nursing knowledge and nursing practice in both the emergency and transport nursing environments

2. The advocacy role the emergency or transport nurse plays in any research study is:
   A. Collection of data according to protocol
   B. Interpretation of data after collection is complete
   C. Protection of patients' rights before and during the research process
   D. Collaboration on the study design with the primary investigator

3. The first step in the research process is:
   A. Obtaining patient consent for data collection
   B. Identifying the research problem or question
   C. Reviewing the current literature related to the research problem
   D. Selecting a research design for the study

4. Which of the following is an example of an instrument that may be used to collect data about a patient's response to a specific research protocol?
   A. NIH Stroke Scale
   B. Pulse oximeter
   C. Cardiac monitor
   D. All of the above

5. When using biophysiological instruments to collect data, the emergency nurse must first evaluate the instrument's:
   A. Battery life
   B. Reliability
   C. Cost
   D. Size

6. In the discussion section of a research report, the researcher:
   A. Tells the reader the significance of the work to nursing practice and links the results with previous studies
   B. Presents the results of the data collection in tables, graphs, or selected reproduction of data collected
   C. Tells the reader about the reliability and validity of the instruments used to collect data
   D. Discusses the definition of the variables that are to be studied during the research process

7. What is the dependent variable in the study, "Does heparin flush or normal saline flush keep an intravenous line patent longer?"
   A. Heparin flush
   B. Normal saline flush
   C. Intravenous line
   D. There is no dependent variable

8. A sample of 513 patients was chosen to evaluate pain medication used to manage fractured arms. Using an exploratory design, the researchers found that only 30% of the patients received any pain medication. What type of statistics did the researchers use to present their results?
   A. Inferential statistics
   B. Descriptive statistics
   C. Correlational statistics
   D. Multiple regression statistics

9. Characteristics of a qualitative research design would include:
   A. Objective systematic process
   B. Rigorous and a controlled design
   C. In-depth, holistic approach
   D. Cause-and-effect relationships

10. Characteristics of an experimental research design include:
    A. Equal group participation
    B. No comparison group
    C. Subjects randomly assigned
    D. Variables not controlled

11. A common pitfall encountered by researchers is:
   A. Building co-worker support for the research project within the emergency department
   B. Providing adequate time to plan and educate all of the affected personnel in the emergency department
   C. Making the entire research process as user friendly as possibly
   D. Choosing an inappropriate research focus for evaluation in the emergency department

12. A difference between clinical problem solving and a research study is:
   A. Clinical problem solving involves a formal plan to solve problems
   B. Clinical problem solving is based upon a specific nursing theory
   C. A research study is concerned with issues of validity and reliability
   D. Clinical problem solving looks for several solutions simultaneously

13. A pharmaceutical company has contracted with the emergency department to evaluate the effectiveness of a new drug. The emergency department researchers are ethically accountable for:
   A. Hiding the disadvantages of the pharmaceutical company's medication
   B. Acknowledging the source of their funding for the research project
   C. Allowing the pharmaceutical company to make all the decisions about the design
   D. Using the funding only if the results please the pharmaceutical company

14. An emergency nurse wants to study the patient's experience related to pain in the emergency department. Which methodology would be most appropriate?
   A. Grounded theory
   B. Ethnography
   C. Phenomenology
   D. Historical

15. Evidence-based clinical practice is:
   A. Derived only from prospective controlled research studies
   B. Composed of uncritically evaluated clinical evidence
   C. An example of how research is utilized in clinical practice
   D. Based on research-guided decision making

ANSWERS

1. **D.** The major purpose of nursing research is to identify and discover what nursing knowledge is. Other purposes include discovering whether nursing care makes a difference, providing scientific explanations of nursing procedures, and helping establish a professional identity for nursing.[1]
2. **C.** One of the most important roles that the emergency nurse plays in the research process—whether or not the nurse is conducting the study—is the protection of human subjects. Emergency department patients comprise a very vulnerable group of people. The emergency nurse may need to act as an advocate, not only to be sure that the patient understands the study, but to support a patient who chooses not to participate.[1,4]
3. **B.** The first step in the research process is identifying the problem or formulating the question. Before one can begin the process, one needs first to identify what is going to be studied. Important determinations to make when identifying a nursing research problem or question include whether the problem or question will add to the body of nursing knowledge, will improve nursing practice, or will provide solutions to explain, describe, identify, or predict behavior.[4]
4. **D.** All of the answers provide instruments that may be used to collect patient data.
5. **B.** The reliability of biophysiological instruments is very important in the collection of data. The instrument must be able to measure accurately what it has been designed to measure. This is very important in the emergency or transport environments, where numerous individuals may use a particular piece of equipment.[2]
6. **A.** The discussion section of a research report should tell the reader about the significance of the research. In addition, particularly in nursing research, there should be a discussion of how the research can be applied to nursing practice.[1-5]
7. **C.** The intravenous line is the dependent variable. The dependent variable is the outcome variable of interest; in other words, the emergency nurse is interested in what will keep the intravenous line patent. The independent variables are the procedures (heparin vs. saline flush) that will be used to keep it patent.[1]

8. **B.** Descriptive statistics, such as the median, mean, and mode, are used to describe what has been found in the research population. In this case, the researchers found that only 30% of the patients with fractured arms received some type of pain medication.[1,4]
9. **C.** A qualitative research design includes systematic, interactive, subjective, in-depth, and holistic characteristics.[1]
10. **C.** The characteristics of an experimental design include random assignment of subjects and control of the independent variable.[1]
11. **D.** Pearls related to research include A, B, and C. A common pitfall encountered by researchers is choosing an inappropriate or ill-defined research question.[11]
12. **C.** A research study is concerned with issues of reliability and validity, looks for several solutions simultaneously, and uses a formal plan of study.[4]
13. **B.** When conducting research with a pharmaceutical company, the researcher is ethically accountable for acknowledging where the funding came from, actively participating in the design of the research, reporting the results accurately, and reporting both the positive and negative results of the study.[12]
14. **C.** Phenomenology provides a framework to study and describe patient experiences.[4,5]
15. **D.** Evidence-based practice looks critically at the evidence and strives to use research in clinical practice. It takes into account the realities of clinical practice, what patients expect from health care, and the resources available to provide the clinical care required.[13]

REFERENCES

1. Polit D, Hungler B: *Essentials of nursing research,* ed 6, Philadelphia, 1995, Lippincott.
2. Semonin Holleran R, editor: *Air and surface transport: principles and practice,* ed 3, St Louis, 2003, Mosby.
3. Mateo MA, Kirchoff KT: *Conducting and using nursing research in the clinical setting,* Baltimore, 1991, Williams & Wilkins.
4. Manton A: Validation of what we do: a word about evidence-based practice, *J Emerg Nurs* 24(1):1-2, 1998.
5. Biros MH, Runge JW, Lewis RJ et al: Emergency medicine and the development of the Food and Drug Administration's final rule on informed consent waiver in emergency research circumstances, *Acad Emerg Med* 5(4):359-368, 1998.
6. *Ethical issues in research involving human participants.* www.nlm.nih.gov/pubs/cbm/hum_exp.html. Accessed October 8, 2004.
7. Cole F: Research. In Jordan KS, editor: *Emergency nursing core curriculum,* ed 5, Philadelphia, 2000, WB Saunders.
8. Thompson C, Walker L: Basics of research (Part 12): qualitative research, *Air Med J* 17(2):65-70, 1998.
9. Rea R, Vancini M, Perdue S: Research in emergency nursing. In Kitt S, Selfridge-Thomas J, Proehl J et al, editors: *Emergency nursing: a physiologic and clinical perspective,* Philadelphia, 1995, WB Saunders.
10. Carlson D, Rouse C: Staff nurses: using research in everyday practice, *J Emerg Nurs* 25(6):564-568, 1999.
11. Panacek E: Basics of research (Part 9): practical aspects of performing clinical research, *Air Med J* 16(1):19-23, 1997.
12. Malone R: Ethical issues in industry-sponsored research, *J Emerg Nurs* 24(2):193-196, 1998.
13. Branson S: Research. In Newberry L, editor: *Sheehy's emergency nursing: principles and practice,* ed 5, St Louis, 2003, Mosby.

CHAPTER 25

EDUCATION: PATIENT, FAMILY, COMMUNITY

REVIEW OUTLINE

I. Teaching and learning process
  A. Identification of learning needs
  B. Assessment of the learner
    1. Readiness to learn
    2. Anxiety level
    3. Capability to learn
    4. Motivation
  C. Establishment of goals
  D. Selection of teaching methods
    1. Verbal
    2. Written
      a. Home care instruction sheets
      b. Patient-specific instructions
    3. Visual aids
    4. Web-based information
    5. Question-and-answer session
    6. Return demonstration
  E. Provision of adequate time
  F. Barriers to teaching and learning in the emergency and transport environments
    1. Pain
    2. Age of the patient
    3. Gravity of the situation
    4. Language and communication
    5. Visual and auditory
    6. Illiteracy
    7. Fear of personal safety, death, long-term consequences of illness or injury
    8. Noise level
    9. Personality factors
    10. Nurses' knowledge deficit

II. Content
  A. Disease, disorder, or injury
    1. Causes
    2. Predisposing and precipitating factors
    3. Expected course
    4. Plan of care
  B. Diagnostic test or procedure
    1. Equipment
    2. Activity
    3. Outcome
  C. Discharge, home care
    1. Equipment and supplies needed
    2. Step-by-step procedure
    3. Specifics regarding medications
    4. Pertinent observations
    5. Appropriate follow-up
    6. Changes requiring immediate intervention
    7. Community resource referral, if indicated
  D. Prevention
    1. Prevention of recurrence
    2. Prevention of infection
    3. General hygiene
  E. Pretransport orientation
    1. Rotary wing
    2. Fixed wing
    3. Ground transport
    4. Other methods of transport
  F. Orientation of patient and family accompanying the patient during transport
    1. Orientation to transport vehicle
    2. Safety briefing
    3. Follow-up visits after the transport

III. Community education
  A. Educational pamphlets
  B. Educational videos
  C. Educational spots on television and radio
  D. Injury prevention
    1. Motor vehicle injuries
    2. Falls
    3. Poisonings
    4. Burns
    5. Recreational injuries
    6. Abuse and assault

7. Suicide
8. Violence
9. Firearm injuries
10. Occupational injuries

E. Health and wellness education
F. Public relations visits
G. Safety presentations
1. Operations around transport vehicles
2. Landing zones

IV. Patient preparation

An important component of emergency and transport nursing is patient, family, and community education. The nurse assumes the role of health teacher in preparing each patient or significant other to provide care on leaving the emergency department. This is a vital nursing task, essential to the practice of emergency nursing. Transport nurses educate patients, families, and communities about the transport process. They also play an active role in community intervention programs.

One must be familiar with the process of teaching and use the time available to prepare the patient for discharge. Ideally, patient teaching begins at the first nurse-patient encounter and continues throughout the patient's stay. Saving all the information until actual discharge can be overwhelming to both patient and nurse. It is much more effective to do teaching in parts so that the patient has time to digest information and ask questions. Discharge is best used as a time of summary and return verbalization of instructions by the patient to ensure understanding. There are a number of obstacles to overcome in preparing patients to care for themselves successfully. The stress of a busy, noisy department can increase the anxiety already felt by the patient, and a high-anxiety level clouds the learning process. The nurse helps to decrease this stress through both verbal and nonverbal means. Simple acts, such as explaining tests and procedures in understandable terms and listening carefully to what the patient has to say, can allay anxiety. Likewise, nonverbal communication in facial expression, touch, and body language is effective.[1]

The vast array of health problems encountered in the emergency and transport settings makes it imperative for the nurse to have a broad range of teaching skills. Whereas the obstetrical nurse or orthopedic nurse usually is dealing with a single issue, the emergency nurse must be able to prepare patients with a variety of health problems for home care.[1]

Issues of importance to be taught during the patient's emergency visit include cause and prevention of the injury or illness and possible complications. Lengthy explanations are not necessary; simple descriptions usually suffice. The patient who understands something about what has happened is more likely to be compliant with treatment and more likely to know how to work toward prevention of a similar episode in the future. This information also assists the patient in recognizing any complications that may arise and in seeking further intervention as necessary.

Obviously, the patient must learn about nursing care measures specific to his or her problem. Discharge instructions given by the physician are not sufficient. Nursing care is best taught by nurses. Items such as wound care, fever control, and walking with crutches are examples of the many things patients must understand in order to get well at home. Also, the nurse must have learned enough about the patient's home situation to help the patient adapt care routines to his or her needs. For example, does the patient with a leg cast have stairs that must be climbed at home? Does the mother of a febrile child have a thermometer, and does she know how to use it? These are nursing problems that need to be solved before the patient leaves the emergency department.

Another educational need the nurse meets in preparing the patient for discharge concerns medications. It is important that the patient understand the expected actions and possible side effects, as well as specifics for taking or using the medication. Reviewing with the patient how to use a suppository, or the importance of taking a particular drug with food, should help ensure that the patient or family will be able to care for him or herself.

Finally, documentation of patient education must be recorded. Many institutions have standardized care instructions, such as wound care and head injury observation. Notation is made that these have been given to the patient. Instructions specific to the individual are written, ideally with a duplicate for the patient to take home. Again, it is important that these instructions are in terms the patient can understand and, of course, they must be legible. The nurse notes on the patient's records exactly who received the instructions and that the receiver verbalized understanding. The chart should be signed by the patient or significant other, verifying this.

One of the primary roles of providing education in transport nursing is teaching those who use a particular mode of transport how to work around it safely, such as how to set up a well-marked, clear landing area. Community outreach programs also afford transport nurses an opportunity to teach about prevention.

Patient teaching in the emergency and transport settings is essential to good care. Patients who leave the emergency department with an adequate understanding of how to care for themselves at home are more likely to recover without complications. Good discharge information often prevents unnecessary return visits and time-consuming phone calls back to the facility.

Community and outreach education help to ensure safe transport operations and to assist in appropriate utilization of resources. Education is a fluid, on-going process in which all emergency and transport nurses must take an active role. Patient and community satisfaction are enhanced when educational needs are met.

REVIEW QUESTIONS

1. An 8-month-old girl is being discharged from the emergency department with bilateral otitis media. In addition to instructions for fever management and medication administration, the nurse tells the mother to:
   A. Weigh the baby daily in the morning before her breakfast
   B. Isolate the baby from other children until the fever is gone
   C. Discontinue formula, substituting clear liquids
   D. Avoid putting the baby to bed with a bottle

2. When providing the baby's mother with information about the antibiotic that has been prescribed for the child, the emergency nurse should:
   A. Use both the generic and commercial name of the antibiotic so the mother will not become confused and give the wrong medication
   B. Use an instruction sheet that assumes that the mother has graduated from a 4-year college to be sure that the problem is covered thoroughly
   C. Use examples to clarify how to administer the antibiotic to the baby, such as syringe administration to a doll
   D. Instruct the mother to return only to her pediatrician for further care, because everything has been done for her child

3. A 32-year-old man is being discharged from the emergency department with a diagnosis of left corneal abrasion sustained at work. He has a patch in place and has been given antibiotic ointment to use. The most important teaching to be done for this patient would be:
   A. Stressing the importance of not driving or operating other machinery while wearing the patch
   B. Teaching him how to apply the ointment to his eyes so that his family will not have to do it for him
   C. Reminding him how long the patch is to be worn and when to follow up with his family doctor
   D. Stressing the importance of wearing goggles at work to prevent recurrence of this injury

4. A 10-year-old boy is being discharged from the emergency department with a right forearm fracture sustained in a fall. A cast has been applied to his arm, and his mother is taught how to do circulation checks every 4 hours until he is seen by the orthopedic surgeon the following morning. The emergency nurse may evaluate the effectiveness of her instruction by:
   A. Asking the mother to read the written instructions back to you or the doctor
   B. Giving the mother a videotape about orthopedic injuries to take home with her
   C. Asking the mother to demonstrate how to do a circulation check on her son's arm
   D. Discharging the mother before evaluating her skills and calling her on the phone later

5. Another bit of advice pertinent for this patient would be:
   A. How to trim excess padding from around the cast
   B. To avoid striking the cast against anything
   C. How to dry the cast if the child gets it wet
   D. That writing on the cast can begin on arrival home

6. A 42-year-old man is being discharged from the emergency department with a diagnosis of low back strain after lifting a refrigerator. His dis-

charge instructions are based on which of the following nursing diagnoses?
A. Pain related to his back injury
B. Activity intolerance related to his back injury
C. Mobility, impaired physical, related to his back injury
D. All of the above would be applicable

7. Methods that the emergency nurse may use to reinforce discharge instructions include:
A. Give only oral instructions when discharging a patient from the emergency department, because most people do not pay any attention to written instructions
B. Tell the patient to call his physician or nurse practitioner if there is anything he does not understand about his care in the emergency department
C. Involve the patient's family or significant others in the discharge instructions that are being given to the patient to further emphasize the information
D. If the patient does not speak English, encourage him to contact a translator when he returns home to explain the instructions to him

8. A 52-year-old woman has been treated in the emergency department for stable angina and is ready for discharge with sublingual nitroglycerin. The most important instruction she receives is:
A. How to take nitroglycerin when she is on vacation in another state or country
B. How to restrict activity when she is having any type of chest pain
C. When to follow up with her private physician after this emergency visit
D. To seek medical attention immediately if pain persists after taking three nitroglycerin tablets

9. Assumptions about adult learners include:
A. The adult learner has no previous experience on which to base her learning
B. Adult learning can be accomplished only through the use of lecture and discussion
C. Adults learn best from problem-centered educational experiences
D. Adults can learn only when they are motivated by a potential salary increase

10. Methods that may be used to enhance teaching and learning in the prehospital and emergency department environments include all of the following except:
A. Lack of privacy
B. Adequate time
C. Well-lit environment
D. Involving the family

ANSWERS

1. **D. Intervention.** Babies who are routinely put to bed with a bottle are more prone to recurrent bouts of otitis media. They often fall asleep in the act of sucking, which increases pressure in the eustachian tubes, inhibiting free drainage. Parents should be encouraged to hold the baby until the bottle is finished. This will prevent prolonged negative pressure in the eustachian tubes, as well as promote bonding between parent and infant.
2. **C. Intervention.** When providing patients and families with discharge instructions, the emergency nurse should use simple, nontechnical terms to describe medications, ensure that the discharge instructions are at an educational level that the patient and family understand (usually from fourth to sixth grade), and offer examples to clarify the instructions.[1,2]
3. **A. Intervention.** When one eye is patched, depth perception is severely altered. To prevent injury to himself and others, the patient should avoid activity in which intact vision is crucial to safety.
4. **C. Intervention.** There are several ways that the emergency nurse could evaluate the effectiveness of her teaching. These include asking the mother questions about the procedure, providing a follow-up call, and having the parent perform a return demonstration of the procedure.
5. **B. Intervention.** A plaster cast is to be kept dry and all padding left as is. A 24-hour drying time is needed, and during that time handling of the cast should be careful and minimal; therefore, writing on it should be deferred until after that time. This patient's age, sex, and mechanism of injury should alert the nurse to the need to stress that the cast is not to be used as a weapon to strike objects or other people. Active children and young men seem prone to this activity and need to be discouraged from it. On impact, the

cast may be damaged, causing further damage to the injured area. Of course, the possibility of harm to other people or objects is obvious.

6. **D. Analysis.** This patient's instructions will include use of medications and nursing comfort measures to be followed at home, as well as prevention of future similar injury. In discussing each of these points with the patient, the nurse is imparting knowledge specific to him and his current problem.
7. **C. Intervention.** Methods that the emergency nurse can use to reinforce discharge instructions include providing written as well as oral instructions, answering and clarifying all questions the patient may have before leaving the emergency department, and providing the instructions in a way the patient may understand (language, visual, etc).[3]
8. **D. Intervention.** Pain not relieved with rest and three successive nitroglycerin tablets may indicate a serious myocardial event. A patient with angina should be reminded when and how to seek help.
9. **C. Intervention.** Adult learners have multiple life experiences, prefer to learn through a number of different types of activities (group and individual), enjoy problem-centered teaching, and are motivated to learn by both intrinsic and extrinsic motivators.[3,4]
10. **A. Assessment.** Lack of privacy is a detractor to the teaching and learning process.

References

1. Rush C: Patient education. In Newberry L, editor: *Sheehy's emergency nursing: principles and practice,* ed 5, St Louis, 2003, Mosby.
2. Duffy M, Snyder K: Can ED patients read your patient education materials? *J Emerg Nurs* 25(4):294-297, 1999.
3. Bracken L, Martinez R: Education. In Jordan KS, editor: *Emergency nursing core curriculum,* ed 5, Philadelphia, 2000, WB Saunders.
4. Krupa D, editor: *Flight nursing core curriculum,* Park Ridge, MD, 1997, Road Runner Press.

PART **TWO**

Prehospital and Transport Issues

CHAPTER 26

Transport Physiology

REVIEW OUTLINE

I. Gas laws[1-3]
   A. Boyle's law: law of gaseous expansion, defines the relationship between gas volume and barometric pressure; gas expands as barometric pressure decreases
   B. Charles' law: defines the relationship between gas volume and temperature; gas volume increases as temperature increases and decreases as temperature decreases
   C. Universal gas law: combines Boyle's and Charles' laws
   D. Henry's law: law of gases in solution, defines the effect of barometric pressure on volume of gas dissolved in fluids; as the pressure of a gas above a liquid increases, more gas is dissolved in the liquid, and as the pressure of a gas above a liquid decreases, the gas comes out of the solution
   E. Dalton's law: law of partial pressures; partial pressure of the gases will change with altitude changes, but the percentage of the gas volume remains constant
   F. Law of gaseous diffusion: gases diffuse from an area of higher concentration to an area of lower concentration

II. The earth's atmosphere
   A. Atmospheric gas composition
      1. Oxygen 21%
      2. Nitrogen 78%
      3. Other gases 1%
   B. Atmospheric gas distribution
      1. Altitude
      2. Latitude
      3. Temperature
      4. Humidity
   C. Physiological zones of the atmosphere
      1. Efficient zone: sea level to 10,000 feet
         a. Oxygen sufficient for human survival
         b. Changes in barometric pressure will change oxygen concentrations, so humans must acclimate to higher altitudes or use supplemental oxygen to prevent problems with hypoxia
      2. Deficient zone: 10,000 to 50,000 feet
         a. Supplemental oxygen required in order to function and remain alive
         b. Barometric pressure drops from 523 mm Hg to 87 mm Hg
      3. Space equivalent zone: 50,000 feet into the outer limits of the earth's atmosphere
         a. Humans must exist in an artificial environment

III. Stresses of patient transport
   A. Barometric pressure changes and physiological changes
      1. Middle ear
      2. Facial sinuses
      3. Teeth
      4. Gastrointestinal tract
      5. Respiratory system
      6. Circulatory system
      7. Extremities
      8. Decompression sickness
      9. Medical equipment considerations
   B. Hypoxia
      1. Hypoxic hypoxia
      2. Hypemic hypoxia
      3. Histotoxic hypoxia
      4. Stagnant hypoxia
      5. Time of useful consciousness (TUC)
   C. Thermal stress
      1. Heat loss
      2. Heat production
      3. Heat conservation
      4. Minimizing heat loss during transport
   D. Gravitational forces
      1. Classification of G (gravitational) forces
      2. Physiological effects
   E. Humidity and dehydration
      1. The transport environment
      2. Physiological effects
   F. Noise
      1. Effects of noise exposure

2. Hearing loss
3. Noise attenuation

G. Vibration
1. Exposure
2. Physiological effects

H. Fatigue
1. Cumulative effects
2. Self-imposed

In order to provide an efficient, therapeutic patient care environment during transport, one must understand characteristics of atmospheric variation associated with flight. The air transport team should develop a practical understanding of physical changes that occur during flight that can create and contribute to physiological stress. It is also important to remember that noise, vibration, heat, cold, and fatigue can impact team members performing ground transport.

Transport team members, whether transporting by air or ground, must understand how and to what extent these stressors can affect the already physiologically compromised patient being transported by fixed-wing or rotary-wing aircraft. In addition, the effect of the transport environment on the team members must be considered to ensure that the team can deliver safe and competent patient care, while anticipating and dealing effectively with those physiological stressors that impact patients, other team members, and themselves.[1]

REVIEW QUESTIONS

You are transporting a patient with an acute anterior myocardial infarction in a fixed-wing aircraft. At 28,000 feet the aircraft experiences a rapid decompression emergency.

1. An oxygen mask should be placed first on:
A. The pilot
B. The patient
C. Yourself
D. Your partner

2. A 25-year-old male with a gunshot wound to the abdomen is being transported by rotor wing at an altitude of 10,000 feet. He begins to complain of severe abdominal pain and nausea. His blood pressure decreases to 80/60 and his heart rate increases to 120 beats per minute. Which of the following would provide an explanation of this patient's symptoms?
A. Compression of gas in the abdomen at altitude causes pressure on the abdominal vasculature, which can increase cardiac preload and precipitate a drop in blood pressure
B. Gas dissolved in the patient's gastrointestinal tract will remain in the digestive fluids and cause severe abdominal pain, nausea, and vomiting
C. Expansion of gas in the abdomen at altitude causes an increase in the ability of the diaphragm to expand, resulting in pain, nausea, and vomiting
D. Expansion of gas in the abdomen at altitude causes distention, which can result in decreased cardiac preload and a drop in blood pressure

3. Which of the following would be the most appropriate intervention for this patient?
A. Descend to 5000 feet as quickly as possible to decrease gas expansion
B. Insert a gastric tube and clamp it to prevent aspiration of stomach contents
C. Insert a gastric tube and leave it unclamped so that gas can escape
D. Remove all of the patient's safety straps so that his abdomen can expand

4. When rapid decompression occurs at 25,000 feet, the transport team members have how much TUC?
A. Less than 15 seconds
B. 20 to 30 minutes
C. 30 to 60 seconds
D. 3 to 5 minutes

5. Which of the following will contribute to hypoxia in transport team members?
A. Smoking cigarettes and drinking alcohol before rotor-wing transport
B. Adequate nutrition and hydration before rotor-wing transport
C. Sleeping 8 hours before rotor-wing transport
D. Dressing appropriately for the outside temperature before transport

6. Two hours after completing a rotor-wing mission, the pilot complains of pain in his left knee. Appropriate actions would include:
A. Range of motion to decrease stiffness
B. Immobilizing the affected limb
C. Administering oxygen by nasal cannula
D. Managing the pain with aspirin

7. The evolution of gas bubbles within the body at high altitudes is best explained by:
A. Boyle's law
B. Charles' law
C. Henry's law
D. Dalton's law

8. The sharp temperature drop associated with a rapid decompression is best explained by:
A. Boyle's law
B. Charles' law
C. Henry's law
D. Dalton's law

A 62-year-old man was found unresponsive in his car in an enclosed garage. He is intubated and transported by helicopter to the closest trauma center.

9. This patient would most likely be suffering from which type of hypoxia?
A. Hypoxic hypoxia
B. Hypemic hypoxia
C. Stagnant hypoxia
D. Histotoxic hypoxia

10. The most common form of hypoxia associated with air transport is:
A. Hypoxic hypoxia
B. Hypemic hypoxia
C. Histotoxic hypoxia
D. Stagnant hypoxia

11. A patient is suspected of having a large right-sided pneumothorax. In order to be transported to a trauma center, the patient must be flown from sea level to 4000 feet in an unpressurized aircraft. The driving force behind volume expansion of the pneumothorax is estimated to be about:
A. 100 mm Hg
B. 10 mm Hg
C. 400 mm Hg
D. 25 mm Hg

12. The limitations of a pulse oximeter to measure a patient's oxygen saturation during transport include:
A. Hypothermia increases the instrument's ability to measure oxygen saturation
B. Digits are always the best place to put the pulse oximeter probe during transport
C. Pulse oximetry accuracy will decline in patients with low-perfusion states
D. Motion does not affect the accuracy of the pulse oximeter during transport

13. After extrication, a pneumatic antishock garment (PASG) is placed on a patient to stabilize a suspected pelvic fracture. On ascent, the patient complains of increased pressure and pain where the PASG has been placed. This is best explained by:
A. Boyle's law
B. Charles' law
C. Henry's law
D. Dalton's law

14. In reviewing the incidence of ear problems among air medical transport team members, it is noted that there is a much higher incidence of barotitis media during the cold winter months when compared with the warmer summer months. This is best explained by:
A. Boyle's law
B. Charles' law
C. Henry's law
D. Dalton's law

15. Barotitis media would most likely occur in which one of the following situations:
A. A rapid ascent from 5000 to 10,000 feet
B. A rapid descent from 25,000 to 20,000 feet
C. A slow descent from 10,000 to 5000 feet
D. A rapid descent from 5000 feet to sea level

16. The noise level within the cabin of a fixed-wing aircraft is measured at 92 dB. The transport team member without hearing protection would exceed maximum recommended daily exposure in about:
A. 16 hours
B. 30 minutes
C. 4 hours
D. 2 hours

17. A transport team member wears a pair of earplugs with a noise attenuation of 15 dB and a helmet with an attenuation level of 25 dB. The level of noise attenuation achieved by this combination would be:
A. 25 dB
B. 15 dB
C. 10 dB
D. 40 dB

A rotary-wing transport team responds to a small rural clinic where they find a 5-year-old boy who was injured in an explosion and subsequent fire. He has sustained second-degree and third-degree burns to approximately 75% of his body surface area. The patient's nasal hairs are singed and he complains of mild shortness of breath.

18. Which of the following mechanisms does not contribute to heat loss?
A. Radiation
B. Conduction
C. Vasoconstriction
D. Evaporation

19. Under which conditions would this patient most likely be exposed to physiological stress associated with decreased humidity?
A. 1-hour flight at 1000 feet in a rotary-wing aircraft
B. 3-hour flight in an unpressurized plane at 5000 feet
C. 1-hour flight in a pressurized plane at 15,000 feet
D. 6-hour flight in a pressurized plane at 25,000 feet

20. The patient must be flown at an altitude of 11,150 feet in an unpressurized aircraft in order to reach a burn unit. The PO_2 at 11,150 feet would be approximately:
A. 18.5%
B. 21%
C. 24%
D. 15.5%

21. Most healthy adults begin to develop signs and symptoms of hypoxia at which altitude:
A. 8000 feet
B. 10,000 feet
C. 16,000 feet
D. 18,000 feet

22. Factors that contribute to a decrease in patient temperature during transport include:
A. Wrapping the patient in a down-filled transport blanket before liftoff
B. Removing all wet clothing before transport in a rotary-wing aircraft
C. Presence of an intact integumentary system before transport
D. Use of neuromuscular blocking agents to manage patient oxygenation

23. Methods to manage motion sickness include:
A. Not eating before taking a rotary-wing flight
B. Taking slow, deep breaths to decrease nausea
C. Making sudden and rapid head movements
D. Blowing warm air on the person's face

24. Positive G forces cause:
A. Blood pooling in the lower extremities
B. Blood pooling in the upper extremities
C. Decreased intravascular pressures
D. Stagnant hypoxia

25. A medical crew member is treated with hyperbaric oxygen for decompression sickness. A serious complication of hyperbaric therapy is:
A. Occasional dry cough
B. Confinement anxiety
C. Generalized seizures
D. Middle ear barotrauma

26. Effects of aircraft vibration on humans include:
A. Enhanced performance effectiveness
B. Increased accuracy of electrocardiographic monitors
C. Decreased patient discomfort
D. Nausea, vomiting, and fatigue

27. What is a Coriolis illusion?
A. A unique cloud formation seen in the night sky over the southern hemisphere
B. Vestibular disorientation resulting from turning one's head in an aircraft that is banking
C. When the dew point temperature equals the outside ambient temperature
D. A false horizon that occurs when a cloud formation is confused with the horizon

28. Why should a patient with decompression illness require a pressurized aircraft for transport?
A. To increase available oxygen to damaged body tissues
B. To prevent additional nitrogen release from body tissues
C. To prevent gut ischemia from gas pressure on the mesenteric artery
D. To prevent a tension pneumothorax

29. Cabin altitude can best be described as:
1. The ambient pressure at which the aircraft is flying equals cabin altitude in an unpressurized aircraft
2. The ambient pressure at which the aircraft is flying equals cabin altitude in a pressurized aircraft
3. The internal pressure within the cabin compartments in a pressurized aircraft
4. The altitude at which the aircraft is flying

A. 1 and 3
B. 2 and 4
C. 2 and 3
D. 1 and 4

30. An example of a self-imposed stressor that may contribute to fatigue in the transport environment is:
A. The duration of the transport shift
B. Working a schedule of only night shifts
C. Eating too much sugar while working
D. Drinking a beer 24 hours before the start of a transport shift

ANSWERS

1. **C. Intervention.** Crew members and patients may become incapacitated within seconds of a rapid decompression. The individual crew members must first supply supplemental oxygen to themselves to ensure that they will be able to assist other crew members and patients in obtaining emergency oxygen supplies.[1,2]
2. **D. Assessment.** As barometric pressure drops, gas in the abdomen expands. This causes reflex venous pooling, resulting in decreased cardiac preload and a drop in blood pressure. Both pain and reflex compensatory mechanisms will increase the patient's pulse rate.[1,2]
3. **C. Intervention.** In order to manage the complications of abdominal gas expansion during transport, the following may be initiated:[2]
   - Insert a gastric tube and leave it unclamped so that gas may escape
   - Descend gradually
   - Loosen safety belts as much as possible to provide patient comfort but not compromise safety
4. **D. Analysis.** TUC at 25,000 feet is 4 to 6 minutes.[1]

Altitude	Expected Performance Time
18,000 feet	20 to 30 minutes
22,000 feet	8 to 10 minutes
25,000 feet	4 to 6 minutes
28,000 feet	2.5 to 3 minutes
30,000 feet	1 to 2 minutes
35,000 feet	30 to 60 seconds
40,000 feet	15 to 20 seconds

5. **A. Evaluation.** Hypoxia is affected by altitude, rate of ascent, individual tolerance, physical fitness, and physical activity. Cigarette smoking and alcohol consumption significantly affect a person's response to altitude, contributing to hypoxia, as well as impairing important transport functions such as being able to see well at night.[1,2]
6. **B. Intervention.** Increasing movement and applying heat packs to the knee would accelerate bubble formation and cause existing bubbles to expand (Charles' law). Splinting the affected limb would help decrease bubble size and formation in the joint, resulting in decreased tissue ischemia. Breathing 100% oxygen will reduce stagnant hypoxia in tissue affected by bubble formation.[1,2]
7. **C. Evaluation.** Henry's law explains that as the pressure of a gas over a liquid drops, the amount of that gas dissolved in the liquid also drops. This leads to gas bubble evolution within the fluid.[1-3]
8. **B. Evaluation.** Charles' law describes the relationship between gas volume and gas temperature. During a rapid decompression, the gas volume within an aircraft cabin is expanding rapidly as it escapes into the outside atmosphere. This rapid volume expansion causes a reciprocal drop in temperature. As the temperature drops, water vapor suspended in the cabin atmosphere forms a fine mist or fog.[1]
9. **D. Assessment.** Histotoxic hypoxia is caused by the cells' inability to accept and utilize oxygen. Causes of histotoxic hypoxia include cyanide poisoning, alcohol ingestion, narcotic overdose, and carbon monoxide poisoning.[1-3]
10. **A. Evaluation.** As altitude increases, the partial pressure of oxygen at the alveolar capillary membrane level drops, leading to hypoxic hypoxia.[1-3]
11. **A. Assessment.** The driving force behind volume expansion is estimated to be 25 mm Hg for every 1000 feet of altitude below 10,000 feet.[1-3]

12. **C. Evaluation.** The accuracy of pulse oximetry is affected by hypothermia, extraneous light, low-perfusion states, and motion.[4]
13. **A. Evaluation.** Boyle's law explains the relationship between the volume of gases trapped in the PASG and changes in barometric pressure.[2]
14. **B. Evaluation.** Charles' law describes the relationship of gas volume and temperature. When atmospheric gases are cooled, they settle and become more concentrated near the surface of the earth. Therefore, altitude changes in cold environments result in larger barometric pressure changes. As a result, signs and symptoms associated with barometric pressure change increase in colder conditions.[1-3]
15. **D. Evaluation.** Barometric pressure changes are greatest at lower altitudes. Because of the relationships between the anatomy of the middle ear, barometric pressure change, and gas volume, barotitis media occurs much more frequently on descent than on ascent.[1,2]
16. **D. Assessment.** Noise levels within many aircraft can cause temporary or permanent hearing loss within a relatively short period.[1,2]
17. **D. Evaluation.** When two noise attenuation devices are worn together, the attenuation levels are additive.[1,2]
18. **C. Assessment.** Vasoconstriction decreases heat loss by restricting the flow of warm blood to the skin and extremities.[1,5]
19. **D. Evaluation.** The humidity inside a pressurized cabin falls rapidly as an aircraft ascends into the cold dry air present at higher altitudes. Exposure to decreased humidity increases as the length of the flight and the altitude increase.[1,2]
20. **B. Evaluation.** The percentage of oxygen in the atmosphere remains constant at 21%. Even though the percentage of oxygen remains constant, the partial pressure of oxygen drops rapidly with increases in altitude (Dalton's law). Decreased partial pressure of oxygen at higher altitudes contributes to hypoxia for crew members and patients.[1-3]
21. **B. Evaluation.** Although hypoxia may begin to affect some physiological functions at only a few thousand feet, actual signs and symptoms of hypoxia are not perceptible in most healthy adults until altitudes of 10,000 feet are reached.[1-3]
22. **D. Assessment.** Factors that contribute to hypothermia during transport include the type of warming devices used to maintain the patient's temperature, the length of exposure, the age of the patient, the injury or illness, hypothermia before transport, and neuromuscular blocking agents, which block the patient's ability to maintain his temperature.[6]
23. **B. Intervention.** Methods to decrease motion sickness include eating a small meal before flying, high-flow oxygen, limiting head movement, visual fixation on a point outside of the aircraft, medications such as scopolamine, and relaxing, which can be accomplished by slow, deep breathing. One study actually found that slow, deep breathing prevented the gastric dysrhythmia that accompanies motion sickness.[1,7]
24. **D. Assessment.** Positive G forces cause blood to be shunted away from the affected body region, so tissues receive less oxygen and become hypoxic. This may lead to stagnant hypoxia.[1,2]
25. **C. Evaluation.** A serious complication of hyperbaric oxygen therapy is generalized seizures. Other less serious complications include middle ear barotrauma resulting in pain and discomfort, confinement anxiety, and occasional dry cough.[8]
26. **D. Evaluation.** The effects of aircraft vibration include nausea, vomiting, and fatigue; increased patient discomfort; interference with the accuracy of patient monitoring equipment; and decrease in crew performance effectiveness.[9]
27. **B. Evaluation.** A Coriolis illusion is caused by abrupt head movement during a constant-rate turn that had existed long enough to stabilize the inner ear. It gives the sensation of motion on another axis. Because of this, an attempt will be made to correct.[2]
28. **B. Intervention.** Transport in a pressurized cabin will prevent further evolution of nitrogen from the body.[2]
29. **A. Evaluation.** Cabin altitude is created by compressing air in the aircraft to obtain a cabin pressure equivalent to 5000 to 8000 feet to prevent hypoxia.[10]
30. **C. Evaluation.** Self-imposed stressors that contribute to fatigue include drug ingestion, either prescribed or over-the-counter; exhaustion, such as not getting enough rest between

flights or shifts; lack of exercise and physical conditioning; alcohol consumption, which should not occur within 12 hours of transport; tobacco use; and hypoglycemia. However, eating too much sugar to make up for missing a meal can actually cause an increase in insulin, which may result in a sudden decrease in blood sugar and hypoglycemia.[2]

REFERENCES

1. Krupa DT, editor: *Flight nursing core curriculum,* Park Ridge, MD, 1997, Road Runner Press.
2. Air and Surface Transport Nurses Association: *Transport nurse advanced trauma course,* ed 3, Denver, 2002, Air and Surface Transport Nurses Association.
3. Semonin Holleran R, editor: *Air and surface transport: principles and practice,* ed 3, St Louis, 2003, Mosby.
4. Thomas F, Blumen I: Assessing oxygenation in the transport environment, *Air Med J* 18(2):79-86, 1999.
5. Browne-Wagner L, Bodenstedt R: Flight physiology. In Department of Transportation: *Air medical crew national standard curriculum,* Pasadena, CA, 1988, American Society of Hospital Based Emergency Air Medical Services.
6. Fiege A, Rutherford W, Nelson D: Factors influencing patient thermoregulation in flight, *Air Med J* 15(1):18-23, 1996.
7. Jokerst M, Fazio R, Stern R et al: Slow deep breathing prevents the development of tachygastria and symptoms of motion sickness, *Aviat Space Environ Med* 27(12):1189-1192, 1999.
8. Plafki C, Peters P, Almeling M et al: Complications and side effects of hyperbaric oxygen therapy, *Aviat Space Environ Med* 71(2):119-124, 2000.
9. Topley DK: Whole body vibration, *Air Med* 5(1):32-37, 1999.
10. Mortazavi A, Eisenberg M, Langleben D et al: Altitude-related hypoxia: risk assessment and management for passengers on commercial aircraft, *Aviat Space Environ Med* 74(9):922-927, 2003.

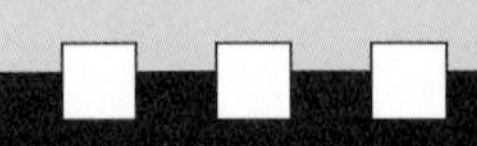

CHAPTER 27

TRANSPORT SAFETY

REVIEW OUTLINE

I. Safety: definition
  A. Practices incorporated into daily operations with the purpose of reducing or eliminating the chance of injury or death to members of the transport team, patients, or other ancillary persons operating around or near the transport vehicle

II. Safety responsibilities
  A. Safety responsibility shared by all members of the transport program
    1. Administrators
    2. Pilots and drivers
    3. Mechanics
    4. Communication specialists
    5. Nursing and medical personnel
  B. Safety is strengthened by
    1. Teamwork
    2. Training
    3. Communication
    4. Crew resource management
    5. Recognizing that people you are working with and people you transport are individuals with worth and dignity[1]
  C. Crew resource management
    1. Preliminary events
    2. Preflight events
    3. Flight-related events
    4. Emergency-related events
    5. Survival-related events
    6. In-flight events
    7. Landing zone issues
    8. Aircraft issues
  D. Components of crew resource management
    1. Teamwork
    2. Communication skills
    3. Decision making
    4. Workload management
    5. Situational awareness
    6. Preparation and planning
    7. Cockpit distraction
    8. Stress management
  E. Components of air medical resource management[2]
    1. Teamwork
    2. Supporting each other
    3. Speaking up when there is a potential problem using a five-step process, being assertive while being respectful
      a. Address person by name
      b. State own emotion
      c. State perceived or real problem
      d. Offer a solution
      e. Obtain recommendation and agreement
    4. Maintaining team situational awareness
    5. Performing team contingency planning
  F. Comprehensive safety program evaluates
    1. Training
    2. Equipment
    3. Policies and procedures
    4. Reporting and examination of incidents or concerns
    5. Communication

III. Safety regulations
  A. Government
    1. Federal aviation regulations (FARs): written and enforced by the Federal Aviation Administration (FAA)
    2. FARs address
      a. Flight operations
      b. Aircraft and equipment operating limitations
      c. Weather requirements
      d. Pilot flight time limitations and rest requirements
      e. Pilot testing and training requirements
      f. Maintenance requirements

3. FAR Part 91: general operating and flight rules for aircraft operating within U.S. airspace
4. FAR Part 135: specifies rules for air taxi and commercial operators; most air medical programs are regulated under this FAR
5. Ground transport
   a. General Services Administration
   b. State and local agency regulations

IV. Safety voluntary guidelines
  A. Association of Air Medical Services
  B. State emergency medical services agencies
    1. State ambulance regulations
    2. Association of Air and Surface Transport Nurses guidelines
    3. Association of Air and Surface Transport Nurses safety paper
  C. Commission on Accreditation of Medical Transport Systems (CAMTS)

V. Safety standards per CAMTS
  A. Policy that addresses right of refusal
  B. Policy to address aircraft and personnel security
  C. Policy to address medical personnel security
  D. Use of the CONCERN Network
  E. Crew work and rest schedules
  F. Hazardous material (hazmat) training
  G. Patient restraints, physical and chemical
  H. Designated safety person for air and ground transport services
  I. Safety committee linked to the committee for quality improvement
  J. Weather minimums

Conditions	**Ceiling**	**Visibility**
Daytime local	500 feet	1 mile
Daytime cross-country	1000 feet	1 mile
Night local	800 feet	2 miles
Night cross-country	1000 feet	3 miles

  K. Weather turn-down policy that requires notification of all programs in service area that a transport was turned down due to weather
  L. Mechanic training and schedule
  M. Database of all helipads
  N. Referral service safety training

VI. Safety risks in the transport environment
  A. Type of mission
    1. Medical
    2. Search and rescue
    3. Trauma
  B. Environmental factors
    1. Terrain
    2. Climate
    3. Population density
  C. Air medical environment
    1. Type of aircraft
       a. Rotary wing
       b. Fixed wing
    2. Single versus multiple engines
    3. Service area of program
    4. Aircraft equipment
       a. Skid height
       b. Flotation devices
       c. Pressurized cabin
       d. Communication equipment
       e. Wire cutters
  D. Ground transport environment
    1. Type of vehicle
    2. Experience of the driver
    3. Equipment
       a. Motor
       b. Headlights
       c. Fluids
       d. Siren
       e. Horn
       f. Radios
       g. Suction
       h. Climate control
       i. Generator

VII. Aircraft safety equipment
  A. Seat belts and restraints
  B. Energy-attenuating seats
  C. Clear head-strike area
  D. Flush-mounted or recessed wall equipment
  E. Halon fire extinguisher
  F. Survival kit
  G. Lighting, cabin and outside of aircraft

VIII. Ground transport safety equipment
  A. Scene lights
  B. Fog lights
  C. Fire extinguishers
  D. Maps
  E. Generator
  F. Ground transport vehicle maintenance
    1. Fluids levels
    2. Visual inspection

   3. Audio inspection
   4. Equipment inspection
   5. Routine maintenance record

IX. Personal safety
   A. Helmets
      1. Lightweight
      2. Custom fitted
      3. Noise reducing
   B. Uniforms
      1. Flame retardant
      2. Cotton underwear
      3. Boots
      4. Gloves
   C. Physical fitness
      1. Yearly audiometric examinations
      2. No alcohol, tobacco, drug use while on duty
      3. Good physical health and agility
      4. Medical screening
      5. Work fitness training
   D. Safety knowledge
      1. Use of fire extinguisher
      2. Location of on-board survival kit
      3. Use of flotation devices
      4. Emergency egress procedures
      5. Emergency locator transmitter location and activation
      6. Fuel shutoff
      7. Battery disconnect
      8. Fuel spillage
   E. Personal survival
      1. Mental and physical preparation
      2. Shelter building
      3. Fire building
      4. Signaling
      5. Obtaining water
      6. Map reading and direction finding
      7. Postaccident incident plan
         a. When to activate the postaccident incident plan
         b. List of personnel to notify in order of priority
         c. Guidelines to follow in attempts to:
            (1) Communicate with aircraft or ambulance
            (2) Initiate search and rescue or ground support
            (3) Resume patient transport per back-up plan
   F. Procedure to secure all documents
   G. Procedure to release information

X. Infection control
   A. Occupational Safety and Health Administration (OSHA) guidelines
   B. Exposure to communicable diseases
   C. Methods to prevent contamination and spread of disease
      1. Standard precautions
      2. Body substance isolation
      3. Vaccinations
      4. Testing and follow-up
   D. Exposure procedures
      1. Reports
      2. Testing
      3. Management for exposures
   E. Right-to-know issues
      1. Federal guidelines
      2. State guidelines
   F. Nursing diagnoses
      1. Anxiety
      2. Fear
      3. Knowledge deficit
      4. Infection, high risk for
      5. Injury, high risk for

XI. Scene safety
   A. Violent situations
      1. Patients
      2. Crowds
      3. Families
   B. Landing zone setup
      1. Adequate space
      2. Free of debris
      3. Appropriate marking
   C. Loading and unloading safety

XII. Patient safety
   A. Securing patient in the aircraft
   B. Securing of medical equipment
   C. Sources of patient discomfort and fear
      1. Fear of flying
      2. Motion
      3. Vibration
      4. Temperature variations
      5. Noise
      6. Atmospheric pressure
      7. Humidity
      8. Confinement
   D. Specific patient populations
      1. Neonates: transport isolettes
      2. Pediatrics: child restraint systems
      3. Combative or confused patients
         a. Physical restraints
         b. Chemical restraints
      4. Prisoners

XIII. Ancillary staff safety
   A. Ancillary staff
      1. Public safety personnel
      2. Hospital staff
   B. Helicopter safety education
      1. Helicopter safety
      2. Hazardous areas
      3. Selection and preparation of a landing area
      4. Communications
      5. "Hot" loading and unloading
      6. Crowd control
   C. Fixed-wing safety education
      1. Avoiding intake and exhaust areas that may still be hot following landing
      2. Avoiding contact with or close proximity to propellers even when shut down
      3. Ambulance safety while on taxiway or airport ramps
   D. Flight teams must assist the pilot when landing in unfamiliar areas by surveying the landing area from above and looking for any unusual circumstances that may cause injury to those on the ground

XIV. Transport vehicle following
   A. Performed by a trained, dedicated communication specialist
   B. Communication specialists' roles
      1. Tracking the aircraft
      2. Monitoring for overdue aircraft
      3. Instituting downed aircraft procedures

XV. Quality management programs for safety
   A. Essential element of a safety program
   B. Documentation of safety issues
   C. Documentation of compliance

XVI. Accreditation of medical transport systems
   A. General standards
      1. Medical
      2. Aircraft or ambulance
      3. Management and administration
   B. Standards for critical care and specialty rotary-wing transports
   C. Fixed-wing standards
   D. Standards for critical care and specialty ground transport

---

Transport team members must recognize the unique hazards found in the hectic and potentially life-threatening environment in which they practice. They must not only recognize hazardous situations but must also possess the skills and knowledge to react decisively to prevent these situations from escalating beyond control. The first step to keeping safe is prevention.[1,3]

The role of the transport team to ensure safety is twofold. The transport team's primary role is to provide the best care possible, given the environment in which they function, to critically ill or injured patients by combining patient care skills with advanced technology. The secondary role of the transport team is to function as a safety advocate and maintain a secure and protected environment for patients, other transport team members, ancillary staff, public service personnel, bystanders, and all others who interact with the transport service. The major concern of every transport service must be safety.

In 2003, air medical transport leaders, care providers, experts, and consultants met in Salt Lake City, Utah, to develop an agenda to address the multiple components of patient transport.[4] Among the most important issues identified was safety. Recommendations included that transport programs must reduce complacency, teach team members that they are accountable for their own safety as well as that of other team members and the patients they care for, develop a strong safety culture, ensure adequate crew rest, send a clear safety message, standardize weather minimums, and encourage referral agencies to promote safe behaviors.[4]

Regardless of the complexities or diverse responsibilities of the transport team, good communication skills, a thorough understanding of vehicle safety and the environment in which the vehicle operates, and knowledge of personal survival skills are essential to providing a safe work environment for transport practice.

REVIEW QUESTIONS

1. Transport program safety is the responsibility of:
   A. The program or administrative director
   B. The designated safety officer
   C. All members of the transport team
   D. The pilot or driver in command

2. A comprehensive safety program evaluates all phases of the transport program except:
   A. Training and retraining of the transport team
   B. Policies and procedures related to vehicle safety
   C. Equipment used during air and ground transport
   D. The status of the patient's U.S. citizenship

3. Which of the following government agencies regulates flight operations?
   A. The National Transportation Safety Board
   B. The FAA
   C. OSHA
   D. The National Institute of Aviation and Health

4. An example of voluntary guidelines for flight safety is:
   A. Association for Air Medical Services (AAMS) weather minimum recommendations
   B. FAA guidelines for weather minimums
   C. OSHA guidelines for the disinfection of equipment
   D. National Transportation Safety Board reporting guidelines for accident investigation

5. *Sterile cockpit* is defined as:
   A. Ensuring that all patient care equipment has been disinfected appropriately
   B. A conversation of a social nature occurring during initial aircraft approach
   C. Conversation with the communication center during the transport process
   D. Conversation restricted to those comments needed for the safe operation of the aircraft on all take-offs and landings

A rotor-wing aircraft was en route to pick up a patient when the aircraft experienced an in-flight emergency requiring an immediate landing. The pilot alerted the medical team to prepare for a hard landing.

6. Which of the following actions should the flight team initiate?
   A. Remove their helmets so that they can assist the pilot in finding a safe place to land
   B. Remove the patient's restraints so that the patient can exit the aircraft after landing
   C. Maintain radio and intercom silence unless instructed by the pilot to talk or contact base
   D. Restrain only equipment that may come loose upon impact

7. The pilot has brought the aircraft to a full stop but has sustained injuries that render him unconscious. Both medical crew members are unharmed. Of the following, which is the greatest danger immediately following impact?
   A. Damage to the radio may complicate rescue efforts and keep the helicopter from being found sooner
   B. The impact may not have been great enough to activate the emergency locator transmitter
   C. The outside temperature of minus 10° F may cause hypothermia to the crew before rescue
   D. Fire is possible because of the presence of fuel and oxygen in rotor-wing aircraft

8. Following the forced landing, what course of action should be taken by the flight team members?
   A. Immediately evacuate the aircraft and meet at a safe distance from the aircraft until it stops running
   B. Shut off the fuel and battery switches, evacuate the aircraft, and meet at a safe distance
   C. Attempt to move the injured pilot from the aircraft to a safe distance
   D. Ensure that the emergency locator transmitter is transmitting, then evacuate the aircraft and meet at a safe distance

9. The number-one killer of people in survival situations is:
   A. Hunger
   B. Thirst
   C. Fatigue
   D. Cold

10. The decision by the flight team to stay at the site or attempt to hike the estimated 40 miles to a known town would likely be made on the strength of the following information:
   A. The appropriately dressed flight team has an adequate survival kit, including a compass, and poor visibility is moving in, making aerial search and rescue difficult. The flight team should begin moving away from the crash site.
   B. The flight team has an adequate survival kit, but has no flares or signaling devices, and

no fresh water. Poor visibility is moving in, making an aerial search and rescue difficult. The flight team should begin moving away from the crash site.
C. The flight team has adequate shelter, water in the form of intravenous fluids, but no food. Poor visibility is moving in. Staying near the crash site may be the best option.
D. The flight team has no survival kit and one member did not dress properly for the cold weather. The pilot is injured and may not survive the night. The flight team should begin moving away from the crash site.

11. When making an emergency landing in the water, the flight team must:
A. Inflate their personal flotation devices before exiting the aircraft
B. Swim away from other team members so rescuers can have more to spot
C. Leave all equipment inside of the aircraft, because it may cause them to sink
D. Let the aircraft fill with water to equalize internal and external pressure

12. A basic skill that all flight team members who are employed by programs that operate or fly over large bodies of water should have is:
A. The ability to swim
B. A knowledge of personal flotation devices
C. Open-sea survival skills
D. The ability to inflate a survival raft

13. Choosing a site for a temporary shelter requires careful consideration. Which of the following sites would make the best choice for a temporary shelter?
A. A site next to the aircraft wreckage
B. A site near some tall dead trees
C. A site at the edge of a fast-moving stream
D. A site near the edge of a clearing of trees

14. Following the forced landing of an aircraft, attempts should be made to contact the hospital base, air traffic control, or flight service on the aircraft radio. If attempts fail, the emergency VHF should be used. This frequency is:
A. 121.5 MHz
B. 151.2 MHz
C. 125.0 MHz
D. 555.5 MHz

15. The most important characteristic in a survival situation is:
A. A variety of life experiences, including survival training
B. The individual's sense of well-being
C. Yearly survival principles practice
D. The individual's will to live

16. Protecting the body from hypothermia is essential for flight personnel working in cold weather. Basic protection begins with the knowledge that most heat is lost through:
A. Arms and hands
B. Feet and legs
C. Head and neck
D. Chest and back

17. The greatest advantage of conducting a missing or overdue aircraft drill is that:
A. The drill approximates the stress that the communication specialist may experience if a real incident were to occur
B. CAMTS accreditation requires it for program accreditation for air and ground
C. The drill allows the program administration an opportunity to see how their personnel would react, especially when they do not know it's a drill
D. The drill can be completed without performing a critique to identify any deficiencies or problems

18. The primary role of a civilian hospital-based air medical transport team in search and rescue is:
A. To use their helicopter to perform the rescue before the search and rescue team arrives
B. To communicate only with their home base communication specialist
C. To transport the rescued patient to definitive care from a safe landing area
D. Not to participate in the search and rescue debriefing because they are not official members

19. The most common cause of death in helicopter crashes is:
A. Rib fractures
B. Skull fractures
C. Pelvic fractures
D. Femur fractures

20. A protocol addressing the response to a hazardous material (hazmat) incident would most likely contain all of the following statements except:

A. The patient must be flown to a center capable of handling hazmat emergencies for primary decontamination
B. A relationship with a local hazmat resource person and center must be established to ensure quick access to information
C. Annual training for air medical personnel and communications specialists must be included in the program's continuing education program
D. Extreme saturation with gasoline or diesel fuel should be handled as a hazmat incident

21. The most important principle in guiding the actions of the transport nurse while working near a hazmat accident area is:

A. Evacuate and treat contaminated individuals quickly
B. Contain the contamination to a designated area for safe disposal
C. Evacuate the surrounding area to prevent further contamination
D. The individual flight nurse's safety is paramount

22. What is considered a significant exposure to blood?

A. Touching dried blood on a piece of equipment without gloves
B. Potentially infectious fluid coming in contact with a mucous membrane
C. Needle stick through a glove in the palm of the transport nurse's hand
D. Blood splash on goggles worn during an intubation procedure

23. The risk for infection after an exposure to blood is determined by:

A. The pathogen involved
B. The amount of virus in the patient's blood at the time of the exposure
C. The type of exposure
D. All of the above

24. Which of the following are examples of appropriate personal protective equipment (PPE) to have in a transport vehicle?

A. Gloves, face shields, masks, and gowns
B. Gloves, impermeable sheets, and aprons
C. Eye protection, masks, and gowns
D. A spray bottle with bleach for spills

25. When cleaning used patient care equipment, the transport team member should wear:

A. Gloves, goggles, and a gown
B. Gloves and goggles only
C. No PPE
D. Goggles and a gown or an apron

26. What type of procedure should the transport team employ to clean reusable patient care items?

A. Reusable items should never be used in the prehospital care environment because of the risk of infection
B. Reusable items should be disinfected on a regular basis, which is recorded and documented
C. Reusable items need to be cleaned only when they come in contact with a potentially infectious substance
D. Reusable items do not require routine cleaning because they pose no threat of exposing patients to disease

27. Can any type of disinfectant be used to clean blood and body fluids out of a helicopter?

A. The chance of disease exposure from fluids in a helicopter is minimal
B. Any solution can be used as long as it will disinfect all the potential organisms
C. Care must be taken with some disinfectants, because they may cause corrosion
D. There are no disinfectants that may be used to clean body fluids from a helicopter

28. The transport team responds to a motor vehicle crash. The patient requires a surgical cricothyrotomy and there is large amount of blood on the road. The transport team should instruct the prehospital providers to:

A. Leave the blood as is, because spills do not need to be removed; the sun and rain will dissipate any infectious agents that may be in the fluid
B. Ask the fire service to spray the area with a fire hose to dissipate the blood
C. Use a 1:100 household bleach solution or approved germicide to clean the fluid
D. Scrub the area with warm soapy water until it is clean

29. The transport nurse suffers a significant exposure to a patient who has been diagnosed with hepatitis C virus (HCV). Postexposure management includes:
   A. Hepatitis B immune globulin or hepatitis B vaccination, or both, and close monitoring of the employee
   B. A 4-week course of zidovudine and lamivudine for the employee
   C. Three to four doses of γ-globulin intramuscularly for the employee
   D. There currently is no recommended postexposure management for HCV

30. Safety evaluation of medical equipment should include all of the following except:
   A. Vibration testing
   B. Electrical safety testing
   C. Monitor screen evaluation
   D. Thermal and humidity conditions

31. Components of scene safety include:
   A. All patients who are victims of penetrating trauma should be searched or their clothes removed because of the risk of weapons
   B. Any patient who is under arrest must receive chemical paralysis and intubation before being transported by the transport team
   C. Running to the scene of the crash or injury after exiting the helicopter without your partner or appropriate safety gear
   D. Not wearing turnout gear if you participate in the extrication, because your flight suit will provide all the protection you need

32. Safety training that should be provided to first responders who use a rotor-wing service should include:
   A. Always approach the aircraft before the pilot or transport team signals you
   B. Remove rescue equipment while the aircraft is lifting off from the landing area
   C. How to walk safely under the tail rotor while the aircraft is running
   D. What types of patients can or cannot be transported safely in a helicopter

International Transport Safety Questions

33. What safety items are twin engine aircraft required to carry when operating long distances off shore (>10 nautical miles off shore)?
   A. Emergency locator transmitter and survival kit
   B. Emergency locator transmitter and life raft
   C. Life raft and life jacket
   D. Life raft and survival kit

34. Which of the following statements is incorrect regarding the emergency locator transmitter?
   A. Signal is transmitted on 121.5 MHz
   B. It is always activated on impact
   C. It may be activated manually
   D. It has a limited time of operation

35. Dangerous goods training for transport team members is to be undertaken:
   A. Upon employment within the orientation period
   B. Once every 5 years
   C. Once every 12 months
   D. Upon employment and then every 2 years

ANSWERS

1. **C. Assessment.** Safe program operations require a commitment by all members of the transport program and are strengthened through teamwork, training, and communication. The total safety approach involves developing meaningful measures of safety and annual reviews.[2]
2. **D. Evaluation.** A comprehensive safety program evaluates vehicle safety, equipment safety, team training, safety policies and procedures, and quality assurance parameters.[2]
3. **B. Assessment.** The FAA is the federal regulation and enforcement agency that oversees all air medical programs.[4]
4. **A. Intervention.** The Association of Air Medical Services is a voluntary organization for the providers of air medical transport services. The association encourages and supports its members in maintaining a standard of performance reflecting safe operations and efficient, high-quality patient care; however, it has no power of enforcement over member programs.[4]
5. **D. Intervention.** *Sterile cockpit* is defined as minimal conversation required to operate the aircraft from engine start-up until a safe cruis-

ing altitude is reached on take-offs and from the beginning of descent until engine shutdown on landings.[5,7]

6. **C. Intervention.** Preparation for a crash should include all of the following: maintain radio and intercom silence unless instructed by the pilot, restrain all equipment, place helmet face shields down, roll down uniform sleeves, locate a preplanned hand position that can act as a reference point when the aircraft lands, and ensure that the patient is restrained appropriately.[2]
7. **D. Assessment.** Fire is the most immediate danger following a forced landing. No one should exit the aircraft until the blades have come to a complete stop.[4,6]
8. **B. Intervention.** Everyone must exit the aircraft as quickly as possible, pausing only to shut off the fuel and battery switches, when possible. Do not attempt to rescue any victims until the danger of fire no longer exists. The crew members should meet at a predestinated rendezvous point near the aircraft.[4,6]
9. **D. Assessment.** The number-one killer of people in survival situations is hypothermia. Hypothermia prevention begins with the proper selection of clothing.[5]
10. **C. Assessment.** Based on the location, the equipment available, and the impending weather, the flight team should stay near the crash site. Survival priorities include checking for injuries and administering first aid, building a shelter, providing warmth, obtaining water, signaling, and direction finding.[1]
11. **D. Intervention.** The flight team should let the aircraft fill with water to equalize the internal and external pressure. Their next step is to unplug, unstrap, exit, and then inflate their life vests.[4]
12. **A. Intervention.** The ability to swim is a basic skill that everyone involved in transport over water must have. Many people have died in survival situations because they could not swim.[1]
13. **D. Assessment.** A temporary shelter situated on the edge of a clearing provides the best visibility. Always scan the area for hazards, which can be found anywhere, and choose a campsite with the fewest hazards. Do not build a shelter beneath a rock bluff, because wind and rain may send rocks and debris into the shelter. Do not build a shelter near tall dead trees that can fall or blow down or may be struck by lightning. Shelters built by a stream may be subject to flooding without warning, and rescuers may not be heard over the noise of running water. Even though the wreckage could be used for shelter, it should be a choice of last resort.[1,2,5]
14. **A. Intervention.** There are two aeronautical emergency frequencies, 121.5 MHz and 243.0 MHz. The emergency locator transmitter transmits on the 121.5 MHz frequency.[6]
15. **D. Evaluation.** The most important characteristic is the will to live, which cannot be learned. In many situations, attitude and sheer willpower have been the most important factors in rescue and survival.[1]
16. **C. Assessment.** Most heat is lost through the head and neck. Therefore, protecting these areas is essential. Hands should be protected because they are needed to perform lifesaving tasks such as building fire and shelter.[5]
17. **A. Intervention.** The greatest advantage of initiating a postaccident incident plan drill is that the communication specialist has the opportunity to experience the stress without a real incident. All personnel should be told that it is a drill, and the drill should be critiqued for deficiencies and problems.[8]
18. **C. Intervention.** Unfortunately, over the years, hospital-based air medical transport team members have died attempting to rescue patients. Without specific search and rescue training, the primary role of the transport team is to transport the patient to definitive care from a safe landing area.[3]
19. **B. Assessment.** Skull fracture is the most common cause of death in helicopter crashes. Although blunt trauma causes many injuries, head injuries that most likely are caused by the collapse of the helicopter cause most deaths.[9]
20. **A. Evaluation.** The primary concern is the safety of the flight team and aircraft in situations in which hazardous materials are known to exist. Patients must never be transported prior to decontamination. A hazmat resource should be available to all programs, as well as yearly training and updating in hazmat responses. Patients contaminated with gasoline or fuel must not be placed in the aircraft until the saturated clothing has been removed.[1]
21. **D. Intervention.** The overriding concern at a hazmat incident, as with any dangerous situation, is the safety of the rescuers. Until properly trained personnel and equipment become available, distance from the accident area is one's greatest ally.[1]
22. **C. Assessment.** A needle stick is considered the most significant exposure to a patient's blood.[9]

23. **D. Assessment.** Most exposures do not result in the health care provider becoming infected, but factors that may determine the risk include:
    - The pathogen involved
    - The type of exposure
    - The amount of blood involved
    - The amount of virus in the patient's blood at the time of exposure[9]
24. **A. Intervention.** The employee must wear PPE, such as gloves, face shield, mask, eye protection, gown, and apron, to prevent the spread of infectious diseases.[10]
25. **A. Intervention.** PPE should be worn when cleaning used patient care equipment. The hepatitis virus can survive for several days in dried blood.[10]
26. **B. Intervention.** Reusable items need to be disinfected on a regular basis, which is recorded and documented on a cleaning schedule. Items need to be cleaned on a scheduled basis, so that all items are accounted for. Floors and walls typically do not pose a serious threat for spreading infectious diseases unless they come in contact with the infectious substance. A regular schedule is helpful, because it can be difficult to be aware of what actually becomes contaminated.[12-14]
27. **C. Intervention.** No, some chemicals can interact with the aluminum alloy of the helicopter. The aluminum alloy is attacked by strong corrosive materials that will decrease the strength of the aluminum. Stress corrosion cracking is rapid and unpredictable.[12-14,15]
28. **C. Intervention.** The area should be cleaned with 1:100 household bleach or an approved disinfectant to protect people from exposure.
29. **D. Intervention.** Unfortunately, there are no current recommendations for postexposure management for HCV. There have been some trials with interferon outside of the United States. However, the Centers for Disease Control and Prevention recommends close monitoring of the exposed employee for development of the disease before any management is initiated.[12]
30. **C. Assessment.** Safety evaluation of medical equipment includes evaluation of electrical safety, vibration, response to hypobaric and rapid decompression, thermal and humidity conditions, and an in-flight evaluation.[16]
31. **A. Intervention.** Components of scene safety include:
    - Wearing appropriate turnout gear to prevent personal injury
    - Conducting a scene survey before exiting the aircraft
    - Watching out for your partner
    - Searching victims of penetrating trauma or removing their clothes to detect weapons
    - Establishing protocols related to the transport of prisoners[14,17,18]
32. **D. Intervention.** Training for first responders should include:
    - How to approach an aircraft safely
    - How to work around aircraft, such as never to walk under the tail rotor
    - What types of patients can be transported safely in the helicopter
    - What to do when the aircraft is departing the scene
33. **C. Intervention.**
34. **B. Intervention.**
35. **A. Evaluation.** Dangerous goods are classified in the Civil Aviation Regulations (Australia) and usually all staff are required to undertake a dangerous goods course.

References

1. North M: Cause factor: human, *Air Med J* 19(1):4-5, 2000.
2. Association of Air Medical Services: *Guidelines for air medical crew education,* Dubuque, IA, 2004, Association of Air Medical Services.
3. Isaacs SM, Saunders CE, Durrer B: Aeromedical transport. In Auerbach PS, editor: *Wilderness medicine,* St Louis, 1995, Mosby.
4. Thomas F, Robinson K, Judge T et al: 2003 Air Medical Leadership Congress: findings and recommendations, *Air Med J* 23(3):20-36, 2004.
5. Association of Air Medical Services: *Minimum quality standards and safety guidelines,* Pasadena, CA, 1994, Association of Air Medical Services.
6. Rouse M: Flight safety and personal survival. In Semonin Holleran R, editor: *Flight nursing principles and practice,* ed 2, St Louis, 1996, Mosby.
7. Krupa D, editor: *Flight nursing core curriculum,* Park Ridge, MD, 1997, Road Runner Press.
8. Semonin Holleran R, editor: *Air and surface patient transport: principles and practice,* ed 3, St Louis, 2003, Mosby.

9. Taneja N, Wiegmann D: Analysis of injuries among pilots killed in fatal helicopter accidents, *Aviat Space Environ Med* 74(4):337-341, 2003.
10. Rogers L, Fiege A: Missing/overdue aircraft: are you prepared? *AirMed* 5(2):24-26, 1999.
11. Kovacs T: A primer on search and rescue, *AirMed* 6(1):20-24, 2000.
12. MMWR: Updated US Public Health Service guidelines for the management of occupational exposures to HBV, HCV, and HIV and recommendations for post exposure prophylaxis, www.cdc.gov. Accessed May 21, 2004.
13. Corriere C, Zarro C, Connelly P et al: A national survey of air medical infectious disease control practices, *Air Med J* 19(1):8-12, 2000.
14. Semonin Holleran R, editor: *Prehospital nursing: a collaborative approach,* St Louis, 1994, Mosby.
15. Austin E, Austin H, McKechinie T: The effect of disinfectants on 2024-T3 aluminum in the air medical helicopter, *Air Med J* 1:57-64, 1993.
16. Hale J, Hade E: Safety evaluation of medical equipment before flight certification, *AirMed* 3(3):42-46, 1997.
17. High K, Yeatmann J: Safety: ground rules for flight crews, *Air Med J* 4(6):28-30, 1998.
18. Air and Surface Transport Nurses Association: *Transport nurse advanced trauma course,* Denver, 2002, Air and Surface Transport Nurses Association.

CHAPTER 28

Patient Care During Transport

REVIEW OUTLINE

I. History
  A. Florence Nightingale
  B. Clara Barton
  C. Military service
    1. World War I
    2. World War II
    3. Korean War
    4. Vietnam War
    5. Global conflicts
  D. Laurette Schimmoler
  E. First hospital-based helicopter program: St. Anthony's Hospital
II. Indications for patient transport
  A. Trauma
    1. Recommendations for helicopter transport of trauma patients
      a. Transport time to trauma center longer than 15 minutes
      b. Ambulance transport impeded because of access
      c. Multiple victims
      d. Time to local hospital by ambulance is greater than time to trauma center by helicopter
      e. Wilderness rescue
    2. Mechanism of injury
      a. Accident speeds over 55 miles per hour
      b. Patient entrapment
      c. Death of another occupant
      d. Falls more than 15 feet
      e. Penetrating injuries
    3. Scoring systems
      a. Trauma score 12
      b. Glasgow Coma Scale (GCS) score less than 10
      c. Baxt Trauma Triage Rule
    4. Specific injuries
      a. Spinal cord injury, or injury producing neurological deficits
      b. Two or more long bone fractures, major pelvic fracture
      c. Major burns
      d. Patient with multiple injuries older than 55 or younger than 12 years of age
  B. Cardiovascular
    1. Need for cardiac intensive care
    2. Need for cardiac catheterization
    3. Need for surgical procedure, such as angioplasty or cardiopulmonary bypass
    4. Need for a specific treatment
      a. Experimental
      b. Medications
      c. Mechanical assist devices
    5. Need for organ transport
  C. Maternal
    1. Placenta previa or abruptio placentae
    2. Fetal distress
    3. Maternal trauma
    4. Prenatal complications, such as diabetes, preeclampsia
    5. Perimortem delivery
  D. Neonatal transport
    1. Age and weight of the infant
    2. Illness
      a. Sepsis
      b. Respiratory distress
      c. Meconium aspiration
      d. Hydrocephalus
      e. Airway abnormalities
      f. Omphalocele
      g. Tracheoesophageal fistula
      h. Diaphragmatic hernia
      i. Persistent pulmonary hypertension
      j. Necrotizing enterocolitis
    3. Injury
    4. Near drowning
    5. Therapeutics
      a. Nitric oxide
      b. Extracorporeal membrane oxygenation
      c. High-frequency ventilation
  E. Pediatric
    1. Respiratory distress

2. Respiratory failure
3. Shock and multiple organ system failure
4. Status epilepticus
5. Asthma and status asthmaticus
6. Multiple organ system failure
7. Multiple trauma
8. Burns
9. Near drowning
10. Poisonings
11. Foreign body aspiration
12. Specialty referrals such as to cardiology, oncology
13. Diabetic ketoacidosis
14. Ruptured appendix
15. Psychosocial issues

III. Pretransport planning and patient preparation and transport
   A. Care based on transport nursing standards of practice (nursing process)
   B. Care based on adult critical care transport standards
   C. Care based on American Academy of Pediatrics standards
   D. Assessment
      1. History
      2. Physical assessment
         a. Primary survey
         b. Secondary survey
         c. Illness or injury survey
      3. Diagnostic
         a. Laboratory evaluation
         b. Radiographic evaluation
   E. Related nursing diagnoses
      1. Infection, high risk for
      2. Altered body temperature, high risk for
      3. Hypothermia
      4. Hyperthermia
      5. Ineffective thermoregulation
      6. Altered tissue perfusion: renal, cerebral, gastrointestinal, peripheral
      7. Fluid volume excess
      8. Fluid volume deficit
      9. Decreased cardiac output
      10. Impaired gas exchange
      11. Ineffective airway clearance
      12. Inability to sustain spontaneous ventilation
      13. Impaired skin integrity
      14. Impaired physical mobility
      15. High risk for peripheral neurovascular dysfunction
      16. Body image disturbance
      17. Pain
      18. Anxiety
      19. Fear
   F. Outcome identification
      1. Based on the patient's problem
      2. Provide direction for the care the patient is to receive
      3. Outcomes are based on a collaborative approach to patient care
   G. Planning
   H. Implementation
      1. Collaborative care interventions, dependent on the patient's age
         a. Airway management
            (1) Basic life support
            (2) Advanced life support
            (3) Rapid sequence induction
         b. Cervical spine immobilization for the injured patient
         c. Breathing or ventilation management
            (1) Ventilators
            (2) Sedation
            (3) Decompression
         d. Circulatory management
            (1) Intravenous (IV) access
            (2) Intraosseous (IO) access
            (3) Monitoring
            (4) Pneumatic antishock garment application
            (5) Urinary catheter
         e. Neurological management
            (1) Cervical spine immobilization
            (2) Traction
         f. Illness or injury specific
            (1) Gastric decompression
            (2) Wound care
            (3) Splinting
            (4) Temperature
      2. Equipment, dependent on the patient's age
         a. Airway
            (1) Pulse oximeter
            (2) End-tidal carbon dioxide ($ETCO_2$) monitor
         b. Breathing
            (1) Ventilator
            (2) Decompression equipment
            (3) Apnea monitor
         c. Circulation
            (1) Intravenous devices
            (2) Cardiac devices

(3) Invasive monitors
(4) Central venous pressure (CVP) monitor
(5) Laboratory values

d. Neurological
(1) Cervical collar
(2) Backboard, adult and pediatric
(3) Extrication boards

e. Temperature
(1) Isolette
(2) Warming devices

f. Transport devices
(1) Stretcher
(2) Car bed
(3) Car seat

3. Medications
a. Neuromuscular blockade
b. Sedation
c. Advanced cardiac life support
(1) Adult
(2) Pediatric
d. Neonatal resuscitation program
e. Medical
(1) Cardiovascular
(2) Gastrointestinal
(3) Pulmonary
(4) Disease related
(5) Other
f. Injury
(1) Head injury
(2) Spinal cord injury
(3) Abdominal injury
(4) Orthopedic injury
(5) Multiple system injuries

4. Pain management
a. Level of pain
b. Medications
c. Alternative care methods

5. Family care
a. Information
b. Additional passengers
c. Safety

I. Invasive monitoring
1. Arterial monitoring
a. Systolic phase
(1) Valves opening
(2) Correlation with electrocardiogram (ECG)
(3) Dicrotic arch
b. Equipment setup
c. Troubleshooting
(1) Dampened waveforms
(2) High digital pressure
(3) Low-flow states

2. Pulmonary artery (PA) catheters
a. Waveform patterns
(1) Right ventricle
(2) PA catheter over-wedged
b. Equipment setup
(1) Leveling of transducer
(2) Zeroing of transducer
(3) Catheter position
(4) Inflating PA balloon
c. Troubleshooting
(1) Right ventricular position and ectopy
(2) Dampened waveforms
(3) High PA digital readings
(4) Treatment of low PA wedge pressure (PAWP) readings
(5) Transport issues

J. Intraaortic balloon pump (IABP)
1. Rationale for use
2. Timing of IABP
a. Triggering
b. Inflation
c. Deflation
3. Transport issues
a. Loss of vacuum
b. Positioning the patient
4. Complications
a. Emboli
b. Thrombus

K. Left ventricular assist device

L. Delayed transport
1. Prolonged patient entrapment
2. Wilderness rescue
3. Limited equipment
4. Inaccurate assessment of illness or injury
5. Development of complications from illness or injury that require transport to another facility

M. Evaluation
1. Ongoing assessment
2. Documentation of care effectiveness
3. Follow-up information

IV. Quality management
A. Standards for critical care and specialty rotor-wing transport
B. Standards for critical care and specialty ground transport
C. Commission on Accreditation of Medical Transport Systems

D. Guidelines for air medical crew education
E. Documentation of care
F. Identification of care
G. Initiation of change

V. Challenges in transport nursing practice
A. Ethical issues (see Chapter 23)
B. Legal issues (see Chapter 23)
C. Stress and stress management
1. Sources of stress
a. Work environment
b. Equipment
c. Age of the patient
d. Death of a patient
e. Death of a co-worker
2. Reactions to stress
a. Acute
b. Chronic
3. Stress management
a. Exercise
b. Diet
c. Emotional care
4. Critical incident stress
a. Hostage situations
b. Excessive violence
c. Suicide or unexpected death of a co-worker
d. Incidents attracting media attention
e. Pediatric patients
5. Critical incident stress management
a. Defusing
b. Debriefing

VI. Follow-up debriefing

According to the *Standards of Flight Nursing Practice,*[1] *Standards for Critical Care and Specialty Rotor-Wing Transport,*[2] and the *Standards for Critical Care and Specialty Ground Transport,*[3] "transport nursing practice involves the nursing process: assessment, diagnosis, outcome identification, planning, implementation, and evaluation."[1-3] However, patient transport is collaborative and not performed by just one type of team. Care of patients begins with obtaining patient information, performing a primary and sometimes a secondary assessment, planning and implementation, and finally evaluating the care provided.

The types of patients encountered depend on the mission of the transport program. Some transport teams are generalists transporting a variety of patients, whereas others perform specialty transports such as neonatal or pediatric. In addition, transport team members collaborate with a variety of others, including physicians, respiratory therapists, and paramedics. The educational preparation for transport is discussed in Chapter 1. A key component of patient transport is anticipation. Transport team members need always to expect the unexpected. The present and potential patient condition requires the transport nurse to have the appropriate equipment and medications available and functioning to prevent any further complication or injury during the transport process.

The family of the ill or injured patient has important needs that the transport team must consider. The stresses of transport on the family include complete separation of the patient and family, transport to an unfamiliar place, risks associated with the transport, and the stress of the transport itself.[4] Most of the time family members cannot accompany the patient because of transport vehicle size, weight limits, and the condition of the patient.

Other issues involved in patient transport include quality management, ethical and legal issues (see Chapter 23), and stress. Stress and stress management are vital concerns in transport nursing practice. There are many sources of stress in the transport environment, including limited space in which to care for patients, malfunctioning equipment, and the age, illness, or injury of the patient. Learning to manage stress keeps transport team members in the prehospital, hospital, and interhospital environments.

This chapter contains review questions that involve issues encountered while providing care during patient transport. In addition, our international transport colleagues have contributed questions. Care of the patient during transport is truly a global experience.

REVIEW QUESTIONS

1. Mr. T is being transferred by ground from a rural emergency department to an academic medical center about 1 hour away. In making the necessary arrangements for transfer, you telephone a ground transport service that can provide the critical care necessary for Mr. T while he is in transit. Which component of the nursing process best describes these actions?
A. Assessment
B. Planning
C. Implementation
D. Evaluation

2. Factors associated with an increased risk for neonatal resuscitation include all of the following except:
   A. History of maternal substance abuse
   B. Previous fetal or neonatal death
   C. History of normal labor and delivery
   D. Prolonged rupture of membranes

3. Which of the following would be an indication for the intubation of a neonate?
   A. Positive pressure ventilation by bag and mask is resulting in good rise and fall of the neonate's chest and the need for assisted ventilation is limited
   B. No meconium is present and the baby has good respiratory effort, muscle tone, and heart rate after stimulation
   C. A neonate with acrocyanosis of the hands and feet whose trunk and mucous membranes are pink and warm after delivery
   D. A neonate who requires epinephrine for resuscitation and intravenous access cannot easily be obtained before transport

4. Which of the following is an indication for use of nitric oxide during neonatal transport?
   A. Persistent pulmonary hypertension of the newborn
   B. Meconium aspiration syndrome
   C. Pneumonia
   D. All of the above

5. The transport nurse is able to determine that the umbilical catheter is correctly placed by:
   A. Obtaining a good blood return after the catheter is inserted
   B. Inserting the catheter until it can no longer be threaded into the umbilical vein
   C. Observing there is no return of free blood once the catheter has been inserted
   D. Inserting the catheter into the thickest-walled vessel that can be visualized

The transport team has been called to transport a 30-week-old infant who is having severe respiratory distress and has been diagnosed with respiratory distress syndrome. Upon arrival at the referring facility, the transport team finds a 3500-g child with rapid grunting respirations, flaring, and sternal retractions. The child has circumoral cyanosis and an oxygen saturation of 88% on 100% oxygen by mask.

6. Preparation of this neonate for transport would include:
   A. Maintaining the child's airway with 100% oxygen by mask
   B. Endotracheal intubation to improve the neonate's oxygenation
   C. Initiating effective bag-valve-mask ventilation for transport
   D. Obtaining a chest radiograph to confirm the referring physician's diagnosis

7. To determine which size endotracheal tube (ETT) this neonate would require, which of the following would be used?
   A. 16 plus the infant's age divided by 4
   B. The diameter of the infant's nares
   C. Width of the infant
   D. Weight of the infant

A 32-week-old infant is being transported to the neonatal intensive care unit after delivery. The mother's membranes had been ruptured for a prolonged period. The neonate is febrile, has a heart rate of 200, and delayed capillary refill (>4 seconds). She is maintaining her airway and has oxygen at 100% by mask. The baby weighs 4.5 kg.

8. The transport nurse would administer a fluid bolus of:
   A. 45 ml of O negative blood
   B. 45 ml of normal saline
   C. 90 ml of normal saline
   D. 45 ml of dextrose and water

9. To evaluate the effectiveness of this neonate's resuscitation, the transport nurse would monitor:
   A. The neonate's brachial and pedal pulses
   B. The neonate's radial and pedal pulses
   C. The neonate's rhythm on the cardiac monitor
   D. The number of diapers the neonate uses

10. The neonatologist with the transport team speaks to the mother and tells her of the gravity of her child's condition. Which nursing diagnosis would be appropriate to plan the care of this infant's mother?
   A. Ineffective breastfeeding, related to the infant being transferred to the neonatal intensive care unit
   B. Ineffective family coping, related to the infant being transferred to the neonatal intensive care unit

C. Fear, related to the infant being transferred to the neonatal unit and the seriousness of the baby's condition
D. High risk for caregiver role strain, related to the neonate being transferred to the intensive care unit

11. The transport team has been called to transport a set of twins who are joined at the thorax. The infants are full term and experiencing no distress. Preparation for transport should include:
A. Ensuring that there is one functioning intravenous line, because the infants would share the intravenous fluids
B. Administering any sedative needed for transport to the stronger of the twins, to evaluate the effectiveness of the medication
C. Placing the conjoined infants at different levels in the isolette to ensure that they do not become hypovolemic
D. Calculating their fluid needs based on their total body weight and administering a share to each infant

12. Which of the following is considered high-priority information by most families of patients transported to intensive care units?
A. To know how the patient will be treated during transport
B. To have their questions answered honestly
C. To know that the transport equipment is as good as that of the hospital
D. All of the above

13. Electromagnetic interference during air transport may affect which of the following patients?
A. One who is being paced with a transcutaneous pacemaker
B. One being monitored with a portable cardiac monitor
C. One with a permanent internal pacemaker
D. One with an arterial line and a portable monitor

A 5-year-old child is involved in a motor vehicle crash. The child has suffered a severe head injury and is to be transported by helicopter to the children's hospital. The parents would like to accompany the child to the hospital in the helicopter.

14. The transport team must consider which of the following when making the decision about whether the parents may accompany the child?
A. Whether the parents can pay for the child's transport
B. Whether the referring hospital will assume liability for the parents' transport
C. Whether the pilot and the other crew members like the parents
D. What effect the parents' presence may have on the child during transport

15. The transport team is unable to let the child's parents accompany them during the transport. What interventions could the transport nurse implement to meet the needs of the parents?
A. Do not allow the family to see the child before transport, because it may upset them to see his injuries
B. Explain to the family that a fixed-wing aircraft is more likely to crash than a helicopter
C. Allow the family to talk to and touch the child before leaving the referring facility for the receiving facility
D. Tell the family to call information for directions to the receiving hospital once the transport vehicle and team have left the hospital

16. Which of the following may be considered a disadvantage of allowing the family to accompany the patient during transport?
A. The family member may be able to provide pertinent medical history about the patient
B. Allowing a family member to ride along promotes a positive image for the program
C. The family member may be able to assist in the care of the patient during transport
D. The family member may suffer from motion sickness during the transport

17. A common complication of manual ventilation during air transport is:
A. Hypocapnia from excessive ventilation
B. No change in the patient's metabolic status
C. Adequate and consistent tidal volumes
D. Reexpansion of a deflated lung after intubation

18. The effects of mivacurium may be increased with the use of:
A. Nitroglycerin
B. Ceftriaxone
C. Gentamicin
D. Heparin

A 3-year-old girl with a history of status epilepticus is being transferred to another facility for care. The child has been intubated with a 4.5 ETT according to the Pediatric Advanced Life Support guidelines and has a peripheral intravenous line infusing normal saline.

19. What additional interventions should the transport team consider to prepare this child for transport?
A. Insert a gastric tube to decompress the child's stomach and prevent possibility of aspiration during transport
B. Change the intravenous fluid to dextrose in water to prevent hypoglycemia during transport
C. Change the air in the endotracheal cuff to normal saline so that there will be no additional pressure exerted on the patient's airway when at a higher altitude
D. Insert an IO needle so that the child has additional intravenous access for medication administration during the transport

20. Delayed transport of a critically ill patient may occur because:
A. The patient was not appropriately insured and the receiving specialty center refused to admit the patient
B. The acuity of the patient's illness was not initially recognized by the referring facility and complications have occurred
C. The referring facility was tired of the patient and his family and referred him to another facility for further care
D. The patient refused to be transferred despite his altered mental status, and the referring facility had to wait until he was no longer responsive

21. An 18-year-old man diagnosed with meningococcal meningitis is to be transferred to another critical care unit by helicopter. He is currently intubated and connected to a ventilator. His oxygen saturation is 88% on 100% oxygen. His vital signs are B/P 86/50, P 110 and regular, with assisted ventilations. Which of the following nursing diagnoses would be most appropriate for the transport nurse to base care on?
A. Gas exchange, impaired, related to inadequate tissue perfusion, as evidenced by his low oxygen saturation
B. Infection, high risk for, related to the medical diagnosis of meningitis, evidenced by his low oxygen saturation
C. Injury, high risk for, related to moving the patient out of the referring hospital, evidenced by his low oxygen saturation
D. Fluid volume overload, related to the patient's medical diagnosis of meningitis, evidenced by his low oxygen saturation

22. A patient with a fractured femur from a small town is being transferred to a regional hospital. He suffered his injury after a boating accident 12 hours previously. When loading him into an unpressurized aircraft, he tells the transport team how great the shellfish was where he had been diving before the accident. What additional information should the transport team collect before transport?
A. His diving profile
B. History of decompression illness
C. Any equipment failure during the diving period
D. All of the above

23. Information that should be communicated to a receiving facility so that a transport decision can be made includes all of the following *except:*
A. Patient's age, weight, and sex
B. The type of insurance the patient has
C. Pertinent patient medical history
D. Diagnosis and current vital signs

24. A source of stress in the transport environment is:
A. Appropriate and functioning equipment in the transport vehicle
B. Good working relationships with one's co-workers and hospital personnel
C. Ample space in the aircraft for patient care and resuscitation during transport
D. Expected death of a pediatric patient during transport

25. An example of an acute reaction to stress is:
A. Chronic illness
B. Anomia
C. Powerlessness
D. Anger

26. An example of stress management after a critical incident would be:
A. Drinking a bottle of beer
B. Taking a brisk walk
C. Smoking a pack of cigarettes
D. Going to a bar for a beer

27. Potential side effects of succinylcholine include all of the following except:
A. Increased intragastric pressure
B. Increase in serum potassium
C. Decreased intraocular pressure
D. Triggering malignant hyperthermia

28. Which of the following is an intubating dose of a nondepolarizing neuromuscular blocking agent?
A. Mivacurium 0.05 mg/kg rapid IV push
B. Mivacurium 0.15 mg/kg rapid IV push
C. Vecuronium 0.05 mg/kg IV push adult
D. Vecuronium 0.25 mg/kg IV push child

29. High-dose methylprednisolone, if administered within 8 hours of injury, has been shown to improve the outcome of spinal cord injury. Some actions of the drug that are thought to facilitate this process include all of the following except:
A. Decreased nerve excitability
B. Restoration of extracellular calcium
C. Inhibition of tissue lipid peroxidation
D. Repression of the release of free fatty acids

30. A relative contraindication to methylprednisolone after spinal cord injury includes:
A. Blunt injury to the spinal cord
B. Spinal cord lesion at the C1 level
C. A negative purified protein derivative test result within the last 7 days
D. History of gastrointestinal bleeding

31. Cyanide toxicity is a potentially lethal side effect of nitroprusside infusion. An acute symptom that should alert the transport nurse to the possibility of cyanide poisoning would be:
A. A GCS of 15
B. Hypertension
C. Seizures
D. ECG changes

32. Current dosage recommendation for the peripheral vasodilator and potent antihypertensive, sodium nitroprusside (Nipride), ranges from 0.3 to 10 mcg/kg per minute for parenteral administration. If your patient weighed 80 kg, the rate of nitroprusside infusion at a dilution of 50 mg in 250 ml 5% dextrose in water would range from:
A. 7 to 240 ml/hr
B. 5 to 89 ml/hr
C. 9 to 142 ml/hr
D. 5 to 71 ml/hr

33. A 78-year-old patient has suffered an acute inferior myocardial infarction that has failed fibrinolytic therapy. He is to be transferred to another facility for rescue angioplasty. However, he has never flown before and is quite anxious. The referring physician is considering midazolam 2 mg IV. A potential adverse effect of this drug the transport team must consider before administration is:
A. It will increase the patient's respiratory rate, requiring that a nonrebreather mask be placed on the patient during transport
B. It will increase his systemic vascular resistance, placing him at risk of increasing his cardiac output and causing bradycardia
C. Midazolam has analgesic effects that will enhance the effects of nitroglycerin and decrease the patient's need for additional morphine for his chest pain
D. Midazolam decreases peripheral vascular resistance, lowering the patient's blood pressure and resulting in hypotension

34. The following statements are true regarding benzodiazepines except:
A. Potential side effects of intravenous midazolam (Versed) are bronchospasm and laryngospasm
B. All benzodiazepines must be administered with caution in elderly, debilitated patients
C. Sedative effects are diminished when benzodiazepines are administered along with narcotics

D. Midazolam is a water-soluble benzodiazepine that is 2 to 3 times more potent than diazepam

35. Flumazenil is to be used with great caution in which type of scenario?
A. Benzodiazepine overdose with respiratory depression
B. Diazepam overdose with alcohol intoxication
C. Midazolam overdose with tricyclic antidepressant ingestion
D. Lorazepam overdose with drug-induced coma

36. Patient anxiety related to air medical transport may be managed by:
A. Administering phenothiazines to decrease symptoms of anxiety about flying
B. Asking the patient about previous flight experience and past reactions to news stories about plane crashes
C. Telling the patient that she is an adult and must learn to cope with these types of stresses because there is no other way to get there
D. Explaining to the patient that he must fly in the smaller aircraft, which is the most difficult one to manage a patient in

The transport team is called to transport a 2-year-old near-drowning victim. The child is currently undergoing full cardiopulmonary resuscitation (CPR). The referring rescue squad has administered the first dose of epinephrine through an IO needle.

37. The second and subsequent epinephrine doses that should be considered for asystolic or pulseless arrest in children, per American Heart Association recommendations, are:
A. 0.2 mg/kg of 1:10,000 solution IV or IO
B. 0.3 mg/kg of 1:1000 solution IV or IO
C. 0.1 mg/kg of 1:1000 solution IV, IO, or ETT
D. 0.1 mg/kg of 1:10,000 solution ETT

38. High-dose epinephrine provides both α- and β-adrenergic agonist effects. Which action is thought to be of primary benefit with attempts at CPR?
A. α-Agonist effect
B. β-Agonist effect
C. Both α-agonist and β-agonist effects
D. Neither α-agonist nor β-agonist effects

Questions 39 through 41 are to be answered using information from the following patient scenario:

During the resuscitation of an elderly female (100 kg) who suffered a cardiac arrest during transport, the following sequence of events ensued. She arrived at the landing zone per basic life squad, with bag-valve-mask ventilations, cardiac compressions, and no intravenous line in place. Her initial rhythm by cardiac monitor was ventricular fibrillation. She was immediately defibrillated with 200, 300, then 360 joules, with no apparent change in her cardiac rhythm.

39. She was intubated immediately by the transport paramedic. How much epinephrine should be administered through the ETT?
A. Epinephrine 1 mg (1:1000)
B. Epinephrine 2 mg (1:1000)
C. Epinephrine 2 mg (1:10,000)
D. Epinephrine 0.1 mg/kg (1:1000)

CPR was continued and intravenous access was obtained. Defibrillation was promptly repeated with 360 joules, again with no change in her cardiac rhythm.

40. The transport nurse administered 300 mg amiodarone IV push without any effect. What other treatment may be considered for this patient's ventricular dysrhythmia?
A. Adenosine 12 mg IV push
B. Atropine 3 mg IV push
C. Bretylium 50 mg/kg IV push
D. Amiodarone 150 mg IV push

41. The patient develops a pulse at a rate of 56 beats per minute and blood pressure of 88/50. What interventions should the transport nurse consider next?
A. Administration of atropine 3 mg IV push
B. Fluid bolus of 200 ml normal saline
C. Epinephrine infusion at 2 to 10 mcg/hr
D. Dopamine infusion at 2 to 10 mcg/hr

42. Indications for sodium bicarbonate during resuscitation include:
A. Uncorrected hypoxic metabolic acidosis
B. Known overdose of tricyclic antidepressants

C. Return of spontaneous circulation postarrest
D. To make the urine acidic in a patient with a drug overdose

43. Administration of 50% dextrose is indicated when:
A. Prehospital adult resuscitation exceeds 30 minutes
B. A whole blood glucose value demonstrates hypoglycemia
C. The patient with an altered mental state may have had a stroke
D. A whole blood glucose assay demonstrates hyperglycemia

44. Adenosine:
A. Should be the first drug administered in wide-complex tachycardia
B. May be used safely in patients with poor left ventricular function
C. Should be administered quickly and followed by a saline flush
D. Is effective in terminating dysrhythmias such as atrial fibrillation or flutter

45. A potential adverse effect of adenosine administration is:
A. Persistent first-degree, second-degree, or third-degree atrioventricular (AV) block
B. Dysrhythmias such as ventricular tachycardia
C. Facial flushing, shortness of breath, and dyspnea
D. Hypoventilation and systolic hypertension

46. Amiodarone facilitates termination of sustained ventricular tachycardia by:
A. Causing coronary artery vasoconstriction and decreasing coronary blood flow
B. Causing peripheral vasoconstriction and increasing systemic vascular resistance
C. Shortening infranodal conduction and lengthening the sinus cycle
D. Prolonging the action potential and retarding the refractory period

47. Serious adverse effects following mannitol administration may include which of the following:
1. Paradoxical increased intracranial pressure (ICP)
2. Seizures
3. Pulmonary edema and heart failure
4. Acute renal failure
A. 1 and 2
B. 2 and 3
C. 1, 2, and 3
D. All of the above

48. The transport team is caring for a 55-year-old man, weighing approximately 80 kg, who was involved in a serious motor vehicle accident and suffered severe head injuries. His neurological examination reveals decerebrate posturing of the extremities and a unilaterally dilated pupil. After initial resuscitation is completed involving immobilization, endotracheal intubation, and oxygenation, as well as intravenous access, medical direction orders mannitol to be administered.
A. Mannitol dosage is 0.25 to 2 g/kg of a 20% solution
B. Mannitol is given in a 50% solution at a dose of 20 to 160 g
C. Mannitol should be administered with an electrolyte solution
D. Mannitol may be administered with fresh frozen plasma

49. Magnesium sulfate may be used to treat which of the following:
A. Third-degree heart block with hypotension
B. Torsades de pointes or refractory ventricular tachycardia
C. Seizures due to a minor head injury
D. Second-degree heart block in an acute myocardial infarction

50. Nursing assessment parameters during the infusion of magnesium for preeclampsia or eclampsia should include which of the following:
1. Fetal heart rate and reactivity
2. Intake and output
3. Deep tendon reflexes
4. Respiratory rate and function
A. 1, 2, and 4
B. 1, 3, and 4
C. All of the above
D. None of the above

51. The transport team is called to transport a 65-year-old female who has been involved in a motor vehicle accident. She has suffered a pulmonary contusion and a moderately severe

head injury. Upon arrival at the referring facility, the transport team finds a patient in severe respiratory distress being treated with a nonrebreather mask. Her oxygen saturation is 80%. The transport team prepares to intubate the patient when her family doctor states that she has cancer and has given him verbal do-not-resuscitate (DNR) orders. He states that the patient must be transported without intubation. The transport team may:
A. Refuse to transport this patient because she has cancer and does want to be resuscitated
B. Transport the patient because the DNR orders are not available in written form
C. Refuse to transport because the physician has given them a verbal order that the patient is not to be resuscitated
D. Attempt to contact the patient's family and wait to see if they will reverse the doctor's verbal order

52. Visualization of only the corniculate cartilages is what grade on the Cormack and Lehane airway classification system?
A. Grade II
B. Grade I
C. Grade III
D. Grade IV

53. Potential adverse reactions associated with intravenous administration of fentanyl (Sublimaze) include:
1. Diaphoresis
2. Hypotension
3. Muscle rigidity
4. Tachycardia
A. 1, 2, and 3
B. 1, 2, and 4
C. 2, 3, and 4
D. All of the above

54. During the active resuscitation phase of a patient exhibiting signs and symptoms of neurogenic shock, hemodynamic effects of phenylephrine (Neo-Synephrine) that may prove beneficial include:
A. α-Agonist, β_1-agonist, and β_2-agonist effects
B. α-Agonist effects, with an increase in heart rate
C. α-Agonist effects, with an increase in systemic resistance
D. α-Agonist and β_1-agonist effects, with an increase in cardiac output

55. Side effects of terbutaline sulfate (Brethine) when used as a tocolytic agent are:
A. Hyperkalemia
B. Bradycardia
C. Hypoglycemia
D. Palpitations

56. Information needed to calculate intravenous medication infusion rates include:
A. Dosage, concentration of medication in solution, and patient's weight
B. Amount of fluid to be infused and patient's weight
C. Concentration in medicine solution and amount of intravenous fluid
D. Dosage and patient's weight

57. If you were asked to start a dopamine infusion at 8 mcg/kg per minute (concentration of 1600 mcg/ml) for a patient weighing 72 kg, the flow rate that you would infuse equals:
A. 27 mcg/min
B. 25.2 mcg/min
C. 21.6 mcg/min
D. 20 mcg/min

58. A 28-year-old male has been involved in a motor vehicle crash. He has sustained a severe head injury and requires intubation and oxygenation. His vital signs are B/P 100/50, P 120, and assisted respirations on the ventilator. The patient is restless and fighting the ETT. Which of the following agents may be used to sedate this patient for safe transport?
A. Vecuronium 10 mg every 20 minutes
B. Succinylcholine 100 mg IV boluses
C. Ketamine 1 to 2 mg/kg as an infusion
D. Etomidate 0.3 mg/kg every 15 to 20 minutes

59. When preparing an obstetrical patient for transport, the transport team should:
A. Place the patient in a right lateral recumbent position
B. Always perform a vaginal examination before transport
C. Place the patient in a left lateral recumbent position

D. Place a stretcher restraint directly over the patient's abdomen

60. Which of the following statements is true regarding heparin administration?

1. Low-dose heparin is effective in prophylaxis of thrombosis

2. High-dose heparin (0.3 units/ml and above) is required once clotting is established

3. Vitamin K is the antidote for heparin overdose

4. Heparin slows the incorporation of new fibrin, preventing clot extension

A. 1 and 2 only
B. 1, 2, and 4
C. 2, 3, and 4
D. All of the above

61. The transport team receives a report about a cardiac patient who is receiving a nitroglycerin infusion. The nurse reports that this patient is receiving an infusion at 32 ml/hr and she is uncertain what this converts to in mcg/min. The concentration of nitroglycerin is 150 mg in 500 ml 5% dextrose in water. What actual dosage of nitroglycerin is the patient receiving?

A. 40 mcg/min
B. 107 mcg/min
C. 150 mcg/min
D. 160 mcg/min

62. Which action is not characteristic of the intravenous infusion of nitroglycerin?

A. Decreases afterload
B. Relaxes smooth muscles
C. Increases cardiac output
D. Decreases preload

63. Which of the following actions are characteristic to both dopamine and dobutamine?

1. Vasoconstriction

2. Positive inotropic action

3. Alpha stimulation

4. Increased peripheral perfusion

5. Increased cardiac output

6. Tachycardia

7. Beta_1 stimulation

8. Increased myocardial contractility

A. 1, 2, 4, and 5
B. 3, 4, 5, and 6
C. 2, 3, and 5
D. 2, 5, and 7

64. Which of the following shock states would be a potential indication for the administration of norepinephrine (Levophed)?

1. Cardiogenic shock

2. Hypovolemic shock

3. Septic shock

4. Anaphylactic shock

A. 1 and 2 only
B. 3 and 4 only
C. 1, 2, and 4
D. All of the above

65. Advantages of using the laryngeal mask airway (LMA) include:

A. Advanced skills are required to use this type of airway
B. Blind insertion can be accomplished only from the front of the patient
C. Endotracheal intubation can be accomplished through the LMA
D. All laryngeal tracheal masks are made from latex

66. The transport team is transporting a man who has suffered 90% total body surface area full-thickness burns of his trunk, arms, legs, and groin, exhibiting significant hypotension. Which alternative site for an oximetry probe is least affected by poor perfusion?

A. Index finger
B. Chest wall
C. Earlobe
D. Great toe

67. Which of the following will not cause changes in the pulse oximetry readings?

A. Carbon monoxide poisoning
B. Anemia
C. Hypovolemia
D. Patient motion

68. All of the following statements are true regarding the accuracy of the pulse oximetry measurements except:

A. You will need to perform arterial blood gas monitoring per needle stick less often, even when the patient's condition is acute
B. You may verify the reading by observing the pulse waveform display

C. Comparing the heart rate displayed on the oximeter and the patient's pulse is a reliable check for accuracy
D. Pulse oximeter readings are generally unreliable during cardiac arrest states because there is no pulse

69. In which of the following clinical situations would $ETco_2$ readings be beneficial in determining ETT placement?
   1. A near-drowning victim with a palpable pulse and blood pressure
   2. A patient who has been under CPR for approximately 15 minutes
   3. A trauma victim with extensive facial injuries and extensive blood in the airway
   4. A patient who has suffered a massive pulmonary embolus
A. 1 and 3
B. 1 and 4
C. 3 and 4
D. All of the above

70. Which of the following is not a common cause of low $ETco_2$ readings?
A. Esophageal intubation
B. Pulseless electrical activity
C. Inadequate chest compressions
D. Tension pneumothorax

71. Which of the following circumstances may cause an inaccurate $ETco_2$ reading when determining tube placement?
   1. Administration of drugs via endotracheal route
   2. $ETco_2$ concentrations during profound shock or CPR
   3. Esophageal intubation of a patient who has been drinking beer
   4. Use on a victim who has aspirated a large amount of blood
A. 1, 2, and 4
B. 1, 3, and 4
C. 1, 2, and 3
D. All of the above

72. A disadvantage of ventilator use during transport is that it:
A. Frees a pair of hands during transport
B. Aids in preventing barotrauma during transport
C. Delivers consistent tidal volumes during transport
D. Causes a loss of the ability to feel lung compliance

73. You are asked to connect a patient suffering from a severe closed head injury to a ventilator, after intubation. Which of the following settings would be appropriate for this patient weighing 185 lb?
A. 100% Fio_2, 700 cc tidal volume (TV), rate 12
B. 100% Fio_2, 700 cc TV, rate 18
C. 100% Fio_2, 1 L TV, rate 16
D. 100% Fio_2, 1.5 L TV, rate 14

74. Which of the following is a relative contraindication to transcutaneous pacing during transport?
A. Unstable drug-induced bradycardia
B. Hypotension due to hypovolemia
C. Prolonged cardiac arrest prior to pacing
D. Symptomatic bradycardia due to hypothermia

75. Which of the following are acceptable methods of determining capture of the transcutaneous pacemaker?
   1. Observe a pacemaker spike followed by a wide QRS complex
   2. Hear blood flow with a Doppler device
   3. Improved level of consciousness
   4. Involuntary arm muscle contraction
A. 1 and 2
B. 1, 2, and 3
C. 2 and 3
D. All of the above

76. Which of the following pad placement positions is recommended for transcutaneous pacing?
A. Apply the anterior electrode to the right lateral aspect of the patient's chest and the posterior electrode over the right scapula
B. Apply the anterior electrode over the right side of the sternum at the fourth intercostal space
C. Apply the posterior pad to the left lateral aspect of the spine at approximately heart level
D. Apply the posterior pad on the left side of the chest in the subclavicular area when using the lateral-to-lateral position

77. A complication associated with transcutaneous pacemaker use during transport that may have lethal complications is:
A. Minor local skin burns from poor, dried electrodes, outdated pads
B. Battery failure in the pacing unit without an alternative power source
C. Continuous capture through multiple-use pads
D. Development of transient hypertension from pacing

78. The transport team is caring for a patient in complete heart block. The patient has received a total of 3 mg of atropine IV push with no change in heart rate or rhythm. You notice that the patient suddenly has a decrease in mental status and becomes hemodynamically unstable with a B/P of 60 systolic, P 30. Which of the following settings would be appropriate to use when initiating transcutaneous pacing?
A. Demand mode, highest output titrating down, rate 60
B. Demand mode, lowest output titrating up, rate 70
C. Asynchronous mode, highest output titrating down, rate 70
D. Asynchronous mode, lowest output titrating up, rate 120

79. Arterial systole begins with the opening of:
A. Mitral valve
B. Tricuspid valve
C. Aortic valve
D. Bicuspid valve

80. The transport team is transporting a 33-year-old male, who is hypovolemic from a pelvic fracture, from a critical care unit to a Level I trauma center. He has a PA catheter in place. His cardiac output is 4 and his CVP reading is 3. His B/P is 96/60, P 110, and R 20. Which of the following findings confirm the clinical picture of hypovolemia?
A. PAWP 12 mm Hg, systemic vascular resistance (SVR) 800
B. PAWP 5 mm Hg, pulmonary vascular resistance (PVR) 400
C. PAWP 5 mm Hg, SVR 1500
D. PAWP 18 mm Hg, SVR 250

81. Following a sharp rise on the arterial pressure waveform, a small dip occurs on the down slope (see figure below). This dip, which marks the onset of diastole and closure of the aortic valves, is called:

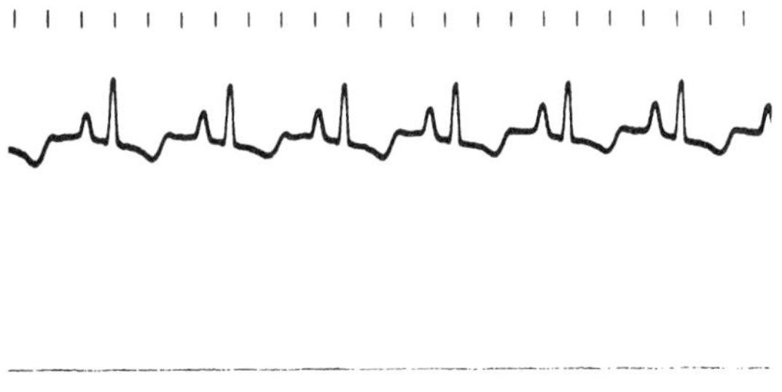

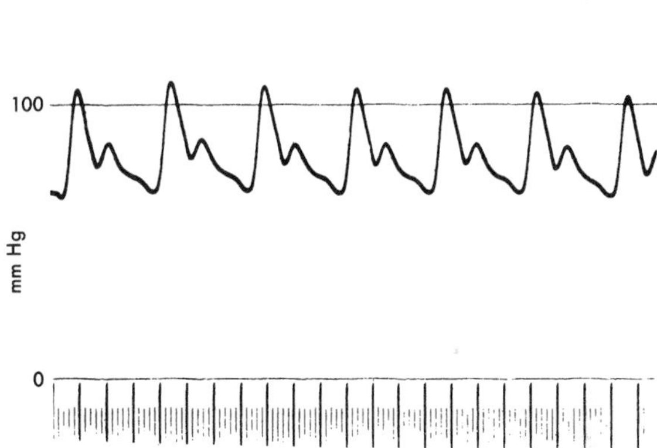

A. Peak systolic pressure
B. Dicrotic notch
C. Diastole
D. Secondary waves

82. Arterial waveforms in the elderly have all the following characteristics except:
A. Dampened dicrotic notch
B. Absent secondary diastolic waves
C. Increased pulse pressure
D. Sharpened dicrotic notch

83. Before any hemodynamic pressure measurements can be obtained, the transport team must position the patient in which manner?
A. Flat supine position without a pillow
B. Head of the bed elevated 90 degrees
C. Head of the bed elevated 60 degrees
D. In a position where the reference point is at the middle of the chest

84. Upon arrival at the referring facility, the transport nurse's assessment findings reveal a dampened arterial waveform and mottling of the extremity distal to the radial arterial line site. Immediate interventions include all the following except:
A. Assess collateral artery for blood flow
B. Flush catheter with saline by syringe
C. Assess intravenous pressure bag for heparin
D. Immediately remove arterial catheter

85. During flight (altitude 8000 ft) the patient's arterial waveform begins to dampen. There are no clinical symptoms, and the patient's vital signs are stable. Which of the following would not contribute to a dampened waveform?
A. A cannula lodged against the arterial vessel wall
B. Air trapped between the transducer and dome diaphragms
C. Stopcocks inadvertently turned in the wrong direction
D. Kinking of the arterial catheter

86. A transport team's assessment of the accuracy of an arterial waveform is performed initially by obtaining a cuff blood pressure reading. A slight difference between the cuff and arterial blood pressure is normally:
A. 5 to 10 mm Hg
B. 11 to 15 mm Hg
C. 16 to 20 mm Hg
D. Over 20 mm Hg

87. During transport, the team notes an increasing heart rate despite the mean arterial pressure (MAP) remaining constant. Which of the following may contribute to these changes?
A. Improper calibration of the equipment
B. Kinked arterial monitoring lines
C. Insufficient pressure in the pressure bag
D. Patient deterioration

88. Ensuring consistency of hemodynamic readings during transport is achieved by taping the transducer to the phlebostatic axis reference point. Which of the following locations serves as this reference point?
A. Second intercostal space at midaxillary line
B. Second intercostal space at anterior axillary line
C. Fourth intercostal space at midaxillary line
D. Fourth intercostal space at anterior axillary line

89. Once the transducer is level with the phlebostatic axis, the transducer must be "zeroed." Before pushing and releasing the auto-zero function button, the stopcock on the transducer must first be open to which port:
A. Patient
B. Flush
C. Air
D. Monitor

90. During flight (altitude 3500 ft), the patient becomes slightly restless. The transport team observes abnormally high digital pressures; however, the waveform remains normal. Troubleshooting focuses on:
A. Ensuring transducer is at phlebostatic axis
B. Checking stopcock positions
C. Aspirating the line for patency
D. Flushing the system

91. Preventing inadvertent tubing separation and accidental blood loss from an arterial line during transport is best achieved with all the following interventions except:
A. Set alarm systems
B. Use Luer-Lok connections
C. Keep connections visible
D. Monitor the MAP

Questions 92 through 94 are to be answered using the following patient scenario:

Upon arrival at the referring facility, the transport nurse assesses a cardiac patient with a PA catheter. The patient is secured to the transport stretcher, and the PA pressure monitoring system has been zeroed, leveled, and calibrated. The system has no air bubbles, and the transducer is set up correctly.

92. When the patient has been placed on the transport stretcher and the monitoring equipment secured and calibrated, the transport nurse observes the following. This waveform is indicative of:

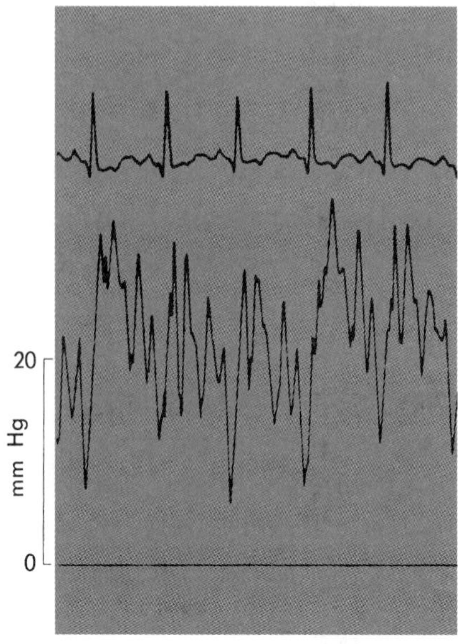

A. A normal PA waveform without interference
B. A pattern of elevated PA pressure
C. A waveform demonstrating excessive catheter movement
D. Normal PAWP waveform

93. The patient simultaneously develops ventricular ectopy during this period. The first intervention the flight nurse should do is:
A. Administer an antidysrhythmic medication
B. Inflate the PA balloon
C. Flush the hemodynamic line setup system
D. Deflate the PA balloon

94. The transport nurse inflates the PA balloon with 2 cc of air, and the following pattern occurs:

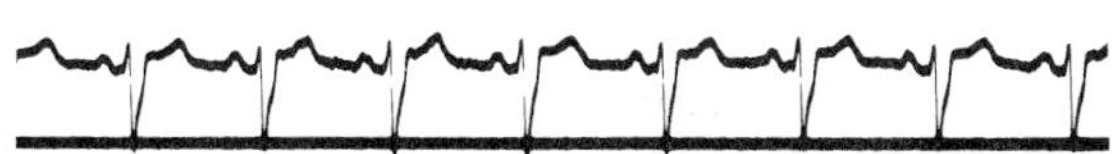

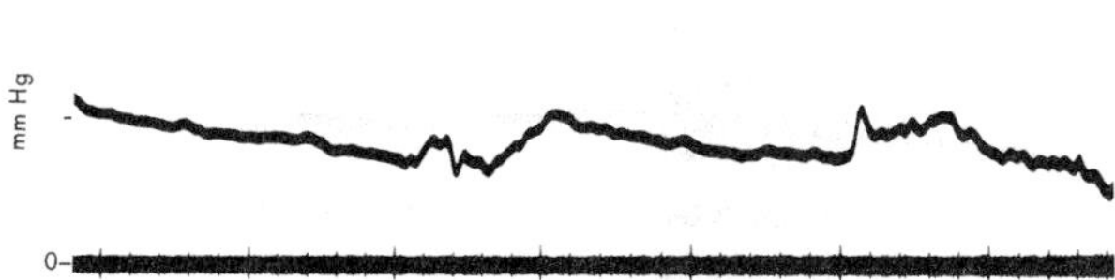

The following immediate action should be taken:
A. Deflate balloon
B. Withdraw PA catheter 5 cm
C. Activate quick-flush device
D. Check stopcocks

95. The transport team is requested for a 66-year-old diagnosed with an acute anterior wall myocardial infarction. During flight, the patient's clinical status deteriorates. The systolic blood pressure falls to 70 mm Hg. The PAWP reading has increased to 20 mm Hg. Which of the following interventions would best assist the patient's hemodynamic status?
A. Administer 500 ml normal saline bolus
B. Administer dopamine infusion
C. Administer 500 ml lactated Ringer's bolus
D. Administer nitroglycerin infusion

Questions 96 through 98 are to be answered using the following patient scenario:

The patient at the referring facility was diagnosed with an acute inferior wall myocardial infarction. Nitroglycerin and dopamine infusions were initiated for hemodynamic support. The referring nurse stated that the arterial line pressure correlates with B/P cuff readings, and the PAWP correlates with the PA end-diastolic (PAD) pressure. Initial ECG assessment revealed sinus rhythm with ST elevation in leads II, III, and aVF. Patient denies chest pain or discomfort. The patient is secured to transport stretcher, and the arterial and PA catheters are properly zeroed.

96. During flight, the patient develops chest pain, diaphoresis, and hypotension. The transport nurse is unable to obtain a PA wedge waveform. An alternative method to assess the patient's fluid volume status is best accomplished by:
A. Arterial diastolic blood pressure
B. PA systolic pressure
C. PAD pressure
D. Arterial systolic pressure

97. The patient continues to experience chest pain, diaphoresis, and hypotension. The PAD pressure is 4 mm Hg. Which of the following interventions may best assist the patient's hemodynamic condition?
A. Increase dopamine infusion
B. Increase nitroglycerin infusion
C. Administer morphine IV push
D. Administer normal saline bolus

98. Upon arrival at the receiving hospital, the patient states his neck feels wet. In assessing the area, the transport nurse finds fluid leaking from the catheter. Three small black bands are noted at the point the PA catheter enters the subclavian introducer. Immediate intervention includes:
A. Flushing the catheter to determine patency
B. Inflating PA balloon to see if the monitor works
C. Advancing PA catheter until the lines disappear
D. Administering the intravenous medications at another site

99. Upon arrival at the referring facility, the transport nurse is unable to obtain a normal PA waveform pattern. The waveform appears dampened. In assessing the flush system, the flush bag device has insufficient pressure. A clot in the catheter is suspected. Corrective measures include:
A. Gentle aspiration followed by gentle flushing
B. Instill 1000 units heparin into the catheter
C. Discontinue and change the flush setup device
D. Reposition the catheter to assess waveform changes

100. The transport team is requested for a patient diagnosed with an anterior wall myocardial infarction. The vital signs have been stable. Cuff blood pressures correlate well with those of the arterial line. PA pressure is 25/10 mm Hg, and PAWP is 11 mm Hg. Due to equipment failure, only one invasive pressure channel is available. Which of the following parameters should be monitored during transport?
A. Central venous pressures
B. Arterial line pressures
C. PA wedge pressures
D. PA pressures

101. Inflating a PA balloon requires how much air?
A. Less than 0.5 cc
B. 0.5 to 1 cc
C. 1.25 to 1.5 cc
D. 1.6 to 2 cc

102. IABP therapy is indicated to:
A. Decrease cardiac afterload
B. Decrease systemic perfusion
C. Increase myocardial oxygen demand
D. Decrease coronary artery perfusion

103. The most commonly used reference point, or "trigger," for inflation and deflation of the IABP is the patient's:
A. T wave of ECG
B. R wave of ECG
C. Slightly before the QRS complex
D. Slightly after the QRS complex

104. Adjusting the inflation time of the IABP corresponds to which segment of the arterial waveform?
A. Peak systolic pressure
B. End-diastolic pressure
C. Systolic upstroke
D. Dicrotic notch

105. Optimal deflation of the IABP occurs:
A. At peak systolic pressure
B. At middiastolic pressure
C. Prior to systolic upstroke
D. At dicrotic notch

106. During transport, the patient with an IABP requests to "sit up a bit" so she can "see the scenery." The patient's vital signs have been stable. Which of the following responses should the flight nurse give the patient?
A. "You'll have to lie flat to prevent kinking of the catheter."
B. "You'll have to lie flat to prevent the catheter from migrating."
C. "You can only have your head raised with pillows."
D. "You can have your head raised less than 15 degrees."

107. The transport team has been requested for a patient with an IABP. The transport nurse can prevent a serious complication of IABP by assessing which of the following?
A. Monitoring the insertion site for infection
B. Preventing complications from immobility
C. Monitoring for signs of improved cardiac function
D. Monitoring the patient's left radial pulse

108. During transport, your assessment of the IABP reveals a loss of vacuum. Indicate the amount of air needed to manually inflate and

deflate the balloon every 5 minutes in order to prevent clot formation.
A. 10 cc of air in a 20 cc syringe
B. Half the total amount of the balloon volume
C. Total amount of the balloon volume
D. Inflation and deflation not necessary due to administration of anticoagulant therapy

A 19-year-old man is the victim of a drive-by shooting. The patient is lying supine on a lawn and is moaning. The patient's skin is pale, cool, and diaphoretic. He has a weak radial B/P of 110 and a respiratory rate of 36. Gunshot wounds are noted to the right upper chest, approximately 2 cm below the clavicle and toward the right upper quadrant.

109. What is the first priority of the transport team when entering the scene?
A. Check the patient's airway for patency
B. Obtain report from the first responders
C. Evaluate the scene for potential hazards
D. Complete a primary assessment in 60 seconds

110. During the primary survey, you note that the patient's respiratory rate is 36 per minute. At what rate should the transport team be concerned about respiratory compromise?
A. 28 to 30
B. 24 to 26
C. 18 to 20
D. 22 to 26

111. During the primary survey, the transport team discovers that the gunshot wound has caused an open pneumothorax (sucking chest wound). At this point the transport nurse would administer oxygen and:
A. Decompress the left chest with a 14-gauge needle
B. Decompress the right chest with a 10-gauge needle
C. Apply a sterile occlusive dressing to the wound
D. Apply a pulse oximetry probe to monitor the SaO_2

112. During the primary survey, which three observations will assist in determining the patient's hemodynamic stability?
1. Skin color
2. Blood pressure
3. Pulse
4. Level of consciousness
A. 1, 2, and 3
B. 1, 3, and 4
C. 2, 3, and 4
D. 1, 2, and 4

113. The patient is combative and uncooperative, requiring restraint for safe transport. The most common type of chemical restraint used by most air medical transport programs is:
A. Leather restraints or police handcuffs attached to the transport stretcher
B. Neuromuscular blockade with concomitant sedation
C. Haloperidol or droperidol intravenously or intramuscularly
D. Morphine or fentanyl intravenously every 60 minutes

A 24-year-old woman was a passenger on a motorcycle that broadsided an automobile at a high rate of speed. The patient was found approximately 40 feet from the accident site. She was not wearing a helmet. Upon initial assessment, she is unresponsive to verbal stimuli, does not open her eyes, withdraws to pain, and is moaning.

114. From the description of this patient, what would her GCS be?
A. 7
B. 8
C. 6
D. 9

115. Oxygenation and ventilation should be accomplished by what method?
A. Oxygen at 15 L/minute per nonrebreather mask
B. Oxygen at 5 L/minute per nasal cannula
C. Endotracheal intubation with 100% oxygen
D. Bag-valve-mask ventilation with room air

116. When securing the airway of a patient with multiple injuries, which additional intervention should be performed?
A. The head should be placed in the sniffing position for better tube placement
B. An additional caregiver is needed to perform spinal immobilization
C. Blow-by oxygen should be administered during the entire procedure

D. An intravenous line should always be inserted before intubation is attempted

117. During transport, the patient's GCS remains 7. Her pulse rate is 64 and her respirations are being assisted at a rate of 24. Her B/P decreases to 88/40. The transport team should:
A. Increase her ventilation rate to 30 to decrease her ICP
B. Initiate a vasoactive medication until her systolic B/P is 100 mm Hg
C. Place the patient in Trendelenburg position to increase her blood pressure
D. Administer isotonic intravenous fluids until an adequate blood pressure is obtained

A 15-year-old male patient dove from a rock approximately 15 feet into a shallow river, hitting his head on the river bottom. Since the dive, he has been unable to move his extremities and has no sensation from the nipple line down.

118. During the primary survey, it is important to expose the patient to:
A. Avoid missing any obvious injuries such as a protruding object or other injuries that may have been missed
B. Obtain intravenous access to administer pain medication during the transport process
C. Mark on the patient the level of sensation that he is able to perceive
D. Induce mild hypothermia, which may protect the spinal cord from swelling and additional injury

119. When securing this injured patient to a backboard, the patient's head should be secured:
A. First before his trunk and extremities
B. Last after his trunk and extremities
C. At the same time as the trunk and extremities
D. Not at all because he is already paralyzed

120. The patient asks if he will ever move again. The transport nurse should:
A. Tell the patient that everything is going to be fine because he is being transported to a Level I trauma center
B. Tell the patient that you will take very good care of him but that he has a serious injury and may never move again
C. Tell him not to worry about it because there are other things he should be concerned about at this time
D. Change the subject by pointing out what equipment is used inside of the aircraft and how rapidly you will get him to the hospital

You arrive at the scene of a motor vehicle accident to find a 68-year-old woman, who was the unrestrained front-seat passenger, in an auto/auto accident. The vehicles have collided in a head-to-head manner, leaving the front ends of both vehicles severely compromised.

121. From the transport team's observation of the crash scene, which injuries would be anticipated based on a frontal and side impact mechanism of injury?
A. Fractured ribs
B. Spinal injury
C. Pelvic fracture
D. All of the above

122. The patient is extricated from the car. Her airway is patent, and high-flow oxygen is administered. She has equal bilateral breath sounds, but no peripheral pulses are palpated. The patient has received 2 L of normal saline, and the transport team decides to infuse O-negative packed red blood cells. Advantages of administering blood during transport include:
A. Delaying the launch of the transport because the blood bank is located some distance from the transport vehicle
B. Clinical evaluation of the amount of significant blood loss is difficult in the transport environment, so deciding when to administer the blood may be difficult
C. Blood resuscitation is indicated after a 2-L bolus of crystalloid in patients with ongoing blood loss to increase oxygen carrying capacity
D. Not all transport teams employ personnel who are familiar with blood transfusion procedures, and patients may be placed at grave risk

123. During transport, the patient is complaining of severe dyspnea. She has no palpable radial pulse; the monitor shows a heart rate of 140. Upon auscultation, breath sounds are found to be absent on the right side. Her neck veins are

slightly distended. The transport nurse should suspect:
A. Cardiac tamponade
B. A simple pneumothorax
C. A tension pneumothorax
D. Hypovolemic shock

124. Predisposing factors to empyema include all of the following except:
A. Multiple chest tube placement
B. Prehospital tube placement
C. Underlying pulmonary damage
D. Persistent pleural effusion

You respond to a construction accident. You arrive to find a 28-year-old male who has sustained a traumatic amputation of his right thumb and a partial amputation of the right index finger by a table saw.

125. An important determinant in the success of reimplantation is:
A. The general health of the patient before the injury
B. The amount of time the amputated part is ischemic
C. How contaminated the amputated part has become
D. The amount of tissue that has been amputated

126. How should the amputated fingers be transported?
A. Immersed in cold, sterile water, sealed in a plastic bag
B. Placed in a bag of ice, wrapped in a moistened dressing, and placed in a basin
C. Wrapped in a moistened gauze, sealed in a plastic bag, which is placed in melting ice
D. Wrapped in a dry sterile dressing and placed dry in a plastic bag

127. During transport, management of severe head injury includes:
A. Administering high-dose glucocorticoids intravenously as soon as possible
B. Hyperventilating the patient at a rate of 30 breaths per minute to decrease the PCO_2 to 30
C. Administering mannitol prophylactically to prevent an increase in ICP
D. Maintaining an adequate blood pressure to maintain adequate cerebral perfusion pressure

Your rotary-wing aircraft has been called to a rural facility to transport a 19-year-old male who was involved in an assault. The injury occurred about 2 hours earlier, and the patient has been diagnosed with a probable diffuse axonal injury. His GCS is 5 (E-1, V-1, M-3). Pupils are midsize and nonreactive to light. The patient has been intubated and is being ventilated manually, has two peripheral intravenous lines at a keep-open rate, and remains in full spinal immobilization.

128. In preparation for transport, the transport team should:
A. Remove the patient's cervical collar and raise the head of the bed 30 degrees to facilitate intracranial blood flow
B. Insert a gastric tube to decompress the patient's stomach and decrease the risk of aspiration during transport
C. Increase the patient's intravenous fluid rate to 100 ml/hr for fluid maintenance and to decrease the patient's intracranial blood flow
D. Decrease the assisted ventilatory rate to 16 breaths per minute to decrease the risk of pulmonary edema

129. The referring facility shows the transport team the patient's cervical spine film. After reviewing the film, the flight nurse should consider all of the following except:
A. The film shows all seven vertebrae without deformity; spinal immobilization may be removed
B. The film does not show all seven vertebrae; spinal immobilization should be maintained
C. The film shows all seven vertebrae without deformity; spinal immobilization should be maintained
D. The film shows deformity; spinal immobilization should be maintained until the patient arrives at the receiving hospital

130. Subcutaneous emphysema on a chest radiograph is:
A. A uniform density indicating a collection of blood

B. Defined as fluid collection in the pleural space
C. Noted as radiolucent pockets or spongy areas
D. Ill-defined, saucer-shaped, nonvascular densities

131. The transport team is reviewing the following cervical spine films of a patient involved in a motor vehicle crash. This film demonstrates:

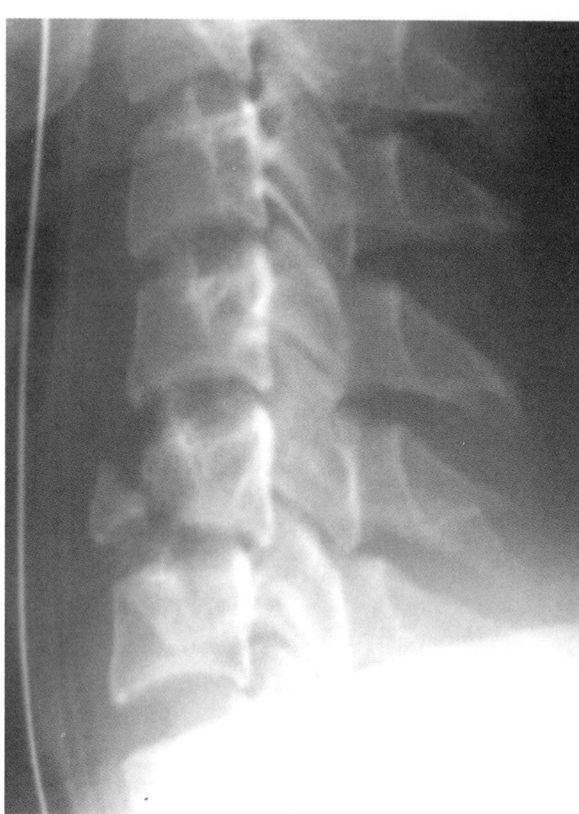

From Mirvis S, Shanmuganathan K: *Imaging in Trauma and Critical Care*, ed 2, Philadelphia, 2003, Saunders.

A. Unilateral facet dislocation
B. Flexion teardrop fracture of C5
C. Normal anteroposterior projection
D. Normal atlantooccipital alignment

132. The transport team is looking at the following films. The referring physician states that based on these views, he feels comfortable removing the patient's cervical collar. The transport team should:

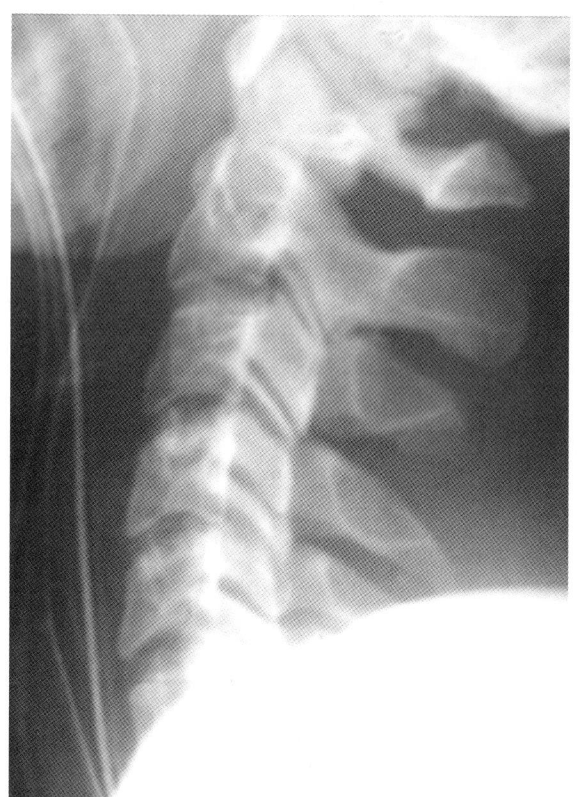

From Mirvis S, Shanmuganathan K: *Imaging in Trauma and Critical Care*, ed 2, Philadelphia, 2003, Saunders.

A. Allow the referring physician to remove the patient's cervical collar based on these views
B. Request that a magnetic resonance imaging scan be performed before the patient is cleared for transport
C. Request an additional view so that the cervical spine can be evaluated adequately
D. Wait to put the collar back on the patient once the patient is in the transport vehicle

133. The radiograph demonstrates:

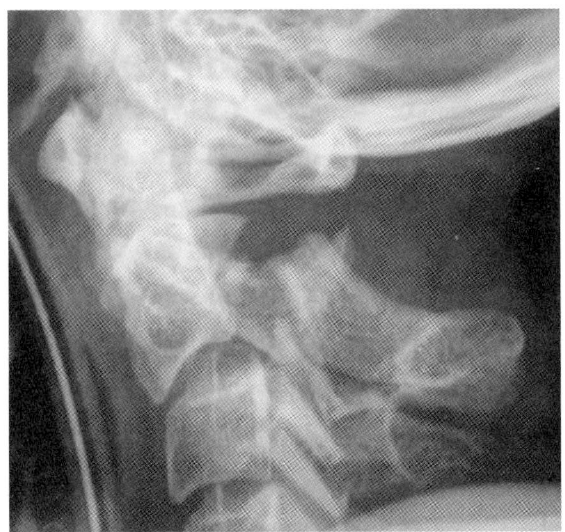

From Mirvis S, Shanmuganathan K: *Imaging in Trauma and Critical Care*, ed 2, Philadelphia, 2003, Saunders.

A. A jumped cervical facet
B. A teardrop fracture
C. An extension sprain
D. A hangman's fracture

134. This chest radiograph demonstrates:

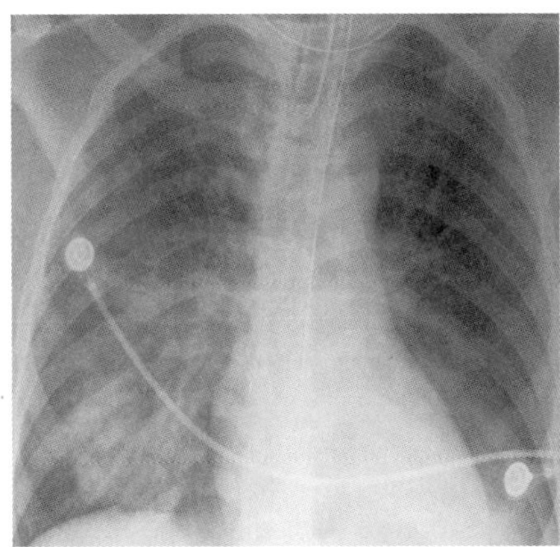

From Mirvis S, Shanmuganathan K: *Imaging in Trauma and Critical Care*, ed 2, Philadelphia, 2003, Saunders.

A. Tension pneumothorax
B. Pulmonary contusion
C. Hemothorax
D. Pneumohemothorax

135. This chest radiograph demonstrates:

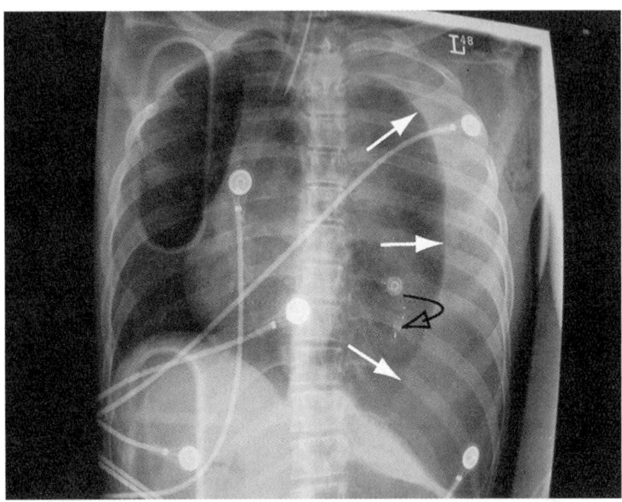

From Mirvis S, Shanmuganathan K: *Imaging in Trauma and Critical Care*, ed 2, Philadelphia, 2003, Saunders.

A. A tension pneumothorax
B. A pulmonary contusion
C. A hemothorax
D. A pneumohemothorax

136. A 33-year-old male with an acute myocardial infarction who has had an IABP inserted is being transported. The rate is 1:2. During transport, his level of consciousness begins to decrease. He has a patent airway and his B/P is 100/78, P 90, R 20, and Sao_2 98%. What may be happening?
A. The patient's myocardial infarction has extended
B. The balloon catheter has migrated upward
C. The balloon catheter has migrated downward
D. It is normal for this occur during transport

137. During transport of a 55-year-old male with an IABP, the transport nurse notices a U shape of the waveform inscribed before the next systolic upstroke. What is the timing problem?
A. Late inflation
B. Early inflation
C. Late deflation
D. Early deflation

138. The transport team knows that when transporting the IABP, the balloon catheter inflation should occur:
A. Before closure of the pulmonic valve
B. Before opening of the pulmonic valve

C. Before closure of the aortic valve
D. Immediately before the aortic valve opens

139. The transport team knows to watch for signs of preload elevation in which patient?
A. The patient in septic shock
B. The patient in neurogenic shock
C. The patient hypovolemic shock
D. The patient in cardiogenic shock

140. The transport team is preparing to transport a 40-year-old female with an acute myocardial infarction. The referring facility has inserted a PA catheter. Her B/P is 100/66, P 66, CVP 16, cardiac output 3.8, PCWP 14. Which of the following treatments is indicated to treat this patient?
A. Nitroglycerin
B. Dopamine
C. Amrinone
D. Insertion of an IABP

141. Which of the following is not an indication for an IABP?
A. Severe left ventricular failure
B. Acute ventricular septal rupture
C. Unstable angina
D. Aortic valve regurgitation

142. During transport of a patient with an IABP catheter that was placed in the left femoral vessel, it is noted that the patient's urinary output has decreased. What should the transport team suspect?
A. Renal failure
B. Possible displacement of the catheter
C. Improper timing of the IABP
D. IABP leak

143. The transport team is transporting a 44-year-old female who has had an IABP inserted. Her vital signs are B/P 86/45, P 70, R 16, and SaO_2 98%. The patient denies chest or other discomfort. The team notes scattered petechiae over her trunk and extremities. What do these findings indicate?
A. Infection
B. Aortic dissection
C. Thrombocytopenia
D. Emboli

144. During transport, the transport team notes brown flecks in the IABP catheter line. What could cause this?
A. A balloon leak
B. A balloon rupture
C. Improper timing
D. This is a normal finding

145. What is the significance of 2,3-diphosphoglycerate (2,3-DPG) in relation to the oxyhemoglobin dissociation curve?
A. It indicates a left shift
B. It causes hemoglobin to hold on to oxygen
C. It causes hemoglobin to release oxygen
D. It has no clinical significance

146. Which of the following arterial blood gas results would you expect to see in a patient with diabetic ketoacidosis?
A. pH 7.40, PaO_2 80, $PaCO_2$ 30, HCO_3 22
B. pH 7.40, PaO_2 90, $PaCO_2$ 50, HCO_3 33
C. pH 7.27, PaO_2 90, $PaCO_2$ 50, HCO_3 20
D. pH 7.20, PaO_2 88, $PaCO_2$ 23, HCO_3 16

147. What is the single most significant predictor of violent behavior during transport?
A. History of substance abuse
B. History of verbal aggression
C. Hypoxic brain injury
D. History of violent behavior

148. A 65-year-old male patient has suffered a myocardial infarction without ST elevation and requires transport to a tertiary center for rescue angioplasty. During flight (altitude 8000 ft), he develops 10/10 chest pain. The first two actions the flight nurse should perform are:

1. Wait for 5 minutes to see if the pain decreases
2. Increase the oxygen to 15 L/min via nonrebreather mask
3. Increase the oxygen to 5 L/min via nasal prongs
4. Administer 2 puffs of nitroglycerin spray
5. Administer 2.5 mg IV morphine sulfate
6. Request medical priority from air traffic control

A. 1 and 6
B. 3 and 4
C. 2 and 5
D. 2 and 4

149. As a flight nurse you are working for an Australian aeromedical organization and are repatriating a U.S. patient to Los Angeles from Australia. The commercial airline operator is British Airways. Over New Zealand airspace, the patient becomes critically ill and a Canadian physician volunteers to assist. If the patient dies, the laws of which country will apply to the patient's death?
A. United States of America
B. New Zealand
C. Australia
D. Great Britain

150. A complete transport record should include a statement that contains which of the following?
A. Mode of transport, air or ground
B. Patient assessment
C. Reason for patient transport
D. All of the above

ANSWERS

1. **B. Intervention.** The nursing process is composed of assessment, planning (identifying and making the appropriate transport arrangements), implementation (transferring the patient), and evaluation.
2. **C. Assessment.** Maternal risk factors associated with an increased need for neonatal resuscitation include age over 35 years, diabetes, hemorrhage, no prenatal care, infection, premature rupture of membranes, and a prolonged labor.[5]
3. **D. Assessment.** Indications for endotracheal intubation of the neonate include the need for tracheal suctioning of meconium, ineffective bag-valve-mask ventilation and, when there is a need, prolonged positive-pressure ventilation, which may be required during transport. In addition, when the infant requires epinephrine for resuscitation, the ETT is a common route of administration.[5]
4. **D. Intervention.** Research and reported cases have demonstrated that patients transported using nitric oxide included those with persistent pulmonary hypertension of the newborn, meconium aspiration syndrome, congenital diaphragmatic hernia, respiratory distress syndrome, congenital heart disease, hypoplastic lungs, and pneumonia.[6]
5. **A. Evaluation.** A good blood return indicates that the umbilical catheter is appropriately placed. The catheter should be inserted only 1 to 4 cm and should be located in the umbilical vein. The umbilical vein is a thin-walled single vessel compared with umbilical arteries, which are thick walled and are paired.[5]
6. **B. Intervention.** Preparation for the transport of this child should include definitive airway management. Based on the child's clinical findings and oxygen saturation, endotracheal intubation before transport would afford the best method of managing this child's airway.[5-7]
7. **D. Intervention.** The approximate size of the ETT is determined by the baby's weight.[5]

Tube Size (mm, inside diameter)	Weight (g)	Gestational Age (wks)
2.5	Below 1000	Below 28
3.0	1000 to 2000	28 to 34
3.5	2000 to 3000	34 to 38
3.5 to 4.0	Above 3000	Above 38

8. **B. Intervention.** The infant should receive 45 ml of normal saline.[5]
9. **A. Evaluation.** The neonate's central and peripheral pulses should be monitored to evaluate the effectiveness of fluid resuscitation.[6-8]
10. **C. Analysis.** Based on the gravity of the child's condition, the mother is probably fearful of whether the child will survive. Many neonatal transport teams carry a camera so that they can leave a picture of the child with the mother, as well as calling the mother when arriving at the receiving facility to help decrease her fear about her child.[5]
11. **D. Intervention.** The intravenous fluids should be calculated based on the total weight of the twins and then divided and a share given to each infant. Each infant should have her own intravenous access. Medication should be given to the weaker or smaller of the twins first, so that its effects can be evaluated. Positioning of the infants in the isolette should ensure that both twins are at the same level to prevent hypovolemia.[5-10]
12. **D. Intervention.**[4]
13. **C. Assessment.** Electromagnetic interference can trigger or inhibit pacemaker output, cause inappropriate programming, and cause permanent function disruption.[11]
14. **D. Assessment and Intervention.** When deciding whether family members should

accompany a child during transport, the flight team needs to consider the size of the transport vehicle, the condition of the child, if the flight program has a protocol to allow someone to ride along, and what effect the presence of the parents would have on the child.[12,13]

15. **C. Intervention.** Nursing interventions for families include speaking to the family before transport, allowing the family to see the child before transport, and providing them with written material about the transport, how to get to the receiving facility, and who to contact on their arrival.[3,12,13]
16. **D. Assessment.** Even though the literature has shown many advantages of allowing family members to accompany patients during transport, there are some significant disadvantages. These include fear of flying which could distract the pilot, motion sickness, interference with patient care, and feeling forced to accompany the patient.[14]
17. **A. Assessment.** Research has shown that bag ventilation contributes to either hypocapnia or hypercapnia because of interruption of ventilation, limited crew members, and the need to interrupt ventilation to perform other treatment modalities.[15-17]
18. **C. Assessment.** The administration of aminoglycoside agents to the patient receiving mivacurium will increase the duration of the neuromuscular blockade. Additional medications that will increase neuromuscular blockade include quinidine, local anesthetics, halothane, procainamide, and lithium.[17-19]
19. **A. Intervention.** A nasogastric tube will decompress the child's abdomen and decrease the possibility of aspiration. Because the child was intubated using Pediatric Advanced Life Support guidelines, the ETT will not have a cuff.[5]
20. **B. Assessment.** Transport of a critically ill or injured patient may be delayed because of prolonged entrapment, lack of rescue equipment and personnel, bad weather conditions, and inaccurate assessment of the acuity of the patient's illness or injury.[20]
21. **A. Analysis.** The most appropriate nursing diagnosis on which to base this patient's care would be gas exchange, impaired, related to his medical diagnosis as evidenced by his low oxygen saturation.
22. **D. Assessment.** Because of the risk of decompression illness, the patient's diving history must be evaluated carefully before transport.
23. **B. Assessment.** The insurance status of the patient should not factor into the decision to transport a patient to the appropriate receiving facility.[20]
24. **D. Assessment.** Sources of stress in the flight and prehospital care nursing environment include lack of space, malfunctioning equipment, difficult work relationships, age of the patient, and death of the patient (expected or unexpected).[13,18,21,22]
25. **D. Assessment.** Stress reactions are classified as either acute or long term. Examples of acute stress reactions include exhaustion, headaches, nightmares, and anger. Long-term stress reactions include chronic illness, alteration in personal finances, anomia, and negative patient interactions.[18,21,22]
26. **B. Intervention.** Stress management after being exposed to a critical incident would include eating an appropriate diet, particularly one high in vitamin B, cutting back on alcohol and cigarettes, and exercise such as a brisk walk.[18,21,22]
27. **C. Assessment.** An adverse reaction to succinylcholine is increased intraocular pressure. Relative contraindications for use should therefore include penetrating eye wounds, eye surgery, and glaucoma.[19,23] Complications such as increased ICP, muscle fasciculations, and cardiac dysrhythmia can be greatly reduced by premedication with lidocaine 1 mg/kg IV push.[19,23]
28. **B. Intervention.** The recommended intubation dose of mivacurium chloride is 0.25 mg/kg (0.15 mg/kg over 1 to 2 minutes). The onset of action, producing intubation conditions is approximately 1.8 minutes.[22] The recommended paralyzing dosage of vecuronium (Norcuron) ranges from 0.04 to 0.1 mg/kg in the child and 0.1 mg/kg in the adult patient.[19,23]
29. **A. Intervention.** Methylprednisolone is a glucocorticoid that is thought to limit secondary injury to the spinal cord by inhibiting lipid peroxidation. This, in turn, helps to limit formation and release of the various deleterious chemicals such as prostaglandins, maintain spinal cord blood flow, decrease nerve degradation, and enhance nerve excitability.[24]

30. **D. Assessment.** Gastrointestinal bleeding is a relative complication associated with glucocorticoid use, but was not found to worsen with administration of this drug. A contraindication is a spinal cord lesion below L-2. Special considerations in methylprednisolone administration include pregnancy, age younger than 13 years, penetrating wounds to the spinal cord, fulminant infection or tuberculosis, human immunodeficiency virus infection, and severe diabetes.[24] Methylprednisolone, which can cause immunosuppression, may worsen these conditions.
31. **B. Assessment.** Although the first clinical indicators of cyanide toxicity may be behavioral, these changes are often attributed to ICU psychosis in the critically ill. A good warning sign of impending toxicity may be hypertension. Unfortunately, this will often trigger staff to increase the nitroprusside infusion to control the rising blood pressure, which rapidly compounds the cyanide accumulation and resultant life-threatening complications.[25]
32. **A. Intervention.** When determining any infusion rate, one must first calculate the concentration of the solution. This solution was made with a dilution of 50 mg of nitroprusside in 250 ml 5% dextrose in water. After dividing 50 mg by 250 ml, a concentration of 0.2 mg/ml, or 200 mcg/ml, was determined. To further calculate the dosage rate in mcg/kg per minute, you must simply multiply the appropriate numbers: 10 mcg × 80 kg × 60 min (multiplying by 60 [minutes] will convert the product to the rate of mcg/hr). Lastly, this total must be divided by the concentration, which is 200 mcg/ml in this example. The entire formula written out would appear as: 10 mcg/kg/min × 80 kg × 60 min/hr ÷ 1 ml/200 mcg = 240 ml/hr.
33. **D. Assessment.** The side effects of midazolam include respiratory depression and decrease in peripheral vascular resistance, which results in hypotension.[19]
34. **C. Assessment.** You may get prolonged respiratory depression when these drugs are combined with other CNS depressants, such as alcohol or barbiturates. An increased sedative and hypnotic effect occurs when combined with fentanyl, narcotic agonists, or analgesics. Benzodiazepines will demonstrate a shorter onset of action and a longer duration of sedation when used in combination therapy.[19]
35. **C. Evaluation.** Flumazenil has a specific warning against its use in multiple drug ingestion, especially if a tricyclic antidepressant is suspected. This warning refers to the adverse effect of seizures brought about in patients treated with flumazenil and that life-threatening seizures can occur in tricyclic antidepressant overdose.[26]
36. **B. Intervention.** Patient anxiety related to flying can be allayed by keeping in mind that:[27]
    - Most patients are more concerned about their medical condition than the flight
    - Asking patients about their previous flight experience and their reactions to plane crashes can help predict their level of anxiety
    - Patients' anxiety levels decrease as the flight progresses
    - Educating patients about the transport environment helps
37. **C. Intervention.** For asystolic, or pulseless, arrest in children, the recommended first dose is IV or IO: 0.01 mg/kg (1:10,000) or ETT: 0.1 mg/kg (1:1000). The subsequent dose may or may not be a higher dose given IV, IO, or ETT: 0.1 mg/kg (1:1000). Higher dose epinephrine may actually cause a worse outcome in pediatric patients. It is important to note that this was found in pediatric arrests that occurred in the hospital.[5,28]
38. **A. Assessment.** The effects of the β-agonist are increased heart rate, increased force of contraction (both of these lead to an increase in myocardial oxygen consumption), and bronchodilation. The α-agonist action results in vasoconstriction, leading to an increase in blood pressure. Several investigators have established that increasing the α-agonist effect (by increasing the dosage of epinephrine) results in improved coronary blood flow, improved cerebral blood flow, and improved rate of resuscitation.[28]
39. **C. Intervention.** The recommended dosage of epinephrine is 1 mg down the ETT every 3 to 5 minutes.[29]
40. **D. Intervention.** An additional dose of amiodarone 150 mg IV push may be administered.[29-31]
41. **B. Intervention.** When a bradydysrhythmia occurs, the cause should be evaluated before

administering medication. Causes of bradydysrhythmia include hypoxia, hypovolemia, and hypothermia. A fluid bolus should be tried first, then atropine or vasoactive drugs considered.[29]

42. **B. Evaluation.** Sodium bicarbonate to alkalinize the urine is indicated if a tricyclic antidepressant overdose has occurred. Sodium bicarbonate may be helpful in cases of documented metabolic acidosis after return of spontaneous circulation.[29]
43. **B. Intervention and Evaluation.** Clinical findings classically associated with hypoglycemia are not adequate to guide the use of glucose in resuscitation. However, research has demonstrated that glucose levels actually rise in long-term adult resuscitation. Because research findings continue to be unclear, it is recommended that 50% dextrose be administered if the patient is hypoglycemic.[29]
44. **C. Intervention.** The starting dose of adenosine is 6 mg, given rapid IV push over 1 to 3 seconds. Because of its extremely short elimination half-life in blood, adenosine must be given very quickly and followed with a saline solution flush to ensure that the drug reaches the AV node. If the first dose is not effective within 1 to 2 minutes, a follow-up dose of 12 mg may be administered.[29]
45. **C. Assessment.** The adverse effects associated with a bolus of adenosine are transient and generally do not require intervention. These side effects have been attributed to a complex interplay of direct effects on organ adenosine receptors, vascular chemoreceptors, and autonomically mediated responses. These side effects have an average duration of less than 60 seconds, and none lasts more than 2 minutes.[29]
46. **D. Intervention.** Amiodarone reduces membrane excitability and facilitates the termination of ventricular dysrhythmia by prolonging the action potential, retarding the refractory period of the myocardial conduction system.[29,30]
47. **D. Evaluation.** All are potential adverse effects following mannitol administration. Paradoxical increased ICP and further deterioration of patient status may be seen, especially if the blood-brain barrier is not intact. Seizures may be secondary to electrolyte imbalances. Pulmonary edema and heart failure can ensue from fluid overload.[17]
48. **A. Intervention.** Mannitol dosage should be from 0.25 to 2 g/kg as a 15%, 20%, or 25% solution, infused over 10 to 60 minutes. When using the higher concentrations, an inline filter may help to prevent unnoticed crystals from entering the patient. Concentrated mannitol is incompatible with both electrolyte solutions and blood products.[17]
49. **B. Intervention.** Magnesium is considered a treatment of choice in patients with torsades de pointes. Hypomagnesemia can precipitate refractory ventricular fibrillation and can hinder the replenishment of intracellular potassium. Magnesium sulfate, 1 to 2 g, is diluted in 100 ml 5% dextrose in water and administered over 1 to 2 minutes for ventricular fibrillation or tachycardia. Magnesium is also used to control seizures in eclampsia and preeclampsia. Magnesium decreases acetylcholine in motor nerve terminals, providing the anticonvulsant property.[17]
50. **C. Assessment.** Fetal heart rate and reactivity may decrease with this drug if used during labor. Intake and output should remain at 30 ml/hr or more, whereby its use is contraindicated in patients with renal disease. A decrease in knee jerk or patellar reflex may signal magnesium toxicity. Lastly, respiratory status must be evaluated continuously and the drug held if the respiratory rate is less than 16 breaths per minute. Also, the respiratory rate and rhythm of the newborn should be monitored closely if magnesium was administered 24 hours or less before delivery.[8,17]
51. **B. Intervention.** The team should transport the patient, because there are only verbal and no written DNR orders. The patient is unable to confirm or deny what her physician has stated. When uncertain, the team should always act in the best interest of the patient.[31,32]
52. **C. Assessment.** The Cormack and Lehane classification system is based on four grades:
    - Grade I: glottis, including anterior and posterior commissures, can be fully exposed
    - Grade II: glottis can be partially exposed
    - Grade III: glottis cannot be exposed; only corniculate cartilages can be visualized
    - Grade IV: glottis, including corniculate cartilage, cannot be exposed[33]
53. **A. Assessment.** Circulatory responses associated with intravenous administration of fentanyl may involve bradycardia, hypotension, circulatory depression, and cardiac arrest.

Potential adverse reactions involving respiratory functions may include muscle rigidity (especially muscles of respiration) following rapid intravenous infusion, laryngospasm, bronchoconstriction, respiratory depression, and respiratory arrest.[17]

54. **C. Evaluation.** Hemodynamic effects of intravenous phenylephrine include:
    - A strong α-adrenergic effect, causing vasoconstriction
    - No β_1 or β_2 stimulation
    - No change in heart rate
    - A slight decrease or no change in cardiac output
    - An essential increase in systemic vascular resistance[17]
55. **D. Assessment.** Side effects of terbutaline include tachycardia, palpitations, transient hyperglycemia, nausea and vomiting, and pulmonary edema.[32,34]
56. **A. Intervention.**[17,35]
57. **C. Intervention.** To determine the flow rate in drops per minute, you would multiply 8 mcg × 72 kg × 60 drops/ml and then divide this total by 1600 (mcg/ml concentration).
58. **D. Intervention.** Vecuronium and succinylcholine are neuromuscular blocking agents, not sedatives. Ketamine may increase ICP. Etomidate decreases cerebral oxygen consumption and ICP.[17,19,35,36]
59. **C. Intervention.** The patient should be placed in a left lateral recumbent position to displace the gravid uterus from the inferior vena cava and increase cardiac output.[18,24]
60. **B. Intervention.** Protamine sulfate is an antidote to heparin.[17]
61. **D. Assessment.** When calculating this dosage, one must first determine the concentration of the nitroglycerin solution,[16] then multiply the concentration times the rate and divide this total by 60 (to determine how much is being delivered per minute).[17,33,35]
62. **C. Evaluation.** Nitroglycerin relaxes all smooth muscles by direct action, with the most prominent effect on vascular smooth muscle. Resulting vasodilation produces lowered peripheral resistance (decreasing afterload), fall in blood pressure, and decreased cardiac output due to reduced venous return to the heart (decreasing preload).[17,35]
63. **C. Assessment.** Both dopamine and dobutamine are positive inotropic agents, increasing cardiac output. Dopamine exerts alpha stimulation, and dobutamine exhibits both alpha and beta$_1$ stimulation. Only dopamine causes vasoconstriction, as well as frequently precipitating tachycardia. Dobutamine, itself, enhances peripheral perfusion and increases myocardial contractility.[17,35]
64. **D. Assessment.** Norepinephrine is one of the most powerful vasoconstrictors because of its potent action on alpha$_1$ receptors. Norepinephrine can be useful in severely hypotensive patients, especially when other agents have failed. It may be particularly helpful in septic shock, when systemic vascular resistance is greatly decreased, and when there is loss of venous tone.[17,35]
65. **C. Intervention.** The advantages of the LMA include:[36,37]
    - Minimal training is needed to use the LMA
    - No manipulation of the cervical spine is necessary for insertion
    - LMAs are not made out of latex
    - Endotracheal intubation can be performed through the LMA
66. **C. Intervention.** In patients with vasoconstriction, the earlobe is the site least affected by poor perfusion. The bridge of the nose would also be a viable choice in this instance. (The side of the foot is usually reserved for a small infant.) The important goals are to select a highly vascular site that is rich in arterial blood and to ensure correct sensor placement so that the light-emitting sensor and light-receiving sensor are opposite each other.[38-40]
67. **B. Assessment.** Abnormal hemoglobins such as carboxyhemoglobin (carbon monoxide poisoning) or methemoglobin cannot be distinguished from oxyhemoglobin by pulse oximeters that use two wavelengths of red light. Anemia itself should not affect oximetric SaO_2 readings. However, hypotensive conditions or other conditions that affect peripheral vascular and tissue perfusion (e.g., hypothermia, vasoactive drug therapy) do adversely affect the accuracy of the pulse oximetry measurement. Motion artifact interferes with the pulsatile signal and results in either false SaO_2 measurements or complete loss of signal.[38-40]
68. **A. Evaluation.** Although it may be used as a screening tool for evaluating patient oxygenation, take care in placing too much reliance on

pulse oximetry when a more inclusive arterial blood sample is indicated. Pulse oximetry alone does not provide information on ventilatory status, as measured by carbon dioxide tension and acid-base balance. Arterial blood gas analysis is the most reliable test for determining the adequacy of respiratory gas exchange.[38-40]

69. **A. Assessment and Intervention.** $ETCO_2$ measurements can be used to confirm ETT placement with virtual certainty in the patient who has not arrested, and who has a pulse and adequate perfusion. Disorders that cause significant ventilation-perfusion mismatch (e.g., massive pulmonary embolism) or that decrease carbon dioxide production (e.g., hypothermia) are accompanied by a low $ETCO_2$ concentration. The $ETCO_2$ readings, in these cases, would therefore be of no use in determining ETT placement.[41]
70. **B. Assessment.** Low $ETCO_2$ readings may be seen in situations prohibiting adequate ventilation or adequate blood flow (e.g., tension pneumothorax, pericardial tamponade), or mismatch between ventilation and perfusion. Pulseless electrical activity in itself is not a cause of low $ETCO_2$ concentrations. Furthermore, if a patient exhibits pulseless electrical activity with an $ETCO_2$ concentration of more than 3%, it is highly likely that the patient has an adequate cardiac output but that the pulse is not palpable due to arterial vasoconstriction.[41]
71. **C. Assessment.** Colorimetric $ETCO_2$ devices contain a pH-sensitive membrane that can be altered by administration of certain drugs via the ETT. If the ETT is positioned properly in the trachea but the blood flow is severely reduced, as during profound shock or CPR, less carbon dioxide will be carried to the lungs, which will result in a low $ETCO_2$ reading. Also, when an ETT has been inserted into the esophagus of a patient who has recently ingested a carbonated beverage, such as beer or soda, the initial $ETCO_2$ reading may appear falsely normal or even high.[41]
72. **D. Intervention.** When using a ventilator, the flight nurse loses the ability to feel the compliance of the patient's lungs. One advantage of using a ventilator is that settings during transport can remain consistent. Manual ventilation with self-inflating bags during transport can lead to unintentional hyperventilation and respiratory alkalosis, resulting in hypotension and cardiac dysrhythmia. Ventilator use will also aid greatly in preventing barotrauma, especially in the pediatric patient, as a result of too-aggressive resuscitation.[42]
73. **C. Intervention.** The fraction of inspired oxygen (FiO_2) is often initiated at 100% in the acutely injured patient and later weaned according to blood gas determination. Tidal volume is the volume of air inspired or expired during a normal breath. During mechanical ventilation, tidal volume is calculated as 10 to 15 cc/kg.[42]
74. **C. Intervention.** External pacing is not indicated in cases in which a prolonged period has elapsed between cardiac arrest and treatment. Pacing here is often ineffective due to the heart muscle's limited response to the electrical stimulation of the pacemaker. External cardiac pacing should not be attempted in patients with hypotension caused by hypovolemia. Pacing is frequently beneficial only when the symptoms are the result of cardiac disturbance.[43-45]
75. **B. Assessment.** When you have obtained capture through the myocardium, you should see a wide QRS complex and a tall, broad T wave appearing with the spike and at the rate set by the pacemaker. During external pacing, you are applying an external electrical source, which is capable of causing contraction not only of heart muscle but also of skeletal muscle. This contraction of skeletal muscle, in and of itself, is not evidence of capture. Effective pacing is best determined by the patient's clinical response evidenced by an elevation of blood pressure, a palpable pulse, improved level of consciousness, and improved skin color and temperature.[43-45]
76. **C. Intervention.** The anterior electrode should be applied over the apex of the heart, avoiding direct placement over the sternum. The posterior pad is placed on the patient's back, avoiding both the spine and the scapula. These bony protrusions increase transthoracic resistance and make pacemaker capture harder to obtain. If you are unable to use the anteroposterior placement of the electrodes, the anteroanterior position may be used. The anterior electrode should be placed on the left side of the chest, midaxillary over the fourth intercostal space, and the posterior pad should be

placed on the right chest in the subclavicular area.[43-45]

77. **B. Evaluation.** Battery failure or general equipment failure can have lethal consequences for the patient who is pacemaker dependent. Skin burns may occur due to poor or dried electrode contact. The battery life of each unit varies somewhat, but in all cases the pacemaker should be plugged into an external power source for prolonged pacing. Failure to capture can be due to numerous factors as follows: the current milliampere (MA) setting may need to be increased, the electrodes may be improperly placed, or during prolonged pacing the myocardium may become desensitized to the current and subsequently may need more current supplied to the muscle. Lastly, during the initial phases of pacing, transient hypotension may occur until the body begins to compensate to the new rate and rhythm. In this event, it may be beneficial to give a fluid bolus and evaluate the response.[43-45]
78. **B. Intervention.** The pacing mode may be demand or asynchronous. The demand mode allows the pacemaker to sense the patient's own rhythm and fire only if the rate falls below the selected pacing rate. The output is usually in milliamperes or voltage. Use the lowest setting possible to obtain capture. If no ventricular capture occurs, the output should be increased sequentially until capture does occur. The pacing rate usually is set from 60 to 80 beats per minute. This rate is selected to ensure adequate cardiac output without the increased myocardial oxygen demands that higher rates would require.[43-45]
79. **C. Assessment.** Arterial systole begins with the opening of the aortic valve and rapid ejection of blood into the aorta. This period is indicated on the arterial waveform as rapid upstroke phase.[46,47]
80. **C. Assessment.** In hypovolemic shock, cardiac output usually will be down slightly due to decreased ventricular filling. SVR will increase. PVR will be normal. CVP and PCWP will be decreased and waveforms usually dampened.[47-49]
81. **B. Assessment.** The dicrotic notch represents the small dip on the downslope of an arterial pressure waveform and marks the end of the ejection period. The dicrotic notch occurs after the T wave on the ECG.[46-49]
82. **D. Assessment.** Answers A, B, and C reflect normal changes in the elderly due to arterial stiffening with increased pulse-wave velocity.[47-54]
83. **D. Intervention.** It is not required that the patient be kept in a flat position when obtaining measurements. As long as the air reference port is level with the patient's midchest, the head of the bed may be elevated to 45 degrees, or the patient placed in a lateral recumbent position.[47-54]
84. **B. Intervention.** A clot in the catheter is suspected if the waveform is dampened and pulses are absent or weak. Flushing the catheter may result in dislodging the clot. Interventions consist of gentle aspiration of the line using a small syringe, then flushing the line with the inline flush device.[47-54]
85. **C. Evaluation.** Stopcocks inadvertently turned will result in loss of waveform. Troubleshooting consists of checking line setup:
    - Adequate pressure in flush bag
    - Absence of bubbles and kinks in the tubing
    - Quick rise to the top of the scale
    - A "square-off" of pattern when triggering the fast-flush device[47-55]
86. **A. Assessment.** A slight difference between arterial and cuff pressures is 5 to 10 mm Hg in the normovolemic patient. Abnormally low readings occur due to decreased flow state, use of pressor drugs, improper calibration, and incorrect transducer placement.[47-54]
87. **D. Assessment.** Clinical findings such as increasing heart rate and consistent MAP are physiological attempts to compensate for an altered perfusion status. If hemorrhage occurs or cardiac output decreases, the body compensates by constricting peripheral vessels to maintain blood pressure. In hemorrhage, the MAP may remain constant, while the pulse pressure narrows. Monitoring both systolic and diastolic pressures aides in assessing changes in perfusion.
88. **C. Assessment.** The fourth intercostal space–midaxillary line serves as the reference point for the level of the transducer, which ensures consistency of hemodynamic readings. For each inch the transducer is away from this point, the difference in values is approximately 2 mm Hg.[47-54]
89. **C. Intervention.** The stopcock located on the transducer must be open to air to negate

the effects of atmospheric pressure, so that the only pressure values that are measured are the ones within the blood vessels or within the heart. Once the digital monitor reading falls to zero, turn the stopcock back to the open position.[47-54]

90. **A. Intervention.** Abnormally high digital pressures with normal waveforms are caused when the transducer falls below the phlebostatic axis reference point. In patients who are diaphoretic or restless, the transducer may slip posteriorly and thereby produce abnormally high digital readings.[47-54]
91. **D. Intervention.** When a patient hemorrhages, the MAP may remain constant, while the pulse pressure narrows. Monitoring both systolic and diastolic pressures aids in assessing blood loss.[47-54]
92. **C. Assessment.** This waveform demonstrates catheter fling that is caused by excessive catheter movement, which could have occurred during transfer or movement of the patient. This will interfere with the transport nurse's ability to monitor the patient.[47-54]
93. **B. Intervention.** Initial action consists of inflating the PA balloon. This serves two functions: it assists decreasing myocardial irritability and subsequently decreases ventricular dysrhythmia, and helps the catheter float with the flow of blood from the right ventricle into the pulmonary artery. It is not uncommon for ventricular ectopy to occur when the catheter tip is in the right ventricle.[47-54]
94. **A. Intervention.** The PA catheter is in an over-wedged pattern. The balloon has been over-inflated, and the pulmonary artery may rupture from the pressure. Corrective measures consist of deflating the balloon, and reinflating slowly, with enough air to obtain PAWP. Flushing of the catheter in a wedge position is associated with PA rupture and hemorrhage.[47-54]
95. **B. Intervention.** Normal PAWP is 8 to 12 mm Hg. Administering a fluid bolus (answers A and C) would only increase a high PAWP and further compromise the hemodynamic status. Administering a nitroglycerin infusion (answer D) could potentially decrease the patient's systolic blood pressure. Initiating dopamine infusion (answer B) will assist in increasing the patient's cardiac output.[47-54]
96. **C. Assessment.** In the absence of mitral valve and pulmonary disease, the PAD pressure value corresponds closely to the PAWP. If PAD and PAWP are similar, then PAD can be substituted for PAWP.[47-54]
97. **D. Intervention.** The patient's PAD pressure is abnormally low. Normal PAD pressures are 8 to 12 mm Hg. Administering a fluid bolus may increase filling pressures and improve cardiac output.[47-54]
98. **D. Intervention.** The PA catheter has black bands that indicate length of insertion. Narrow black bands represent 10-cm lengths, and wide black bands indicate 50-cm lengths. The normal subclavian insertion site markings are approximately 45 to 50 cm. It appears that during transport the catheter was inadvertently pulled out (catheter marking showing three narrow bands at subclavian insertion site).[47-54]
99. **A. Intervention.** Most often fibrin at the tip of the catheter is the cause for waveforms to become dampened. The incidence of thrombus formation is increased in patients with low cardiac outputs. Careful aspiration, followed by gentle flushing, usually corrects this problem.[47-54]
100. **D. Assessment.** Spontaneous migration of the PA catheter toward the peripheral pulmonary bed may occur. Migration of catheter into a wedge position will result in pulmonary infarct. Continuous monitoring of PA pressures is important to detect a PA wedge waveform.[47-54]
101. **C. Intervention.** It should take 1.25 to 1.5 cc of air to wedge a PA catheter. Any amount less than this indicates that the catheter is too far into the pulmonary artery.[47-54]
102. **A. Intervention.** IABP therapy actually decreases afterload. Before systole, balloon deflation creates a vacuum-like effect in the aorta, thereby increasing forward propulsion and decreasing afterload.[55,56]
103. **B. Assessment.** The most commonly used reference point or "trigger" for inflation and deflation of the IABP is the R wave of the patient's ECG.[55,56]
104. **D. Assessment and Intervention.** IABP inflation is shown, ideally, by a small box on the ECG paper before the dicrotic notch. This results in changing the typical U-shaped dicrotic notch to a sharp V shape (see below).[55,56]

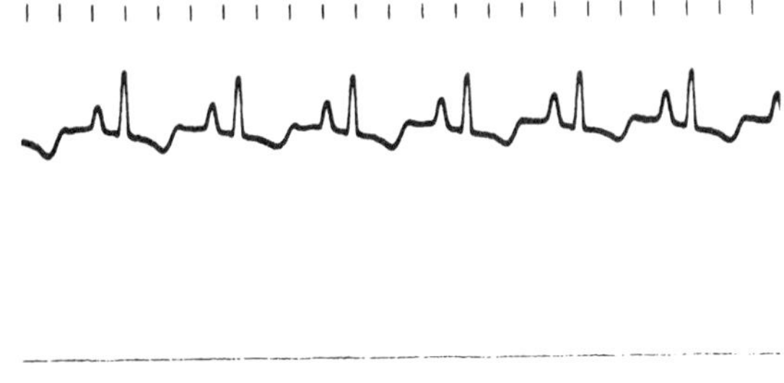

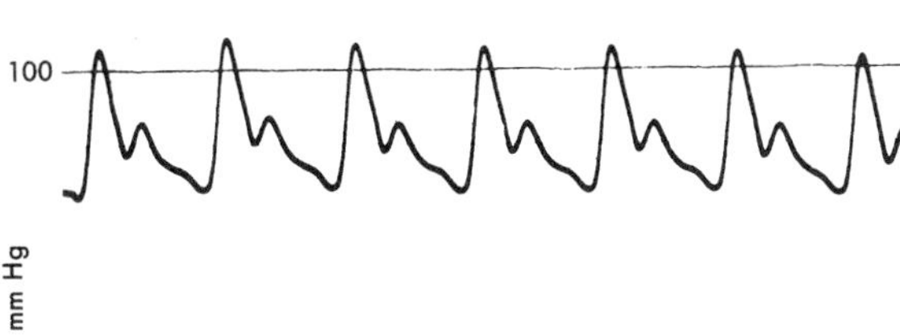

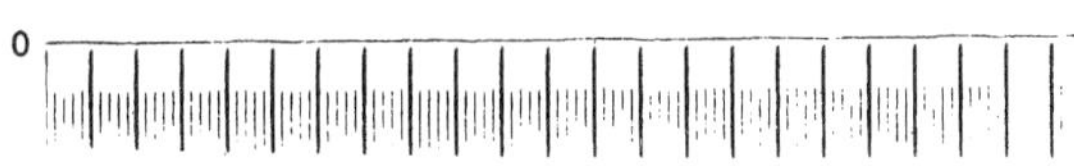

105. **C. Assessment.** IABP deflation occurs just before the aortic valve opens. This occurs immediately before the upstroke on the arterial waveform. See the figure below for safe and unsafe timing for counterpulsation.[55,56]

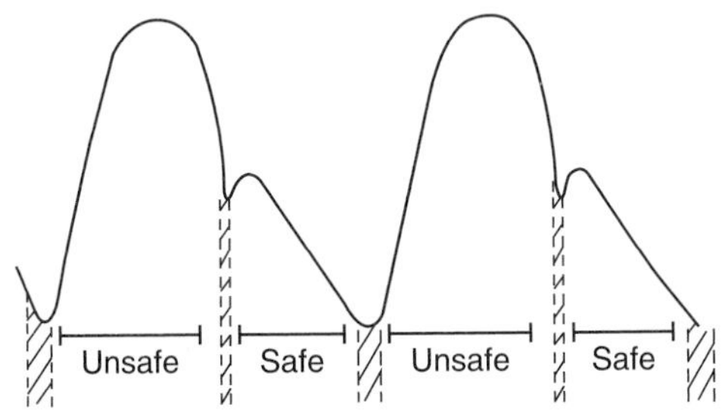

From Quaal S: *Comprehensive intraaortic balloon counterpulsation,* ed 2, St Louis, 1993, Mosby.

106. **D. Intervention.** For patient comfort, the head of bed can be elevated to less than 45 degrees. This prevents kinking and migration of the IABP catheter.[55,56]

107. **D. Assessment.** A major complication of IABP is ischemia of limb or compromised renal circulation. The catheter may trigger thrombus formation, occluding the femoral artery. Migration proximally occludes the subclavian artery, or distally the renal circulation. Dysrhythmia can affect timing of IABP; however, it is not a major complication.[55,56]

108. **B. Intervention.** To prevent clot formation along the dormant balloon, it is necessary to inflate and deflate with one half of the total amount of the balloon volume. Assess for causes of loss of vacuum: large leak caused by loose connections, loss of power source, or empty carbon dioxide–helium tank.[55,56]

109. **C. Assessment.** In the prehospital setting, it is important to assess the scene itself. The nurse can gather many important clues from the scene that may influence the entire assessment. It is also the first priority to protect the emergency responders and the patient from further injury. If necessary, the patient should be moved to a safe area before treatment is initiated.[18,57]

110. **A. Assessment.** The patient's chest should be exposed and visually inspected to assess ventilatory exchange. Airway patency does not ensure adequate ventilation. The nurse should suspect respiratory compromise if the patient's respiratory rate is more than 28 to 30 breaths per minute.[18,57]

111. **C. Intervention.** With a sucking chest wound, air passes from the atmosphere through the chest wall, into the pleural space, and out again with a loss of thoracic pressure. If the diameter of the hole is greater than two thirds of the diameter of the trachea, there is preferential flow of air through the chest wall defect, which is the path of least resistance. The occlusive dressing prevents the atmospheric air from passing through the chest wall.[18,57-59]

112. **B. Assessment.** Three initial observations can give the nurse information regarding the patient's hemodynamic stability.
    - Level of consciousness: as a person's blood volume decreases, cerebral perfusion is impaired, affecting level of consciousness
    - Skin color: in persons of fair skin color, an ashen, gray face and pale, white extremities are ominous signs of hypovolemia; in persons of color, paleness of the mucous membranes is a sign of shock

- Pulse: as the shock state progresses, the peripheral pulses become weak and thready[18,57]

113. **B. Intervention.** The most common chemical restraints used in air medical transport programs are paralytic medications, intubation, and concomitant benzodiazepine administration. Narcotics are used infrequently because of potential respiratory depression and hemodynamic instability.[60]
114. **A. Assessment.** The GCS provides a means to quantitatively measure the patient's best response in three areas:
Eye opening
Spontaneously 4
To verbal stimuli 3
To pain 2
No response 1
Best verbal response
Oriented and converses 5
Disoriented and converses 4
Inappropriate words 3
Incomprehensible sounds 2
No response 1
Best motor response
Obeys commands 6
Localizes to pain 5
Withdrawal 4
Flexion-abnormal 3
Extension 2
No response 1
TOTAL (3 to 15 points)[18,57,60]
115. **C. Intervention.** A patient with a GCS score of 8 is considered to be in coma and should have his or her airway protected. Also, emergency treatment of the patient with a serious head injury is aimed at protecting the brain from further insult by maintaining adequate cerebral oxygenation and preventing systemic hypotension.[18,57,58]
116. **B. Intervention.** The potential for concomitant cervical spine injury is a major concern for the patient requiring an airway procedure. For orotracheal intubation, two-person in-line manual cervical immobilization should be used.[18,57]
117. **D. Intervention.** At no time should fluids be withheld from a hypotensive patient with a head injury. If the mean arterial pressure is allowed to drop, a resultant drop in cerebral blood flow will occur, leading to cerebral anoxia.[61]
118. **A. Assessment.** Due to lack of sensation, a result of the spinal cord injury, the patient will be unable to know if he is injured below his spinal cord lesion. The flight nurse must expose the patient to do a thorough assessment.[18,57]
119. **B. Intervention.** The trunk of the body and the extremities should be secured to the board first with manual stabilization of the head, because tightening of straps may cause movement of the body. Secure the head last, using a towel roll or commercial device to control lateral movement.[18,57]
120. **B. Intervention.** A spinal cord injury, which causes a permanent disability, is extremely frightening to the patient and his or her support group, and has a profound impact on their lives. If there is a deficit, caregivers should provide positive support but not offer false hope.[18,57,58]
121. **D. Assessment.** Autopsy findings, observations by trauma surgeons, and data collected from crash tests with anthropomorphic dummies have provided a correlation between mechanisms of injury and groups of common injuries. Patterns found with frontal and side impacts include clavicle fractures, rib fractures, flail chest, pulmonary contusions, lacerated liver or spleen, cervical spine fracture, cerebral contusion or hemorrhage, femur fracture, and pelvic fracture.[35]
122. **C. Intervention.** An important advantage of blood given during transport is early increase in the patient's oxygen-carrying capacity, unlike the effect achieved from giving crystalloids. However, administration of blood by untrained personnel or delay in transport to obtain the blood are not advantageous.[58,62,63]
123. **C. Assessment.** Tension pneumothorax is a clinical diagnosis. It is characterized by respiratory distress, tachycardia, hypotension, tracheal deviation, unilateral absence of breath sounds, neck vein distention, and cyanosis as a late manifestation.[59]
124. **B. Assessment.** Risk factors for empyema include pneumonia, wound infection, and effusion.[59]
125. **B. Evaluation.** The longer the time the part is ischemic, the less the chance of reimplantation being successful.[18,57,59]

126. **C. Intervention.** Cooled tissue is more resistant to ischemia because of its slowed metabolic rate. Freezing the amputated part should be avoided, because the expansion associated with the formation of ice crystals results in cellular damage.[35]
127. **D. Intervention.** Maintaining an adequate blood pressure to maintain adequate cerebral perfusion pressure is critical in the patient with a head injury.[61]
128. **B. Intervention.** Vomiting in a fully immobilized patient will increase the possibility of aspiration. Gastric decompression may reduce the chances of vomiting and improve ventilation.[35]
129. **A. Assessment and Intervention.** A lateral cervical spine film, in and of itself, is not conclusive to rule out a spinal injury in a patient with a head injury.[35,57,58]
130. **C. Assessment.** Subcutaneous emphysema is noted on the radiograph as radiolucent pockets or spongy areas in the soft tissue.[57]
131. **B. Assessment.** This radiograph demonstrates a lateral view of a flexion teardrop fracture of C5.

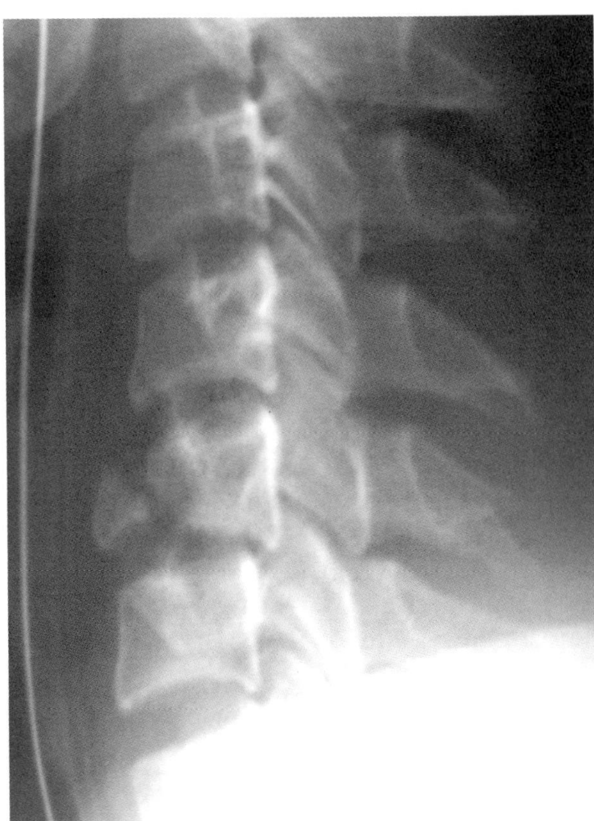

From Mirvis S, Shanmuganathan K: *Imaging in Trauma and Critical Care*, ed 2, Philadelphia, 2003, Saunders.

132. **C. Intervention.** This film includes only to the top of C6, and it is inadequate to fully assess the cervical spine. An additional view should be obtained to evaluate this patient's cervical spine.

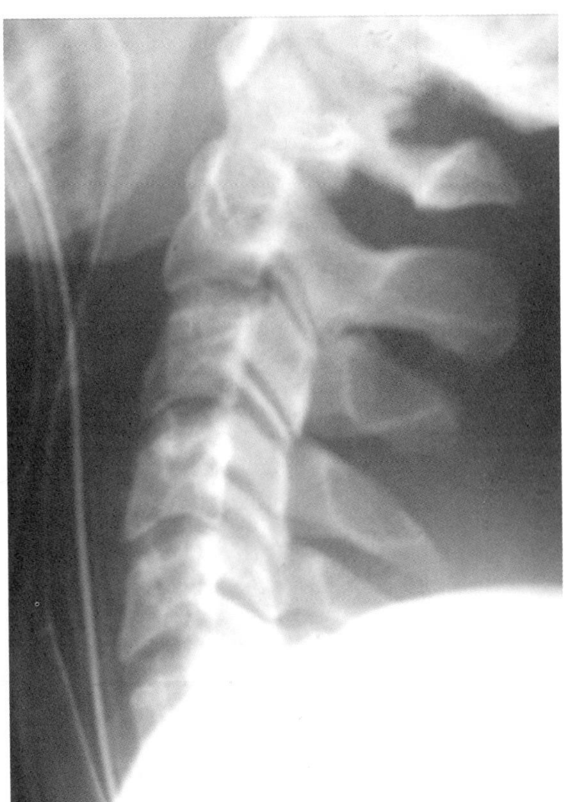

From Mirvis S, Shanmuganathan K: *Imaging in Trauma and Critical Care*, ed 2, Philadelphia, 2003, Saunders.

133. **D. Assessment.** This radiograph demonstrates a hangman's fracture.

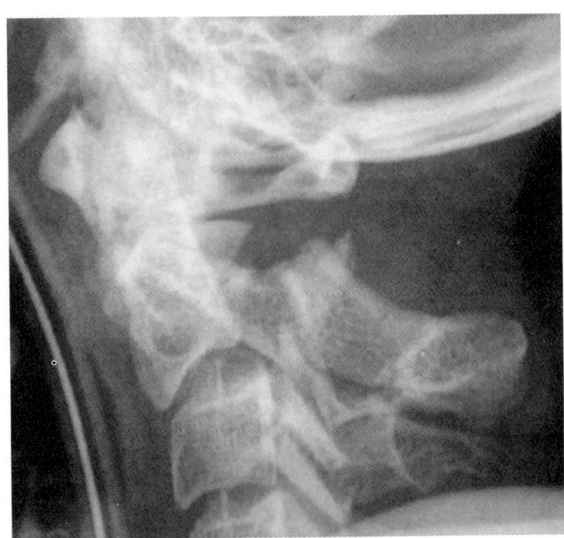

From Mirvis S, Shanmuganathan K: *Imaging in Trauma and Critical Care*, ed 2, Philadelphia, 2003, Saunders.

134. **B. Assessment.** This radiograph demonstrates a pulmonary contusion with left lower lobe atelectasis.

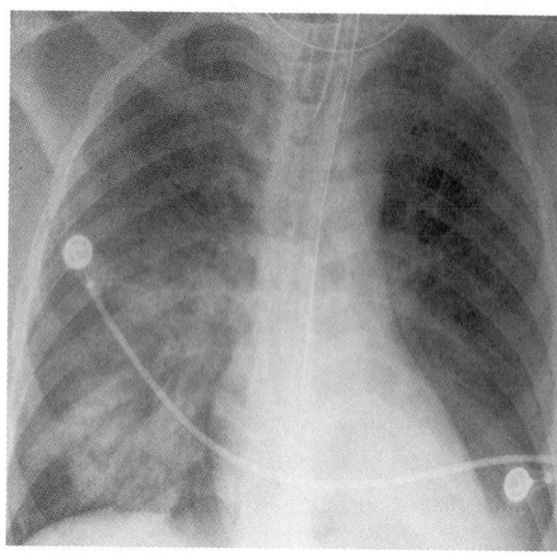

From Mirvis S, Shanmuganathan K: *Imaging in Trauma and Critical Care*, ed 2, Philadelphia, 2003, Saunders.

135. **A. Assessment.** This radiograph demonstrates a tension pneumothorax.

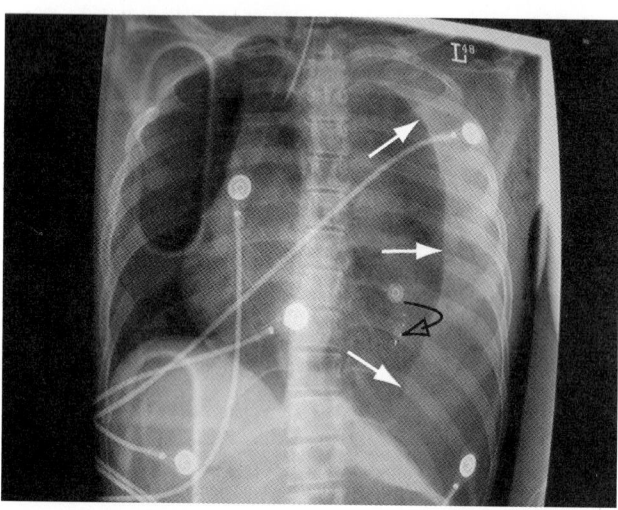

From Mirvis S, Shanmuganathan K: *Imaging in Trauma and Critical Care*, ed 2, Philadelphia, 2003, Saunders.

136. **B. Assessment.** If the IABP catheter is inserted too far, it can occlude blood flow to the brain and affect the patient's level of consciousness. If it is not inserted far enough, it can affect blood flow to the renal arteries and cause a decrease in urinary output.[64]
137. **D. Assessment.** Early deflation results in a premature termination of diastolic augmentation, which is then followed by aortic pressure equilibration back to baseline before the next systole. It is seen as a U rather than V shape on the waveform just before next systolic upstroke.[64]
138. **C. Assessment.** Inflation should occur before closure of the aortic valve. Deflation should occur immediately before the aortic valve opens.[64]
139. **D. Assessment.** The patient in cardiogenic shock will have an increase in preload.[64]
140. **C. Intervention.** Amrinone will decrease preload and afterload and increase contractility, which will increase cardiac output.[64]
141. **D. Analysis.** Aortic valve regurgitation is a contraindication for IABP use. Indications include:
    - Unstable angina
    - Cardiogenic failure
    - Severe left ventricular failure
    - Acute ventricular septal rupture[64]
142. **B. Analysis.** A decrease in urine output could indicate that the intraaortic balloon catheter has migrated downward and is cutting off blood flow to the renal arteries, thereby decreasing urinary output. To prevent this, elevate the head of the stretcher no more than 30 degrees. Make sure that the IABP catheter is secure and the patient's leg remains straight.[55,56]
143. **C. Assessment.** Petechiae or ecchymosis could indicate thrombocytopenia. Check platelet count if possible and discontinue heparin use if anemia is found or suspected.[55,56]
144. **B. Assessment.** Small brown or rust-colored flecks indicate IABP catheter rupture and the catheter should be removed immediately.[55,56,64]
145. **C. Analysis.** 2,3-DPG is a compound present in red blood cells that facilitates oxygen dissociation with hemoglobin. In other words, it pushes oxygen off of hemoglobin toward the tissue.[63]
146. **D. Analysis.** A patient with diabetic ketoacidosis would probably be in metabolic acidosis with respiratory alkalosis.
147. **D. Assessment.** One of the most significant predictors is a history of previous violent behavior.[18]
148. **D. Intervention.**[18]
149. **B. Analysis.**[18]
150. **D. Intervention.**[18]

REFERENCES

1. Hepp H: *Standards of flight nursing practice,* St Louis, 1995, Mosby.
2. Air and Surface Transport Nurses Association: *Standards for critical care and specialty rotor wing transport,* Lexington, KY, 2002, Myers Printing.

3. Air and Surface Transport Nurses Association: *Standards for critical care and specialty ground transport,* Lexington, KY, 2003, Myers Printing.
4. Fulz J: Air medical transport: what the family wants to know, *J Air Med Transport* 12:431-435, 1993.
5. Kattwinkel J, editor: *Textbook of neonatal resuscitation,* ed 4, Chicago, 2000, American Academy of Pediatrics.
6. Jesse N, Drury L, Weiss M: Transporting neonates with nitric oxide: the 5-year Shands Cair experience, *Air Med J* 23(1):17-19, 2004.
7. Hazinski M, editor: *Pediatric advanced life support,* Dallas, 2002, American Heart Association.
8. Task Force on Interhospital Transport: *Guidelines for air and ground transport of neonatal and pediatric patients,* Elk Grove Village, IL, 1999, American Academy of Pediatrics.
9. Aoki B, McCloskey K: *Evaluation, stabilization, and transport of the critically ill child,* St Louis, 1992, Mosby.
10. DeBoer S, Jaracz G, Lass N: Did you bring two isolettes? Transport of conjoined twins, *Air Med J* 18(1):35-37, 1999.
11. Gordon R, O'Dell K: Permanent internal pacemaker safety in air medical transport, *J Air Med Transport* 11:22-23, 1991.
12. Perez L, Alexander D, Wise L: Interfacility transport of patients admitted to the ICU: perceived needs of family members, *Air Med J* 22(5):44-48, 2003.
13. Brown J, Tompkins K, Chancy E et al: Family member ride-alongs during interfacility transport, *Air Med J* 17(4):169-173, 1998.
14. Semonin Holleran R: Transporting the family by air, *Pediatr Emerg Care* 19(3):211-214, 2003.
15. Erler C, Rutherford W, Fiege A et al: Monitored arterial and end-tidal carbon dioxide during inflight mechanical ventilation, *Air Med J* 15(4):171-176, 1996.
16. Martin S, Agudelo W, Oshsner M: Monitoring hyperventilation in patients with closed head injury during air transport, *Air Med Transport* 16(1):15-18, 1997.
17. *Mosby's drug consult 2005,* St Louis, 2005, Mosby.
18. Semonin-Holleran R, editor: *Air and surface patient transport: principles and practice,* ed 3, St Louis, 2003, Mosby.
19. Walls R, Luten R, Murphy M, Schneider R: Manual of emergency airway management, Philadelphia, 2004, Lippincott Williams & Wilkins.
20. Air and Surface Transport Nurses Association: *Transport nurse advanced trauma course,* ed 3, Denver, 2002, Air and Surface Transport Nurses Association.
21. Mitchell J: Comprehensive traumatic stress management in the emergency department, *Leadership Manag* 1:3-14, 1991.
22. Kalaine S: Critical incident stress management: taking care of our own, *AirMed* 5(6):34-36, 1999.
23. Munford B: Practical pharmacology of neuromuscular blockaude, *Air Med J* 17(4):149-156, 1998.
24. Nayduch D, Lee A, Butler D: High-dose methylprednisolone after acute spinal cord injury, *Crit Care Nurse* 14(4):69-78, 1994.
25. Hall VA, Guest JM: Sodium nitroprusside–induced cyanide intoxication and prevention with sodium thiosulfate prophylaxis, *Am J Crit Care* 2:19-27, 1992.
26. Kriegsman W, Peppers M: Flumazenil for benzodiazepine overdose, *Emergency* 1:21-26, 1994.
27. Demmons L, Cook E: Anxiety in adult fixed-wing air transport patients, *Air Med J* 16(3):77-80, 1997.
28. Perondi M, Reis A, Paiva E et al: A comparison of high-dose epinephrine in children with cardiac arrest, *N Engl J Med* 350(17):1722-1730, 2004.
29. Kloeck W, Cummins R, Chamberlain D et al: *ILCOR advisory statements: special resuscitation situations,* Dallas, 1999, American Heart Association.
30. Dries D: Recent progress in adult cardiac life support, *Air Med J* 19(2):36-46, 2000.
31. Cummins R, editor: *Advanced life support,* Dallas, 2001, American Heart Association.
32. Williams A: The dilemma of DNR orders, *AirMed* 4(4):9-10, 1998.
33. Duchynski R, Brauer K, Hutton K et al: The quick look airway classification, *Air Med J* 17(2):46-50, 1998.
34. Krupa D: *Flight nursing core curriculum,* Park Ridge, MD, 1997, Roadrunner Press.
35. Alspach JG, editor: *AACN core curriculum for critical care nursing,* ed 5, Philadelphia, 1998, WB Saunders.

36. Bobek E, Zinc B: Airway management of neurologic emergencies, *Air Med J* 18(2):68-72, 1999.
37. Martin S, Ochsner M, Jarman R: The LMA: a viable alternative for securing the airway, *Air Med J* 18(2):89-92, 1999.
38. DeJarnette R, Rouse M, Holleran R: Pulse oximetry during helicopter transport, *Air Med J* 12:93-96, 1993.
39. Meade D, Farrell K: Pulse oximetry in the field, *J Emerg Med Serv* 3:50-57, 1994.
40. Thomas F, Blumen I: Assessing oxygenation in the transport environment, *Air Med J* 18(2):79-86, 1999.
41. Ornato JP, Peberdy MA: Prehospital end-tidal carbon dioxide monitoring, *J Emerg Med Serv* 8:140-148, 1993.
42. Rouse MJ, Branson R, Semonin Holleran R: Mechanical ventilation during air medical transport: techniques and devices, *J Air Med Transport* 12:5-8, 1992.
43. Wertz E: External cardiac pacing, *Emergency* 4:53-56, 1994.
44. Haught J: Catching up with cardiac pacing, *Emergency* 4:40-43, 1993.
45. Dennison RD: *Pass CCRN!,* ed 2, St Louis, 2000, Mosby.
46. Dailey E, Schroeder JS: *Techniques in bedside hemodynamic monitoring,* ed 5, St Louis, 1994, Mosby.
47. Ahrens TS: *Hemodynamic waveform recognition,* Philadelphia, 1993, WB Saunders.
48. Proehl J, editor: *Emergency nursing procedures,* ed 3, Philadelphia, 2004, WB Saunders.
49. Logston Boggs R, Wooldridge-King M, editors: *AACN procedure manual for critical care,* ed 2, Philadelphia, 1993, WB Saunders.
50. Woods SL, Mansfield L: Effect of patient position upon the pulmonary artery wedge pressures in non acutely ill patients, *Heart Lung* 5(1):83-90, 1976.
51. Baele PL: Continuous monitoring of mixed venous oxygen saturation in critically ill patients, *Anesth Analg* 61(6):513-517, 1982.
52. Hardy J, Ward DR, Gilliliau R: Fatal pulmonary hemorrhage complicating Swan-Ganz catheterization, *Surgery* 91:24, 1982.
53. Bongard FS, Sue D: *Current critical care diagnosis and treatment,* Norwalk, CT, 1994, Appleton & Lange.
54. Visalli F, Evans P: The Swan-Ganz catheter: a program for teaching safe, effective use, *Nursing* 11(1):42-47, 1981.
55. Wojner AW: Assessing the five points of the intraaortic balloon pump waveform, *Crit Care Nurse* 14(3):48-52, 1994.
56. Quall SJ: *Comprehensive intraaortic balloon pumping,* ed 2, St Louis, 1993, Mosby.
57. Semonin-Holleran R, editor: *Prehospital nursing: a collaborative approach,* St Louis, 1994, Mosby.
58. Emergency Nurses Association: *Trauma nursing core course,* Des Plaines, IL, 2000, Emergency Nurses Association.
59. Snow N: Tube thoracostomy in the air medical setting, *Air Med J* 5(3):54-57, 1999.
60. Brauer K, Hutton K: Chemical restraints in the air medical transport environment, *Air Med J* 16(4):105-107, 1997.
61. Letarte P, Shea J, Dries D: Management of head injury in the field environment, *Air Med J* 18(2):73-78, 1999.
62. Berns K, Zietlow S: Blood usage in rotor-wing transport, *Air Med J* 17(3):105-110, 1998.
63. Macnab A, Pattman B, Wadsworth L: Potentially fatal hemolysis of crossmatched blood during interfacility transport: standards of practice for safe transport of stored blood products, *Air Med J* 15(2):69-72, 1996.
64. Darvovic DO, Franklin CM: *Handbook of hemodynamic monitoring,* Philadelphia, 1999, WB Saunders.

CHAPTER 29

CAMTS Standards

REVIEW OUTLINE

I. History of Commission on Accreditation of Medical Transport Systems (CAMTS)
  A. Air medical accidents and fatalities and concern about these led to development of CAMTS
    1. Increased number of air medical transport accidents and fatalities in 1980s
    2. Public scrutiny of industry
    3. Federal Aviation Administration scrutiny of industry
  B. Commission on Accreditation of Air Medical Systems (CAAMS) development
    1. Seven original organizations
      a. American College of Emergency Physicians
      b. Association of Air Medical Services
      c. National Association of Air Medical Communication Specialists
      d. National Association of EMS Physicians
      e. National EMS Pilots Association
      f. National Flight Nurses Association (now Air and Surface Transport Nurses Association)
      g. National Flight Paramedics Association
  C. CAMTS
    1. Name change in 1997
    2. Multiple-association membership (examples)
      a. Emergency Nurses Association
      b. Association of Critical Care Nurses
      c. Fixed Wing Transport
      d. Emergency Medical Systems Educators

II. CAMTS standards
  A. General standards
    1. Medical section
      a. Medical direction and clinical supervision
        (1) Staffing
        (2) Training
      b. Commercial escorts
    2. Aircraft and ambulance section
      a. Medical configuration
      b. Operational issues
      c. Aircraft and ambulance equipment
      d. Communications
    3. Management and administrative section
      a. Management and policies
      b. Utilization review
      c. Quality management
      d. Infection control
  B. Rotary-wing standards
    1. Certificate of aircraft operator
    2. Weather and weather minimums
    3. Pilot staffing and training
    4. Maintenance
    5. Helipad and refueling
    6. Community outreach
  C. Fixed-wing standards
    1. Certificate of the aircraft operator
    2. Aircraft
    3. Weather and weather minimums
    4. Pilot staffing and training
    5. Maintenance
    6. Community outreach
  D. Ground interfacility standards
    1. Vehicles
    2. Driver qualifications
    3. Maintenance and sanitation
    4. Mechanics
    5. Policies

III. Accreditation process
  A. Program information form
  B. Site surveyors
  C. Site visit
  D. Board deliberations
  E. Accreditation decision
  F. Continuous quality improvement

REVIEW QUESTIONS

1. Recommended weather minimums for rotary-wing operations include:
A. Daytime local 1000-foot ceiling and 3 miles visibility
B. Night local 1000-foot ceiling and 1 mile visibility
C. Day local 500-foot ceiling and 1 mile visibility
D. Night cross-country 800-foot ceiling and 2 miles visibility

2. Which is an example of a frequently cited contingency when a program has been evaluated according to CAMTS standards?
A. Head-strike areas in the aircraft are clear of equipment
B. There is a back-up source of oxygen available in the aircraft
C. Clinical education and experience is not documented by staff
D. There is a documented annual postincident accident drill

3. The role of the medical director in a transport program should include:
A. The medical director has no input into the personnel who provide patient care during transport
B. The medical director is not required to provide care to critically ill or injured patients
C. The medical director is not responsible for the quality management program used by the transport program
D. The medical director sets the criteria for the appropriate use of red lights and sirens during ground interfacility transports

4. According to CAMTS, the definition of a critical care mission is:
A. The transport team must have either a registered nurse or physician as the primary care provider
B. The transport team must have either a registered nurse or critical care paramedic as the primary care provider
C. The transport team must be composed of the appropriate staff for the type of mission and the scope of practice of the medical director
D. There is no fixed definition of critical care transport, leaving each program to establish its own definition

5. Good faith in accreditation requires that a program seeking accreditation:
A. Hire additional staff before a site visit with the intention of terminating their employment after the site visit
B. Attempt to discourage open communication between CAMTS by threatening staff with reprisals
C. Have transport program commitment to comply with the CAMTS standards once they have completed the accreditation process
D. Deceive the public about the meaning and limitations of CAMTS accreditation

ANSWERS

1. **B.** Recommended weather minimums for rotary-wing operations include:

Conditions	**Ceiling**	**Visibility**
Daytime local	500 feet	1 mile
Daytime cross-country	800 to 1000 feet	1 mile
Night local	800 feet	2 miles
Night cross-country	1000 feet	3 miles

2. **C.** Examples of frequently cited contingencies include:
   - Head-strike area in the aircraft is violated by equipment
   - Equipment is not secured appropriately
   - There is no back-up oxygen source available in the aircraft
   - The fire extinguisher is not easily accessible
   - Staff education and clinical experience is not documented
3. **D.** The role of the medical director in a transport program includes:
   - Active involvement in the quality management program
   - Active involvement in the hiring, evaluation, and firing of transport personnel
   - Development of guidelines that state when medical control should be consulted
   - Education and training of other medical control physicians who may be used by the transport team
   - Setting criteria for the use of lights and sirens during interfacility ground transports

4. **A.** The current definition of a critical care mission is that the medical team at a minimum must consist of a specially trained physician or registered nurse as a primary care provider. In the fifth edition of the CAMTS standards, there is information about an alternative to this requirement.
5. **C.** A transport program seeking accreditation must engage in the accreditation process in good faith. The program will not deceive the public about the meaning and limitations of accreditation, will allow open communication by personnel, and will commit to comply with the standards.

Additional Readings

Commission on Accreditation of Medical Transport Systems: *Accreditation standards,* ed 6, Anderson, SC, 2004, Commission on Accreditation of Medical Transport Systems. www.CAMTS.org. Accessed October 11, 2004.

Frazer E: Policy changes, *Air Med J* 22(5):16, 2003.

CHAPTER 30

TRANSPORT OPERATIONS

REVIEW OUTLINE

- I. Components of program operations[1-3]
  - A. Transport mission statement
    - 1. Types of patients transported by the service
    - 2. Acuity of patients transported
    - 3. Type of transport vehicles used
  - B. Personnel
    - 1. Medical director
    - 2. Medical control physicians
    - 3. Program director or clinical manager
    - 4. Clinical coordinator or chief transport nurse
    - 5. Continuous quality improvement coordinator
    - 6. Director of safety operations
    - 7. Transport staff
    - 8. Vehicle operators
      - a. Pilots
      - b. Drivers
    - 9. Communication specialists
  - C. Standards and regulations
    - 1. Commission on Accreditation of Medical Transport Systems (CAMTS) standards
    - 2. Federal Aviation Administration
    - 3. Federal airway regulations (FARs)
    - 4. National Transportation Safety Board
    - 5. Health Insurance Portability and Accountability Act (HIPAA)
    - 6. Emergency Medical Treatment and Active Labor Act (EMTALA)
  - D. Policies and procedures
    - 1. Patient care protocols
    - 2. Program operations
    - 3. Safety
    - 4. Mass casualty plan
  - E. Operational readiness
    - 1. Personnel and vehicle assignments
    - 2. Downtime
    - 3. Maintenance
    - 4. Weather restrictions
    - 5. Public relations
    - 6. Premission briefing
    - 7. Postmission briefing
    - 8. Unusual occurrences
      - a. Continuous quality improvement
      - b. Safety
    - 9. Equipment checklists
- II. Crew training and continuing education requirements
  - A. Mission of transport program
  - B. Scope of practice
  - C. State regulations
  - D. Resources
  - E. CAMTS standards
  - F. Monitoring
  - G. Competency evaluation
  - H. Crew resource management (CRM)
- III. Fiscal resources
  - A. Patient transport estimates
  - B. Patient payer mix
  - C. Utilization review
  - D. Contractual agreements
  - E. Budget development
  - F. Billing and collection guidelines
- IV. Total quality management program (TQMP)
  - A. Clinical care and procedure protocols
  - B. Support services
    - 1. Recruitment
    - 2. Training and education
    - 3. Medical direction
    - 4. Human resources
    - 5. Maintenance
    - 6. Safety
    - 7. Information systems
    - 8. Research
    - 9. Purchasing
    - 10. Materials management
    - 11. Communications
  - C. Guidelines and standards
    - 1. Air and Surface Transport Nurses Association standards
    - 2. CAMTS standards

3. Department of Transportation
4. American College of Surgeons
5. American College of Emergency Physicians
6. EMTALA
7. HIPAA
8. Joint Commission on Accreditation of Healthcare Organizations
9. Occupational Safety and Health Administration

D. Identification of quality indicators
1. Airway management
2. Fluid resuscitation
3. Technology use
4. Arrests during transport

E. Data analysis
1. Transport charts
2. Control charts
3. Pareto charts
4. Cause-and-effect diagrams
5. Brainstorming

F. Total quality improvement (TQI) committee
1. Medical director
2. Communication
3. Root cause analysis
4. Loop closure

V. Safety program
A. Vehicle operations
1. Aircraft
2. Ground vehicles
B. Helipad operations
C. Landing zone preparation
D. Biohazard materials safety
E. Employee safety
F. Emergency medical services safety
G. Hospital employee safety

VI. Marketing
A. Marketing and planning personnel
B. Use of current marketing theories
C. Customer satisfaction
D. Evaluation: TQI
E. Outreach education

VII. Strategic planning
A. Program quality
B. Personnel growth and development
C. Injury prevention and safety
D. Education and research
E. Marketing
F. Communications
G. Technology

REVIEW QUESTIONS

1. The HIPAA privacy rule:
A. Ensures that patients are allowed less control over their health information
B. Allows any pharmaceutical company access to patient information, especially that of critically ill patients
C. Enables patients to make informed choices as to how their individual health care information may be used
D. Allows release of all health care information to those who are involved in making a transport decision

2. Protected health information may be disclosed by the transport team without individual authorization in all of the following situations except:
A. Reporting disease, injury, and vital events
B. Referral for a potential funded research study
C. Reporting child abuse or neglect to the appropriate agency
D. Reporting an incident to the US Food and Drug Administration (FDA) related to safety or quality

3. The definition of *local flying area* is determined for the program by:
A. The Part 135 certificate holder
B. The program management
C. The base hospital referral area
D. The local flight standards district office

4. A "sterile" cockpit is maintained below predetermined altitudes to:
A. Allow the transport team to prepare mentally for the flight
B. Allow the pilot to transmit and receive vital flight information
C. Prevent critical information from being heard by the pilot
D. Prevent other air operators from hearing critical mission information

5. Cellular phones are:
A. Acceptable for use to provide patient information during flight
B. Prohibited during any phase of air medical transport
C. Acceptable for use when flying in a low cell-volume area

D. Prohibited for use when the aircraft is airborne

6. CRM is a critical component of transport operations. The transport nurse's role in CRM must include:
A. Remaining quiet during all phases of the patient flight, because transport is still a relatively new role for nurses
B. Remaining alert, situationally aware, and communicating safety issues during the flight
C. Remaining quiet about safety concerns so as not to disturb the pilot during the flight
D. Remaining isolated in the crew cabin so as to ensure that all of their attention is directed toward the patient

7. CRM is required for safe operations. Listening is key to effective CRM. In order to be an effective listener, a transport team member must do all of the following except:
A. Stop talking when another team member is talking
B. Put other team members at ease when they are talking
C. Remove distractions such as television during the conversation
D. Never disagree with the team member who is speaking

8. TQMP used in transport programs should include:
A. Review only of patient records that have identified divergence from selected practice standards
B. Review only of patient care issues related to the mission of the transport program
C. Provision of a method to share issue analysis through continuous communication and feedback
D. Collection of data so that team members who have made mistakes can be identified and appropriately disciplined

9. The principle behind the creation of a control chart is:
A. To identify which of multiple issues should be addressed first in a quality improvement program
B. To look at variation as well as seek and track special causes when evaluating quality indicators
C. To identify the cause and effect of a specific customer complaint in order to develop an action plan
D. To monitor quality improvements that have been put in place and determine their success

10. Which of the following is an example of a public relations initiative that may be used by a transport program?
A. Public speaking
B. Web site
C. Ride-along program
D. All of the above

ANSWERS

1. **C.** HIPAA privacy rule:[4]
   - Gives patients more control over their health information
   - Sets boundaries on the use and release of health records
   - Establishes appropriate safeguards that most health care providers and others must put into place to protect the privacy of health information
   - Holds violators accountable with civil and criminal penalties
   - Strikes a balance between the public health and patients' right to privacy
   - Enables patients to make informed choices based on how their health care information may be used
2. **B.** Protected health information may be disclosed without individual authorization in the following circumstances:[4]
   - Reporting of disease, injury, or vital events
   - Conducting public health surveillance, investigations, or interventions
   - Reporting child abuse or neglect
   - Reporting a person subject to the jurisdiction of the FDA concerning quality, safety, or effectiveness of an FDA-related product or activity
   - Reporting a person exposed to a communicable disease or who may be at risk of contracting or spreading a disease or condition, when legally authorized to notify the person as necessary to conduct a public health investigation
   - Reporting an individual's employer, as needed, for the employer to meet the requirements of the Occupational Safety and Health

Administration, Mine Safety and Health Administration, or a state law

3. **A.** The Part 135 certificate holder determines the program's local flying area.[3]
4. **B.** The use of "sterile" cockpit on take-off and landing allows the pilot to receive and transmit critical information without interference and ensure transport safety.[1,4]
5. **D.** Use of cell phones is prohibited when the aircraft is airborne, as stated in the Federal Communications Code of Regulations #47, parts 20-39, section 22.925, October 1, 1996.
6. **B.** CRM has been used to improve the operation of transport teams. CRM was developed in 1979 in response to a National Aeronautics and Space Administration workshop that examined the role that human error plays in air crashes.[5] CRM emphasizes the role of human factors in high-stress, high-risk environments. John K. Lauber, a psychologist member of the National Transportation Safety Board, defined CRM as "using all available sources—information, equipment and people—to achieve safe and efficient flight operations."[6,7]
7. **D.** Transport team members should be allowed to disagree. However, they must first listen to each other. Recommendations follow:[8]
   - Stop talking while the team member is talking.
   - Put the other team member at ease by paying attention to what is being said.
   - Remove distractions such as TVs and radios when people are talking.
   - Look at the person speaking and give acknowledgment.
   - Stop talking.
8. **C.** The TQMP implemented in transport programs should include:[1-4]
   - 100% clinical chart review, not just patient care records that diverge from accepted program standards. This practice will encourage clinical analysis so that all transport team members can learn from each other and recognize the value of everyone who is a member of the transport system.
   - All aspects of the transport system should be reviewed and evaluated including patient care issues, safety issues, maintenance, information systems, and communications.
   - TQMP must have a method that ensures continuous communication and feedback related to program issues. This is one of the most frequently overlooked components. How does the program ensure that the "loop" is closed? For example, are issues discussed in staff meetings, communicated through e-mail, or covered by continuing education?
   - The focus of TQM is improvement, not punishment. Mistakes are made in practice, but the people in the program need to learn from these and identify ways to improve, which will improve the quality of patient transport overall.
9. **B.** Several approaches may be used to analyze data. These include:[1]
   - Run charts depict events on the y-axis and are graphed against a time span on the x-axis. Run charts can be used to track improvements that have been put into place to measure success.
   - Control charts are created to look at variation, seeking special causes and tracking common causes.
   - Pareto diagram: diagrams data so that the issues that need to be addressed first are more easily identified.
   - A cause-and-effect diagram can identify the causes and effects of a particular issue so that an action plan can be developed.
10. **D.** Examples of public relations marketing initiatives that may be used by transport programs include:[2]
    - Free advertising in newspapers, television stations, and radio stations
    - Author papers in journals and newsletters
    - Trade shows
    - Public speaking
    - Outreach programs that provide education
    - Web site
    - Ride-along programs
    - Promotional products

References

1. Arndt K: *Standards for critical care and specialty rotor-wing transport,* Denver, 2003, Air and Surface Transport Nurses Association.
2. James S: *Standards for critical care and specialty ground transport,* Denver, 2002, Air and Surface Transport Nurses Association.
3. Association of Air Medical Services: *Guidelines for air medical crew education,* Alexandria, VA, 2004, Association of Air Medical Services.
4. Department of Health and Human Services, Centers for Disease Control and Prevention: HIPAA Privacy Rule and Public Health, *MMWR* 4(11):1-24, 2003.

5. Cooper GE, White MD, Lauber JK: *Resource management on the flight deck: proceedings of a NASA/Industry Workshop*, NASA Conference Pub No CP-2120, Moffett Field, CA, 1980, NASA-Ames Research Center.
6. Lauber JK: Cockpit resource management: background and overview. In Orlady HW, Foushee HC, editors: *Cockpit resource management training: proceedings of the NASA/MAC workshop*, NASA Conference Pub No. 2455, Moffett Field, CA, 1980, NASA-Ames Research Center.
7. Wiener EL, Kanki BG, Helmreich RL: *Cockpit resource management,* San Diego, 1993, California Academic Press.
8. Dr. Philip Humbert: *Top 10 tips for effective listening for greater success and influence!,* www.superperformance.com/effectivelistening.html. Accessed October 13, 2004.

PART **THREE**

Critical Care Interventions

CHAPTER 31

INVASIVE INTERVENTIONS

REVIEW OUTLINE

I. Indications for invasive interventions
  A. Advanced airway management
    1. Difficult airway
      a. Digital intubation
      b. Laryngeal mask airway (LMA)
      c. Intubating laryngeal mask airway (ILMA)
    2. Failed airway
      a. Needle cricothyrotomy (percutaneous transtracheal ventilation)
      b. Surgical cricothyrotomy
      c. Retrograde intubation
      d. Combitube
      e. Pharyngeal tracheal lumen airway
  B. Ventilation management
    1. Needle thoracostomy
    2. Tube thoracostomy
  C. Circulatory management
    1. Pericardiocentesis
    2. Seldinger technique
    3. Open thoracotomy
    4. Venous cutdown

II. Complications
  A. Failure to complete the procedure
  B. Bleeding
  C. Anatomical injury
  D. Pain
  E. Infection

III. Procedure preparation
  A. Invasive airway management
    1. Indications
      a. Failed airway management
    2. Contraindications
      a. Lack of advanced airway management skills
      b. Lack of equipment
      c. Lack of an alternative airway
    3. Procedures
      a. Needle cricothyrotomy
      b. Four-step cricothyrotomy
      c. Surgical cricothyrotomy
    4. Complications
      a. Esophageal intubation
      b. Dysrhythmias
      c. Vomiting and aspiration
      d. Bleeding
      e. False passage
  B. Ventilation management
    1. Indications
      a. Tension pneumothorax
    2. Complications
      a. Infection at the insertion site
      b. Pneumothorax
      c. Inappropriate placement
    3. Procedures
      a. Needle decompression
      b. Chest tube thoracotomy
    4. Complications
      a. Infection
      b. Injury to the intercostal vessels
      c. Damage to the great vessels
      d. Injury to the lungs
      e. Intraabdominal placement
      f. Subcutaneous placement
  C. Circulation management
    1. Indications
      a. Peripheral and central line access
      b. Insertion of invasive lines
      c. Enlarging existing central line access
      d. Relieving cardiac compression
    2. Procedures
      a. Seldinger technique
      b. Pericardiocentesis
    3. Complications
      a. Bleeding
      b. Pneumothorax
      c. Infection
      d. Pain
      e. Incorrect insertion

REVIEW QUESTIONS

A 23-year-old male is involved in a head-on motor vehicle collision. He was the unrestrained driver of a small older vehicle without airbags that was struck by a sport utility vehicle. He has suffered massive facial trauma from hitting his face on the steering wheel and has a great deal of blood in his airway. His Glasgow Coma Scale score is 7. Oral tracheal intubation attempts have failed to secure the patient's airway.

1. Which of the following procedures should be considered to manage this patient's airway?
   A. Nasotracheal intubation
   B. Insertion of a Combitube
   C. Digital manual intubation
   D. Surgical cricothyrotomy

2. The advantage of a needle cricothyrotomy over a surgical cricothyrotomy in an emergency situation is:
   A. A needle cricothyrotomy procedure requires more equipment than a surgical cricothyrotomy
   B. This procedure can be performed in both adult and pediatric patients
   C. A surgical cricothyrotomy is simpler to perform than a needle cricothyrotomy
   D. There is more of a risk of tracheal erosion and glottic stenosis with the former

3. One of the most common complications of surgical cricothyrotomy is:
   A. Tracheoesophageal fistula
   B. Correct tube placement
   C. Swallowing problems
   D. Hematoma formation

During transport, a morbidly obese male patient who has suffered an acute myocardial infarction suffers a cardiopulmonary arrest. Several attempts are made at oral tracheal intubation, without success. An LMA is inserted.

4. Indications for the use of an LMA in emergency airway management include:
   A. Inability to open the patient's mouth
   B. Need for high pulmonary inflation pressures
   C. Inability to visualize the patient's larynx
   D. Ability to ventilate a patient with a bag-valve-mask device

5. When ventilating a patient with percutaneous transtracheal ventilation, the nurse should:
   A. Provide oxygen at more than 50 pounds per square inch (PSI) to adults
   B. Allow patient exhalation for 4 seconds
   C. Provide oxygen at more than 30 PSI for pediatric patients
   D. Allow oxygen jet to insufflate the lungs for 20 seconds

An 18-year-old male is involved in a skier-to-skier collision. He is complaining of severe right-sided chest pain and difficulty breathing. A chest radiograph demonstrates a pneumothorax larger than 30%.

6. Before inserting a chest tube, the practitioner should:
   A. Insert a curved clamp and tunnel downward into the chest cavity
   B. Use a trocar device to direct the chest tube into the pleural cavity
   C. Insert a gloved finger into the thoracic cavity and perform a digital examination
   D. Secure the tube to the skin with a purse-string suture through the incision site

7. Confirmation of correct tube placement includes all of the following except:
   A. Palpation of the tube in the subcutaneous tissue
   B. Audible air movement with inspiration and expiration
   C. Free-flow drainage of blood or fluid from the chest tube
   D. Condensation on the inside of the chest tube

8. Which of the following can assist in the identification of an unexpected air leak in a chest drainage system?
   A. Checking and loosening all equipment connections
   B. Observing fluctuations during respirations
   C. Continuous bubbling in the water-sealed chamber
   D. Absence of drainage ports at the chest tube insertion site

9. Which of the following is the best approach to use when performing an emergency pericardiocentesis?
   A. Insertion of a needle at a 90-degree angle between the xiphoid process and the left

costal margin, directing the needle toward the right shoulder
B. Insertion of the needle perpendicular to the skin in the left fifth intercostal space, medial to the border of cardiac dullness
C. Insertion of the needle 1 cm lateral and in the intercostal space below the apical beat, within the area of cardiac dullness, aiming toward the right shoulder
D. Insertion of the needle at a 45-degree angle between the xiphoid process and the right costal margin, directing the needle toward the left shoulder

10. Which is the most common dysrhythmia associated with pericardiocentesis?
A. Atrial fibrillation
B. Ventricular tachycardia
C. Bradycardia
D. Premature ventricular contractions

11. When inserting a central line into a tortuous vessel, which guidewire should be used?
A. J-shaped wire
B. Straight wire
C. C-shaped wire
D. O-shaped wire

12. Complications that may occur with the insertion of a femoral venous line include all of the following except:
A. Bowel perforation
B. Deep vein thrombosis
C. Local hematoma
D. Brachial plexus injury

13. When removing the wire through the needle during insertion of a central line, resistance is encountered. What should be done next?
A. Pressure should be applied until the wire comes out through the needle
B. There is no need to remove the wire, because most catheters can be threaded over both the needle and the wire
C. The needle and the wire should be removed as a unit to prevent shearing of the wire
D. A bolus of heparin may be administered to make the wire move more easily from the needle

14. The preferred site for venous cutdown in the pediatric patient is:
A. External jugular vein
B. Saphenous vein
C. Cephalic vein
D. Basilic vein

ANSWERS

1. **D. Intervention.** Digital manual intubation and insertion of a Combitube are methods used to manage a failed airway in a deeply comatose patient. Nasotracheal intubation is generally contraindicated in patients with facial fractures because of the risk of insertion into the cranial cavity. Indications for surgical cricothyrotomy include maxillofacial injuries and cervical spine instability.[1]
2. **B. Analysis.** Advantages of a needle cricothyrotomy over a surgical cricothyrotomy include the following: (1) the procedure is faster to perform, (2) it requires fewer instruments, (3) it causes less tracheal erosion and glottic stenosis, and (4) a needle cricothyrotomy can be performed in a patient of any age.[2]
3. **D. Assessment.** Common complications of surgical cricothyrotomy include bleeding, hematoma formation, prolonged procedure time, incorrect tube placement, unsuccessful tube placement, and subcutaneous emphysema. Infrequent late complications include tracheoesophageal fistula and glottic stenosis. Swallowing problems have been reported only with tracheotomies.[1]
4. **C. Assessment.** Indications for the use of an LMA for emergency airway management include inability to intubate endotracheally or to ventilate with a bag-valve-mask device. Contraindications include inability to open the patient's mouth, vomiting, and the need for high pulmonary pressures for ventilation.[1]
5. **B. Intervention.** When using jet ventilation, the nurse should: provide oxygen at no more than 50 PSI for adults and 30 PSI for children, allow insufflation of the patient's lung for 1 second, and allow exhalation for 4 seconds.[2]
6. **C. Intervention.** Before a chest tube is placed, a gloved finger should be inserted and a digital examination should be performed. A trocar device should not be used, because it can cause serious pulmonary injury. The tube should not be secured until it is in place.[2]
7. **A. Assessment.** Palpation of the chest tube in the subcutaneous tissue indicates that the tube is not in the pleural cavity.[2]
8. **C. Assessment.** Indications of an unexpected air leak include bubbling in the water-seal chamber. Air in the pleural space causes intermittent bubbling. Constant or massive bubbling

may indicate a bad connection. The air vents should be inserted completely into the pleural cavity, and tightened connections will prevent air leakage. [3]

9. **B. Intervention.** Research using both echocardiography and cadavers has demonstrated that the parasternal approach is less likely to cause injury to the right atrium or cause a pneumothorax, when the needle is inserted perpendicular to the skin, in the left intercostal space, medial to the border of cardiac dullness.[1]
10. **D. Assessment.** Various dysrhythmias can occur during a pericardiocentesis, but the most commonly reported is premature ventricular contractions.[1]
11. **A. Intervention.** A straight wire is indicated when inserting a central line into a vessel with a linear configuration. Included are those used to enlarge a preexisting line, such as a rapid infusion catheter. A J-shaped wire is indicated when inserting a central line into a tortuous vessel, which would allow it to flex when coming into contact with the vessel wall.[1]
12. **D. Analysis.** General complications that may result from central venous line insertion include air embolus, local hematoma, generalized sepsis, osteomyelitis, and catheter malposition. Specific complications related to insertion of a femoral venous line may include bowel and bladder perforation, deep vein thrombosis, and psoas abscess.[1]
13. **C. Intervention.** The wire and needle should be removed as a unit to prevent shearing of the wire and a wire embolism.[1]
14. **B. Analysis.** Even though venous cutdowns are no longer taught routinely in invasive skills laboratories, the technique still has some value when central line placement or other attempts at intravenous access have failed. Clinical indications include venous access in infants and in hypovolemic shock when vessels have collapsed. The saphenous vein is large enough to cannulate in most pediatric patients, and it has an anatomically predictable location, which will result in fewer complications and more success in cannulation.[1]

References

1. Roberts JR, Hedges J, editors: *Clinical procedures in emergency medicine,* ed 4, Philadelphia, 2004, WB Saunders.
2. Wraa C, editor: *Transport nurse advanced trauma course,* ed 3, Denver, 2001, Air and Surface Transport Nurses Association.
3. Mims B, Toto K, Luecke L et al: *Critical care skills: a clinical handbook,* Philadelphia, 2004, WB Saunders.

CHAPTER 32

PHARMACOLOGY

REVIEW OUTLINE

I. Basic pharmacology principles
   A. Pharmacokinetics
      1. Bioavailability
      2. How drugs cross barriers
      3. Absorption
      4. Distribution
      5. Metabolism
      6. Elimination
   B. Pharmacodynamics
      1. Drug receptors
      2. Drug potency
      3. Drug efficacy
   C. Routes of administration
      1. Parenteral
      2. Intramuscular
      3. Sublingual
      4. Subcutaneous
      5. Rectal
      6. Nasal
      7. Dermal
   D. Pharmacological complications
      1. Overdosage
      2. Underdosage
      3. Wrong medication prescribed
      4. Allergies
      5. Side effects
II. Selected medications
   A. Neuromuscular blocking agents
      1. Depolarizing
      2. Nondepolarizing
   B. Induction agents used in the emergency department
      1. Etomidate
      2. Propofol
   C. Opioid analgesics
      1. Morphine sulfate
      2. Fentanyl
      3. Codeine
      4. Hydrocodone
      5. Hydromorphone
   D. Nonsteroidal antiinflammatory drugs (NSAIDs)
      1. Ibuprofen
      2. Ketorolac
   E. Antihypertensive agents
      1. Beta-blockers
      2. Calcium channel blockers
      3. Angiotensin converting enzyme (ACE) inhibitors
   F. Cardiac glycosides
      1. Digitalis
   G. Vasodilators
      1. Nitroglycerin
      2. Nitroprusside
   H. Vasopressors
      1. Dopamine
      2. Dobutamine
      3. Levophed
   I. Antibiotics
   J. Antiviral agents
   K. Psychiatric medications
   L. Sedatives
   M. Antianxiety medications

REVIEW QUESTIONS

1. Pharmacokinetics refers to:
   A. What a drug does to the body
   B. The various administration routes of a drug
   C. The biotransformation of a drug
   D. What the body does to a drug

2. Pharmacodynamics refers to:
   A. What a drug does to the body
   B. The various administration routes of a drug
   C. The biotransformation of a drug
   D. The chemical structure of a drug

3. The reason for large differences in the pharmacological effect between oral and intravenous doses is due to:

A. The difference between the solubility of the oral and intravenous preparation of the drug
B. The first-pass hepatic effect
C. Irritation of the gastrointestinal (GI) mucosa by the drug
D. Changes in the pH of the drug in the stomach

4. A drug which is an agonist will:
A. Undergo no change as a result of the first-pass hepatic effect
B. Bind to a specific receptor, stimulate that receptor, and produce an effect
C. Slow respirations and heart rate
D. Cause an increase in plasma concentrations of similar drugs

5. A drug which is an antagonist will:
A. Undergo no change as a result of the first-pass hepatic effect
B. Have a longer duration of action than an agonist
C. Prevent natural substances from stimulating receptors
D. Cause an increase in plasma concentrations of similar drugs

6. Which of the following neuromuscular blocking drugs is considered an agonist?
A. Vecuronium
B. Pancuronium
C. Rocuronium
D. Succinylcholine

7. Adverse side effects of succinylcholine include all of the following except:
A. Renal failure
B. Cardiac dysrhythmias
C. Hyperkalemia
D. Myoglobinuria

8. Succinylcholine use in burn patients is of concern and in some instances should be avoided because of:
A. An increased risk of infection and delayed wound healing
B. The risk of associated inhalation injury
C. An associated increase in serum potassium
D. The possibility of airway obstruction from increased pulmonary secretions

9. The brief duration of action of succinylcholine (3 to 5 minutes) is due to:
A. Metabolism in the liver by cytochrome P-450 enzymes
B. Hydrolysis by plasma cholinesterase
C. Metabolism by alcohol dehydrogenase
D. Conjugation by glutathione

10. Induction agents used in the emergency setting are primarily for:
A. Analgesia
B. Management of hypotension
C. Sedation
D. To induce unconsciousness

11. The following drugs are induction agents, all of which enhance γ-aminobutyric acid (GABA), the major inhibitory neurotransmitter in the central nervous system (CNS). Which drug, because of its side effect profile, would least likely be used in the emergency department?
A. Propofol
B. Midazolam
C. Etomidate
D. Ketamine

12. Of the following induction agents, which maintains hemodynamic stability as well as provides a cerebroprotective effect?
A. Midazolam
B. Etomidate
C. Ketamine
D. Thiopental

13. This induction agent directly relaxes bronchial smooth muscle, producing bronchodilation. It is the induction agent of choice for patients with bronchospasm who require tracheal intubation.
A. Ketamine
B. Midazolam
C. Etomidate
D. Thiopental

14. All induction agents share one common potential side effect that varies with the particular drug, the patient's underlying physiological condition, and the dosage and speed of injection of the drug. This potential side effect is:
A. Tachycardia and increased myocardial oxygen demand
B. Myocardial depression and hypotension
C. Transient increase in intracranial pressure (ICP)
D. Hallucinations

15. This prototype opioid agonist is the one with which all other opioid analgesics are compared.

It is well absorbed after intramuscular administration, with onset of effect in 15 to 30 minutes and a peak effect in 45 to 90 minutes. The duration of action is about 4 hours.

A. Fentanyl
B. Meperidine
C. Morphine
D. Methadone

16. Morphine is used often in pulmonary edema management. The primary beneficial action of morphine in this setting is due to:

A. The interaction of morphine at the μ (mu) receptor to produce respiratory depression
B. Sensitization of the myocardium to catecholamines
C. Blocking of angiotensin II formation, by which morphine affects the renin-angiotensin system and decreases blood pressure
D. Morphine's effect of decreasing sympathetic nervous system tone to peripheral veins, resulting in venous pooling and subsequent decreases in venous return

17. A patient receives 10 mg of morphine IV for analgesia for a kidney stone. Within 15 minutes of receiving the morphine, the pain is significantly reduced but the patient develops a reddened area along the length of the vein into which the morphine was administered. The skin of the face, neck, and upper chest become flushed and warm. What action should be taken next?

A. Continued observation
B. Administer diphenhydramine 25 mg IV and inform the patient of a suspected morphine allergy
C. Start a second IV and prepare for volume resuscitation
D. Prepare for possible intubation

18. This synthetic opioid analgesic, like morphine, is an opioid agonist at μ (mu) receptors. Its pharmacological effects resemble morphine; however, it is about one tenth as potent. It is structurally related to atropine and causes tachycardia, unlike other opioid analgesics. Prolonged use can result in the accumulation of an active metabolite, which may produce seizures and delirium.

A. Codeine
B. Hydromorphone (Dilaudid)
C. Meperidine (Demerol)
D. Fentanyl

19. Naloxone:

A. Is a pure μ (mu) receptor agonist
B. Is a pure μ (mu) receptor antagonist
C. Is effective orally
D. Produces no hemodynamic effects

20. Which statement regarding benzodiazepines is false?

A. Benzodiazepines produce anxiolysis, sedation, and amnesia
B. Benzodiazepines exert an anticonvulsant effect
C. Benzodiazepine dosages should be decreased in the elderly
D. Benzodiazepines have analgesic properties

21. Which of the following statements relative to the effects of benzodiazepines is true?

A. The combination of opioids and benzodiazepines can result in a greater decrease in blood pressure than that seen with either drug alone
B. The incidence of phlebitis is similar for diazepam and midazolam
C. Diazepam is 2 to 3 times more potent than midazolam
D. Benzodiazepines produce minimal respiratory depression

22. The sedative effect of benzodiazepines is increased by all of the following except:

A. Calcium channel blockers
B. Alcohol
C. Tricyclic antidepressants
D. Antihistamines

23. Flumazenil:

A. Is a useful benzodiazepine agonist used specifically for the management of anxiety
B. Binds to the benzodiazepine receptor competitively inhibiting benzodiazepines
C. Is in an emerging class of anxiolytic agents, with only minimal potential for abuse, and does not react with other CNS depressants
D. Is used only IV to produce sedation, relieve anxiety, and decrease the ability to recall events of that day

24. The class of drugs that inhibit the enzyme cyclooxygenase is important in the relief of:
    A. Anxiety through the GABA receptor complex
    B. Subjective pain at the level of the CNS
    C. Objective pain arising from stimulation of peripheral nerve endings
    D. Pain by rapid hydrolysis of acetylcholine at the neuromuscular junction

25. This prototype of the NSAIDs relieves pain by inhibiting prostaglandin production locally and inhibiting prostaglandin synthesis in the hypothalamus, effectively relieving fever.
    A. Ibuprofen
    B. Acetaminophen
    C. Naproxen
    D. Aspirin

26. Prostaglandins are synthesized from interaction of arachidonic acid by the cyclooxygenase enzymes (COX-1 and COX-2). Prostaglandins are required for normal physiological functions including all of the following except:
    A. Inhibit gastric acid secretion
    B. Maintain renal tubular blood flow and tubular function
    C. Play an important role in platelet aggregation
    D. Increase spasm in bronchial and ileal smooth muscle

27. Concerning cyclooxygenase, which of the following statements is false?
    A. All NSAIDs equally affect COX-1 and COX-2 enzymes
    B. COX-2 is responsible for the production of prostaglandins associated with inflammation
    C. Inhibition of COX-1 is associated with stomach damage, leading to ulcers and kidney damage
    D. Newly developed COX-2 inhibitors do not cause stomach and kidney damage

28. The only NSAID that can be prescribed with absolute safety with respect to the renal system is:
    A. Aspirin
    B. Acetaminophen
    C. Ibuprofen
    D. Naproxen

29. Which of the following statements concerning aspirin toxicity is false?
    A. A child is more likely than an adult to die from an overdose of aspirin
    B. Some patients develop asthma that is triggered by aspirin
    C. Rarely, massive GI bleeding occurs in patients on long-term aspirin therapy
    D. Vitamin C (ascorbic acid) given IV is used to achieve acidic urine, which promotes excretion of salicylic acid in overdose situations

30. Ketorolac is a NSAID with potent analgesic effects but only moderate antiinflammatory activity when administered IM or IV. Ketorolac 30 mg IM produces analgesia equivalent to:
    A. Morphine 0.5 mg
    B. Morphine 1 mg
    C. Morphine 5 mg
    D. Morphine 10 mg

31. COX-2 inhibitors are used in the management of painful joint inflammation associated with various kinds of arthritis. Based on recent studies, COX-2 inhibitors may become important for which of the following?
    A. Management of precancerous intestinal polyps for preventing colon cancer and Alzheimer's disease
    B. Management of melanoma and other forms of skin cancer
    C. Management of multiple sclerosis
    D. Management of cardiac disease and hypertension

32. This class of antihypertensive agent is often a first-line treatment. The drugs work by inhibiting cardiac stimulation and decreasing renin production in the kidney.
    A. Beta-blockers
    B. ACE inhibitors
    C. Calcium channel blockers
    D. Alpha-blockers

33. Beta-blockers may worsen the health status of patients with certain conditions. In which of the following conditions can beta-blockers be used safely?
    A. Asthma
    B. Angina
    C. Peripheral vascular disease
    D. Diabetes

34. Which of the following statements concerning beta-blockers is false?
    A. All beta-blockers are derivatives of isoproterenol
    B. Beta-blockers are classified as partial or pure agonists on basis of absence of intrinsic catecholamine or sympathomimetic activity
    C. Can worsen lung disease, especially with nonspecific blockers and a history of chronic obstructive pulmonary disease or bronchospasm
    D. Bradycardic effects seldom respond to atropine

35. Calcium channel blockers are used in the management of hypertension, dysrhythmias, heart failure, angina, and cerebral vasospasm. They act primarily by:
    A. Increasing the entry of calcium into smooth muscle thereby lowering vascular tone
    B. Blocking the release of calcium from heart muscle thereby lowering cardiac output
    C. Decreasing the entry of calcium into smooth muscle thereby lowering vascular tone
    D. Increasing the entry of calcium into the heart muscle thereby decreasing the force of contraction

36. Calcium channel blockers are particularly useful in the management of angina. The Prinzmetal form of angina:
    A. Is accompanied by bradycardia
    B. Occurs at rest
    C. Does not respond to calcium channel blockers
    D. Occurs with atrial fibrillation

37. When administering potassium chloride to a patient who is also receiving the calcium channel blocker verapamil, which of the following statements is true?
    A. Hyperkalemia is more likely to occur
    B. Hypokalemia is more resistant to management
    C. Hypercalcemia is more likely to occur
    D. Hypercalcemia is more resistant to management

38. Nimodipine is a calcium channel blocker that is highly lipid soluble. Due to its lipid solubility nimodipine:
    A. Has a longer duration of action than other calcium channel blockers
    B. Is more sensitive to cardiac calcium channels than vascular calcium channels
    C. Crosses the blood-brain barrier
    D. Has an unpredictable duration of action profile requiring closer monitoring

39. ACE inhibitors frequently are used to manage chronic hypertension. Angiotensin II is:
    A. A potent vasodilator
    B. An enzyme that inhibits the formation of angiotensin
    C. An enzyme that inhibits renin
    D. A potent vasoconstrictor

40. ACE inhibitors represent a major advance in the management of all forms of hypertension because of their potency and minimal side effects. Which of the following would benefit from the use of ACE inhibitors?
    A. Patients with chronic obstructive pulmonary disease
    B. Nursing mothers with hypertension
    C. Patients with diabetic renal disease
    D. Patients with hyperthyroidism

41. Which of the following side effects is most often seen with ACE inhibitors?
    A. Depression and insomnia
    B. Cough and upper respiratory congestion
    C. Sexual dysfunction
    D. Bronchospasm

42. This class of drugs is used to manage heart failure by increasing contractility of the myocardium, thus improving cardiac output. Unfortunately, there is a small difference between therapeutic and toxic dosages.
    A. ACE inhibitors
    B. Beta-blockers
    C. Calcium channel blockers
    D. Cardiac glycosides

43. In patients taking cardiac glycosides, which class of medication, if taken concurrently, would increase the likelihood of developing digitalis toxicity?
    A. Loop diuretics
    B. NSAIDs
    C. Potassium-sparing diuretics
    D. Beta-blockers

44. The most common digitalis-induced dysrhythmia is:
    A. Sinus tachycardia
    B. Bradycardia

C. Premature ventricular contractions
D. Atrial fibrillation

45. Digoxin is used to manage atrial flutter and fibrillation. The mechanism by which digoxin exerts its effect is:
A. Decreasing the automaticity of the SA node
B. Slowing the conduction of impulses through the AV node
C. Decreasing conduction through the bundle of His
D. Delaying conduction through the Purkinje network

46. Nitroglycerin is a vasodilator used to produce peripheral pooling of blood and decreased cardiac ventricular wall tension. Which of the following statements regarding nitroglycerin is false?
A. Nitroglycerin acts primarily on the capacitance (venous) vessels
B. Nitroglycerin is capable of producing methemoglobinemia
C. Nitroglycerin may increase ICP in patients with decreased intracranial compliance
D. Nitroglycerin increases myocardial oxygen demand

47. Sodium nitroprusside, like nitroglycerin, is a potent vasodilator. It differs from nitroglycerin in that:
A. Sodium nitroprusside does not cause methemoglobinemia
B. Sodium nitroprusside generates nitric oxide, an endogenous vasodilator
C. Nitroprusside decreases both preload and afterload
D. Nitroprusside does not cause increased ICP

48. Dopamine is a naturally occurring catecholamine derived from the amino acid tyrosine and is the chemical precursor of norepinephrine. In addition, dopamine:
A. Is a transmitter confined to the CNS
B. Decreases renal blood flow
C. Stimulates only dopamine$_1$ receptors
D. Stimulates dopamine, alpha, and beta receptors

49. Dobutamine is a synthetic catecholamine administered at 2 to 10 mcg/kg per minute. Dobutamine also:
A. Exhibits little vasoconstrictor activity
B. Precipitates cardiac dysrhythmias at therapeutic dosages
C. Stimulates dopamine$_1$ receptors
D. Is a coronary vasoconstrictor

50. Which of the following catecholamines is the most potent activator at beta$_1$ and beta$_2$ receptors?
A. Dopamine
B. Dobutamine
C. Isoproterenol
D. Epinephrine

ANSWERS

1. **D.** Pharmacokinetics is the quantitative study of the absorption, distribution, metabolism, and excretion of a drug and its metabolites. Pharmacokinetics, therefore, refers to what the body does to a drug.[1]
2. **A.** Pharmacodynamics is the study of the intrinsic sensitivity or responsiveness of receptors to a drug and the mechanisms by which these effects occur. Thus pharmacodynamics refers to what the drug does to the body. The responsiveness of receptors varies among patients. As a result, at similar plasma concentrations of drug, some patients show a therapeutic response, others show no response, and in others toxicity develops.[1]
3. **B.** The first-pass hepatic effect refers to the process of drug absorption from the GI tract and transport to the liver via the portal venous blood system. The drug then undergoes metabolism, which often inactivates drugs before they reach the systemic circulation. As an example, an intravenous dose of morphine has an effect 6 times stronger than that of the oral dose, because oral morphine is almost completely inactivated by the liver.[2]
4. **B.** Any compound, natural or synthetic, which binds to a specific receptor and produces a biological effect by stimulating that receptor is called an *agonist.*[2]
5. **C.** Drugs that produce their action not by stimulating receptors but by preventing natural substances from stimulating receptors are called *antagonists.*[2]
6. **D.** Succinylcholine mimics the action of acetylcholine and, therefore, is considered an agonist. The others interfere with the actions of acetylcholine and are considered antagonist. Because succinylcholine mimics the actions of acetylcholine, it is referred to as a *depolarizing agent.* Nondepolarizing agents interfere with the actions of acetylcholine.[1]

7. **A.** Renal failure is not considered an adverse side effect of succinylcholine. Myoglobinuria reflects skeletal muscle damage associated with succinylcholine-induced fasciculations and is seen in pediatric patients, but for unknown reasons rarely occurs in adults.[1]
8. **C.** Under normal circumstances the serum potassium level may increase by 0.5 mEq/L with the administration of succinylcholine, associated with normal muscle membrane depolarization. In burn victims the increase in serum potassium may approach 5 to 10 mEq/L, precipitating hyperkalemic dysrhythmias or cardiac arrest due to increased receptor density and membrane sensitivity. This situation becomes clinically significant 24 hours after the burn and lasts an indefinite period, depending on the clinical course. The percentage of body surface area burned does not determine the magnitude of the hyperkalemia. Significant hyperkalemia has been reported with as little as 10% total body surface area burned.[3]
9. **B.** Succinylcholine is hydrolyzed by plasma cholinesterase almost immediately following administration. Only a small amount of succinylcholine actually reaches the neuromuscular junction. The speed of onset and brief duration make succinylcholine the ideal neuromuscular blocking agent for patients with a full stomach. Favorable intubation conditions occur faster, reducing the likelihood of pulmonary aspiration. Alcohol dehydrogenase is the enzyme responsible for alcohol metabolism. Normally the substance glutathione, produced by the liver, conjugates toxic metabolites of acetaminophen. When the amount of glutathione available for conjugation is exceeded, the unconjugated metabolites then bind to and destroy liver cells. Hepatic microsomal enzymes, including cytochrome P-450 enzymes, are crucial for the oxidation and resulting metabolism of many drugs.[2]
10. **D.** In the emergency setting, induction agents are used to induce unconsciousness to facilitate endotracheal intubation. Rapid sequence intubation requires administration of a potent induction agent followed immediately by a rapid-acting neuromuscular blocking agent to induce unconsciousness and motor paralysis, respectively, for tracheal intubation. Patients who are chemically paralyzed following rapid sequence intubation must also be sedated to prevent awareness.[3]
11. **A.** Propofol may cause significant decreases in systemic blood pressure sufficient to decrease cerebral perfusion pressure. The blood pressure effects of propofol may be exaggerated in hypovolemic patients, elderly patents, and patents with compromised left ventricular function caused by coronary artery disease.[1,3]
12. **B.** Etomidate has become a very popular induction agent because of its cerebroprotective effect and its unique propensity to maintain hemodynamic stability. Etomidate exhibits the best balance of utility and safety of all the induction agents under consideration.[3]
13. **A.** Ketamine, because of its pharmacological profile, should be considered the induction agent of choice for patients who are hypovolemic or hypotensive without evidence of serious head injury, and for patients with hemodynamic instability due to cardiac tamponade or intrinsic myocardial disease but without ischemic heart disease.[3]
14. **B.** Myocardial depression and hypotension are common potential side effects of all induction agents.[3]
15. **C.** Morphine is the prototype opioid agent and produces analgesia, euphoria, sedation, and a diminished ability to concentrate. Other sensations include nausea, a feeling of body warmth, heaviness of the extremities, dryness of the mouth, and pruritus. The cause of pain persists, but morphine and other opioid analgesics raise the pain threshold and modify the perception of noxious stimulation such that it is no longer experienced as pain. Morphine administered intravenously has an onset of action within minutes, and it peaks within 10 to 15 minutes, with a duration of action similar to that seen with intramuscular administration.[1]
16. **D.** By decreasing venous return, cardiac output and blood pressure decrease, decreasing left ventricular workload. There is also a decreased vulnerability to ventricular fibrillation with morphine, due to morphine-induced bradycardia from vagal stimulation in the CNS and, perhaps, a slowing of cardiac impulse conduction through the SA and AV nodes of the heart.[1]
17. **A.** In some patients, morphine causes cutaneous blood vessels to dilate, caused by the release of histamine. Localized cutaneous evidence of histamine release, especially along the vein into which morphine is injected, does not represent an allergic reaction to morphine. Overall, the

incidence of true allergy to opioid medications is uncommon, although there have been documented cases. More often, predictable side effects of opioid analgesics, such as localized histamine release, orthostatic hypotension, and nausea and vomiting, are misinterpreted as an allergic reaction.

18. **C.** Meperidine, in addition, does not cause miosis but rather tends to cause mydriasis, reflecting its modest atropine-like actions. A dry mouth also reflects the atropine-like effect of meperidine.[1]
19. **B.** Naloxone is a pure μ (mu) opioid receptor antagonist with no agonist activity, used to manage opioid overdose and to reverse opioid-induced ventilatory depression. The higher affinity of naloxone for the opioid receptors results in displacement of the opioid agonist from the μ receptor. Naloxone does not activate the μ receptor, and antagonism occurs. Because naloxone has a short duration of action, it is often necessary to repeat the dose or to give a continuous infusion to avoid recurrence of respiratory depression of ventilation.[1]
20. **D.** Benzodiazepines have no analgesic properties. They exert, in varying degrees, five principal pharmacological effects: sedation, anxiolysis, anticonvulsant actions, spinal cord–mediated skeletal muscle relaxation, and anterograde amnesia (acquisition of new information). Stored information (retrograde amnesia) is not affected by benzodiazepines.[1]
21. **A.** Opioid analgesics and benzodiazepines can have a synergistic hemodynamic effect, which results in a greater decrease in blood pressure when used in combination than that seen with either drug alone. Pain at the injection site is common with diazepam and the incidence of phlebitis is high. Midazolam is 2 to 3 times more potent than diazepam, and respiratory depression is a potential side effect of benzodiazepines. The main hemodynamic effect of midazolam is a reduction in systemic vascular resistance.[1]
22. **A.** Calcium channel blockers do not increase the sedative effect of benzodiazepines. Alcohol, tricyclic antidepressants, antihistamines, and opiate analgesics increase the sedative effects of benzodiazepines.[2]
23. **B.** Flumazenil is a benzodiazepine antagonist that reverses the action of benzodiazepines involved in recall, psychomotor impairment, and sedation. It has no effect on opiate overdose. In addition, flumazenil has been used in the management of alcohol intoxication, hepatic encephalopathy, seizure disorder, and to facilitate weaning off mechanical ventilation.[4]
24. **C.** NSAIDs interfere with the conversion of arachidonic acid to prostaglandins. Prostaglandins sensitize pain receptors to mechanical and chemical stimulation. By blocking cyclooxygenase, these mediators are not produced. Therefore, objective pain, pain arising from stimulation of peripheral nerve endings, is not felt. Opioid analgesics interfere with the subjective pain at the level of the CNS. Because they work at the level of the CNS, they often produce sedation as a side effect. Nonsteroidal agents typically produce no sedation and can be very effective in relieving some types of pain.[2]
25. **D.** Aspirin is the prototype NSAID, causing a decrease in the peripheral synthesis of prostaglandins and acting on the nervous system at the level of the hypothalamus. Acetaminophen is believed to act principally by inhibiting prostaglandin synthesis in the CNS. The extent of its activity in the periphery is unclear. Acetaminophen has very weak antiinflammatory action.[2,4]
26. **D.** The NSAIDs, including aspirin, all inhibit the COX-1 and COX-2 enzymes. The positive result is a dramatic reduction of joint inflammation, pain, and platelet aggregation. On the negative side, most of the side effects of the NSAIDs are due to their disruption of the prostaglandins' widespread physiological functions. In the stomach, prostaglandin (PGE-2) inhibits acid secretion and has a protective effect on the mucosa. Therefore the effect of NSAIDs in the stomach is gastritis and peptic ulceration. When renal circulation is impaired, prostaglandins are important in maintaining renal tubular blood flow and tubular function. NSAIDs administered to the elderly and those with poor renal function may result in nephrotoxicity.[5]
27. **A.** Several COX-2 inhibitors are now available which exhibit little or no activity against COX-1. The first two COX-2 inhibitors to become available are celecoxib (Celebrex) and rofecoxib (Vioxx).[2] However, recent research has demonstrated some significant risk factors with these medications and their use in selected patient populations. Vioxx has been removed. It is important to evaluate current recommendations before using these medications.

28. **A.** There is general agreement that no NSAID other than aspirin can be prescribed with absolute safety with respect to adverse renal effects.[1]
29. **D.** In acidic urine, salicylic acid is unchanged and therefore diffuses back into the blood. Vitamin C maintains an acidic urine when taken in large doses and can therefore delay the excretion of salicylic acid. Intravenous sodium bicarbonate can counter the metabolic acidosis associated with salicylate overdose and produce an alkaline urine that hastens the excretion of salicylate. Long-term aspirin ingestion can cause the loss of 10 to 30 ml of blood daily from GI irritation. This loss may lead to iron deficiency anemia in women with heavy menses. Rarely, massive GI bleeding occurs in patients on long-term aspirin therapy. The Poison Prevention Packaging Act of 1970 required that orange flavored baby aspirin (81-mg tablets) be limited to 36 tablets per bottle and that safety caps be used. Fatalities among children have been dramatically reduced since that time.[2]
30. **D.** Morphine 10 mg or meperidine 100 mg. An important benefit of Ketorolac-induced analgesia is the absence of ventilatory or cardiovascular depression.[1]
31. **A.** High levels of COX-2 in intestinal polyps are believed to promote mutation of polyps to cancerous tissue. COX-2 inhibitors may blunt the progression of Alzheimer's disease. This role is suggested by recent studies in which patients who received NSAIDs seemed to have slowed disease progression.[2]
32. **A.** Beta-blockers are often prescribed as the first drug for management of hypertension. Hypertensive patients with high plasma renin levels, younger white patients, are especially responsive to beta-blockers. Beta-blockers are also indicated for patients with coronary artery disease, and beta-blockers have been shown to have a protective effect against sudden death in individuals who have had a heart attack.[2]
33. **B.** Beta-blockers are used to manage angina and certain dysrhythmias. Blockade of beta receptors can compromise cardiac function, induce bronchospasm, and inhibit peripheral vasodilation. Hypoglycemia normally elicits the discharge of epinephrine. The effects of this released epinephrine will not be noticed easily in a patient who is taking a beta-receptor blocking drug. These drugs impair glycolic control in diabetic patients taking insulin or oral hypoglycemic agents.[2]
34. **D.** Excessive bradycardia or decreases in cardiac output due to drug-induced beta blockade should be managed initially with atropine. If ineffective, isoproterenol in dosages sufficient to overcome competitive beta blockade is appropriate. Dobutamine and calcium glucagon may also be used to reverse myocardial depression.[1]
35. **C.** Calcium channel blockers decrease the entry of calcium into smooth muscle and thereby lower vascular tone, an action that reduces peripheral resistance and blood pressure. Cardiac function is also depressed because of reduced intracellular calcium.[2]
36. **B.** Prinzmetal angina is the result of decreased oxygen supply to cardiac muscle which occurs at rest and may be caused by coronary artery spasm without vessel blockage. The management goal for angina is to decrease the heart's workload, thus decreasing its need for oxygen.[4]
37. **A.** Calcium channel blockers slow the inward movement of potassium ions. Hyperkalemia can occur in patients being treated with verapamil; it may occur after an amount of exogenous potassium much smaller than the usual has been infused to manage hypokalemia.[1]
38. **C.** Nimodipine is highly lipid soluble, which facilitates its entrance into the CNS, where it blocks the influx of extracellular calcium ions necessary for contraction of large cerebral arteries. Nimodipine is approved to manage cerebral vasospasm following a subarachnoid hemorrhage. This action alleviates the cerebral ischemia that can follow a stroke and, by maintaining blood flow, protects the brain from deterioration.[1,2]
39. **D.** Angiotensin II is a potent vasoconstrictor and is formed by the conversion of angiotensin I by ACE. When this enzyme is inhibited, the amount of angiotensin II formed is decreased. The ACE inhibitors also block the degradation of bradykinin and thus increase the amounts of this important vasodilator peptide. The net effect of ACE inhibitors is to decrease peripheral vascular resistance.[2]
40. **C.** ACE inhibitors increase renal blood flow and delay the progression of diabetic renal disease. ACE inhibitors can cause fetal and neonatal problems and should not be administered to pregnant women.[1,2]
41. **B.** Cough, upper respiratory congestion, rhinorrhea, and allergy-like symptoms are the most

common side effects of ACE inhibitors. ACE inhibitors are free of many of the side effects associated with other antihypertensive drugs, including depression, insomnia, and sexual dysfunction. Other adverse effects, such as congestive heart failure, bronchospasm, bradycardia, and exacerbation of peripheral vascular disease, are not seen with ACE inhibitors. Similarly, metabolic changes induced by diuretic therapy, such as hypokalemia, hyponatremia, and hyperglycemia, are not observed.[1]

42. **D.** The cardiac glycosides, digoxin and digitoxin, interfere with the movement of sodium ions across cardiac cell membranes. As a result, increased amounts of calcium ions become available to react with contractile proteins to generate a greater force of myocardial contraction.[1]
43. **A.** The most frequent cause of digitalis toxicity in the absence of renal dysfunction is the concurrent administration of diuretics that cause potassium depletion.[2]
44. **B.** Bradycardia is the most common digitalis-induced dysrhythmia, although other changes in heart rate are possible. Other adverse reactions include weakness, fatigue, and fainting. Visual disturbances such as dimness of vision, double vision, blind spots, flashing lights, or altered color vision also occur. Psychiatric disturbances range from mood alterations to psychoses or hallucinations.[2]
45. **B.** By slowing conduction of impulses through the AV node, digoxin protects the ventricles from overstimulation. The short-term therapeutic goal is not to slow the atrial rate, but to produce a partial heart block that allows fewer impulses from the atria to stimulate the ventricles to beat. Many patients experience spontaneous conversion to normal sinus rhythm after a few days of treatment.[2]
46. **D.** Nitroglycerin improves cardiac output, relieves pulmonary congestion, and decreases myocardial oxygen demand. Nitroglycerin primarily decreases preload (venous return to the heart) and relieves pulmonary edema. Nitroglycerin is capable of producing methemoglobinemia, a condition of interference with oxygen carriage in the blood and release of oxygen to tissues.[2]
47. **C.** Sodium nitroprusside, unlike nitroglycerin, produces direct venous (preload reduction) and arterial (afterload reduction) vasodilation.[1]
48. **D.** Depending on the dosage, dopamine stimulates dopamine receptors (0.5 to 3 mcg/kg per minute IV) in the renal vasculature to produce renal vasodilation, thus increasing renal blood flow; $beta_1$ receptors (3 to 10 mcg/kg per minute IV) in the heart; and alpha receptors (more than 10 mcg/kg per minute IV) in the peripheral vasculature. Dopamine is a transmitter in both the central and peripheral nervous systems.[1]
49. **A.** In contrast to dopamine, dobutamine does not have any clinically important vasoconstrictor activity, and calculated systemic vascular resistance is usually not altered greatly. Dobutamine does not stimulate $dopamine_1$ receptors, but renal blood flow improves as a result of drug-induced increases in cardiac output. Cardiac dysrhythmias are unlikely at therapeutic dosages, presumably because of the absence of endogenous catecholamine release. Dobutamine, but not dopamine, is a coronary artery vasodilator.[1]
50. **C.** Isoproterenol is the most potent activator of all the sympathomimetic agents at $beta_1$ and $beta_2$ receptors, being 2 to 3 times more potent than epinephrine and at least 100 times more potent than norepinephrine. In clinical dosages, isoproterenol lacks any α-agonist effects. The clinical uses of isoproterenol include administration of an aerosol to produce bronchodilation, continuous infusion of 1 to 5 mcg/min to increase heart rate in the presence of heart block, and continuous infusion to decrease pulmonary hypertension. More-specific β_2-adrenergic agonists have largely replaced isoproterenol as a bronchodilator.[1]

References

1. Stoelting RK: *Pharmacology and physiology in anesthetic practice*, Philadelphia, 1999, Lippincott Williams & Wilkins.
2. Clark J, Queener S, Karb V: *Pharmacologic basis of nursing practice*, St Louis, 2000, Mosby.
3. Walls R, Luten R, Murphy M et al: *Manual of emergency airway management*, Philadelphia, 2000, Lippincott Williams & Wilkins.
4. Grajeda-Higley L: *Understanding pharmacology: a physiologic approach*, Stamford, CT, 2000, Appleton & Lange.
5. McGavock H: *How drugs work: basic pharmacology for healthcare professionals,* Oxon, UK, 2003, Radcliff Medical Press.

CHAPTER **33**

INVASIVE MONITORING

REVIEW OUTLINE

I. Indications for invasive monitoring in the emergency department and during patient transport
   A. Oxygenation
   B. Cardiac status
   C. Neurological status
   D. Fluid resuscitation
   E. Pharmacological management

II. Complications of invasive monitoring
   A. Bleeding
   B. Infection
   C. Inaccurate readings
   D. Dysrhythmia
   E. Thrombus
   F. Embolus
   G. Pneumothorax
   H. Pulmonary infarction

III. Invasive monitoring that may be used in the emergency department or during patient transport
   A. Direct arterial blood pressure monitoring
   B. Central venous pressure monitoring
   C. Pulmonary artery pressure monitoring
   D. Intracranial pressure monitoring

IV. Age-related changes
   A. Pediatric patients
      1. Because of the anatomical differences between pediatric and adult patients, invasive monitoring should be initiated only by those with expertise in the management of critically ill or injured children
      2. Appropriate size equipment must be available for any invasive procedures performed
      3. Growth and development must be considered when performing invasive procedures on a newborn, infant, or child
   B. Elderly patients
      1. Cardiovascular changes related to age: for example, atherosclerosis and tortuous vessels need to be considered before performing invasive interventions
      2. Decreased sensation and blood flow to the extremities may place the elderly patient at risk for additional problems, such as infection or ischemic injury, with some invasive monitoring
      3. Preexisting medical problems and medications may interfere with the insertion and use of invasive monitors

V. Nursing diagnosis
   A. Fluid volume deficit related to blood loss
   B. Infection related to invasive monitoring
   C. Pain related to the insertion of catheters or equipment needed to perform invasive monitoring

---

REVIEW QUESTIONS

A 62-year-old female has been brought to the emergency department with profound hypotension. She has had a cough and fever for several days. Her blood pressure is 80 mm Hg by palpation. The emergency physician has decided to place an arterial line to monitor her blood pressure while administering fluids and vasoactive medications to manager her blood pressure and sepsis.

1. Which of the following tests should be performed before insertion of an arterial line into the radial artery?
   A. Homans' sign
   B. Allen's sign
   C. Romberg's sign
   D. Deep tendon reflexes

2. When zeroing a transducer system, the emergency nurse should:
   A. Leave the cap on the top of the zero reference stopcock on so that sterility of the system can be maintained

B. Turn the stopcock off to the monitor and open the system to air so that it can be zeroed
C. Zero the monitor-transducer according to the manufacturer's instructions
D. Leave the stopcock open to air and open the system between the transducer and the patient

3. After the radial arterial line has been inserted, the emergency nurse notices that there is a difference between the arterial blood pressure reading and the blood pressure obtained by cuff. Which of the following may help explain this discrepancy?
A. Edema and obesity may interfere with the arterial line's ability to accurately measure the patient's blood pressure
B. Atherosclerotic changes in elderly patients may cause systolic cuff pressures to be higher than arterial line readings
C. Dysrhythmias will not affect arterial pressure readings, unlike a pressure measured by a cuff
D. A correctly fitting cuff can measure blood pressure directly

4. The arterial waveform becomes dampened. What interventions may the emergency nurse perform to determine if the arterial line is functioning properly?
A. Promptly remove the arterial line to prevent ischemic injury to the artery
B. Forcefully flush the arterial catheter with saline or heparin to be sure that it is still functioning
C. Adjust the pressure scale higher to ensure that the monitor can make the waveform appear larger
D. Reposition the patient's wrist while watching to see if there is improvement in the waveform

5. The phlebostatic axis is located at the:
A. Xiphoid process and the second intercostal space
B. Fourth intercostal space and the midportion of the anteroposterior chest
C. Subclavian vein below the clavicle at the third intercostal space
D. Second intercostal space and the midportion of the anteroposterior chest

6. Pulmonary capillary wedge pressure is elevated in all of the following except:
A. Left ventricular failure
B. Fluid overload
C. Hypovolemia
D. Ischemia

7. A pulmonary artery catheter has been inserted in an elderly trauma patient to monitor fluid resuscitation while the patient waits for a bed in the critical care unit. The trauma intensivist has ordered a pulmonary artery wedge pressure reading every hour. The emergency nurse should perform the following in order to ensure patient safety during wedging:
A. Inflate the balloon with a minimum of 5 to 10 cc, similar to the amount of air needed to inflate an endotracheal tube
B. Keep the catheter wedged for no longer than 10 to 15 seconds to prevent injury to the artery
C. Flush the catheter with 10 ml of normal saline while it is in the wedged position to keep it clear
D. Inflate the balloon with 5 ml of normal saline in order to wedge it and obtain a reading

8. Normal cerebral perfusion pressure is:
A. 70 to 100 mm Hg
B. 0 to 15 mm Hg
C. 30 to 60 mm Hg
D. Over 150 mm Hg

9. When an intracranial pressure monitor is placed, the emergency nurse must remember that:
A. A subarachnoid bolt allows withdrawal of cerebrospinal fluid (CSF), because it is located below the arachnoid membrane
B. Any patient who requires neuromuscular blocking agents or sedation will not benefit from intracranial pressure (ICP) monitoring
C. ICP monitors are closed systems and should not be attached to continuous flush systems
D. CSF must be drained any time the ICP is elevated, no matter the cause of the elevation

10. A 17-year-old male who was not wearing a helmet sustained a head injury when he fell off his bike. His computed tomography scan demonstrated a severe closed head injury. An intraventricular catheter has been inserted by the neurosurgical resident to drain CSF and manage the patient's increasing ICP. Which of the following nursing diagnoses would be the most appropriate on which to base this patient's care while he is in the emergency department?

A. Infection, potential for, related to the insertion of the intraventricular catheter and drainage of the CSF to manage the patient's ICP
B. Pain related to the insertion of the intraventricular catheter while in the emergency department
C. Altered nutrition related to the body's requirements and increased metabolic rate
D. Anxiety related to the insertion of the intraventricular catheter while in the emergency department

ANSWERS

1. **B. Assessment.** Before insertion of an arterial line, collateral circulation should be assessed. Performing the Allen's sign test does this. Both the radial and ulnar arteries are occluded, and the patient is asked to make a tight fist to squeeze blood from the hand. The patient is then instructed to relax the hand, and compression of the ulnar artery is relaxed. Color should return within 5 to 10 seconds. If not, that radial artery should not be used.[1,2]
2. **C. Intervention.** The following steps should be completed when zeroing a monitor and transducer:[3]
   - Remove the cap from the top of the zero reference stopcock; system sterility must be maintained
   - Turn the stopcock off to the patient and open it to air
   - Zero the monitor and transducer according to the manufacturer's recommendations; this is very important, because there will be variance among equipment
   - Turn stopcock off to air and open between the transducer and the patient and replace the occlusive cap
3. **B. Assessment.** An arterial line can measure blood pressure directly. A blood pressure cuff compresses the brachial artery, causing pulsatile turbulent blood flow through the compressed artery, which creates vibrations and Korotkoff sounds that are detected with a stethoscope. If the patient has atherosclerotic changes, it may cause the systolic cuff readings to be higher than those of the arterial line.[3]
4. **D. Intervention.** Methods to troubleshoot dampened waveforms include:[3,4]
   - Assess the patient first, then take a cuff blood pressure to determine if the machine is functioning correctly
   - Make sure the pressure scale is set appropriately to the patient's expected pressure readings
   - Assess that the system is functioning properly
   - Remove any unnecessary stopcocks and excessive tubing
   - Check to see if the catheter is kinked
5. **B. Assessment.** The phlebostatic axis is the reference point from which pressure measurements are made and is approximately at the level of the atria. It is located at the intersection of the fourth intercostal space and the midportion of the anteroposterior chest.[3]
6. **C. Assessment.** Pulmonary capillary wedge pressure is elevated in left ventricular failure, constrictive pericarditis, mitral stenosis, mitral regurgitation, fluid overload, and ischemia. It is decreased with hypovolemia or vasodilating medications.[2]
7. **B. Intervention.** To wedge a pulmonary artery catheter, the following steps should be followed:[3]
   - Inflate the balloon with no more than 1.5 cc of air unless otherwise directed by the manufacturer of the catheter
   - Do not keep the catheter wedged for longer than 10 to 15 seconds
   - Do not wedge the catheter unnecessarily
   - Do not flush the catheter when it is wedged
   - Do not inject the catheter with fluid
8. **A. Assessment.** The cerebral perfusion pressure (CPP) is calculated by:

   CPP = mean arterial pressure (MAP) - ICP

   Normal cerebral perfusion pressure is 70 to 100 mm Hg and intracranial pressure is 0 to 15 mm Hg.[3,4]
9. **C. Assessment.** Subarachnoid bolts do not allow for drainage of CSF because of their location. Indications for ICP monitoring include the inability to asses the patient's neurological status because of sedation, analgesia, or neuromuscular blocking agents. CSF should be drained only when there is a sustained increase

in ICP. Nursing care such as suctioning will cause a transient increase in ICP. It is imperative that emergency nurses realize that ICP monitoring is a closed system and is not connected to a continuous flush system as are arterial lines. They should generally be flushed when needed by those who are experienced and with preservative-free saline.[3,4]

10. **A. Analysis.** Infection is one of the major and serious complications of intraventricular catheter insertion and could lead to increased mortality and morbidity in this patient.

References

1. Darovic GO: *Hemodynamic monitoring: invasive and noninvasive clinical applications*, Philadelphia, 1995, WB Saunders.
2. Alspach JG: *AACN core curriculum for critical care nursing*, Philadelphia, 1998, WB Saunders.
3. Mims BC, Toto KH, Luecke L et al: *Critical care skills*, Philadelphia, 2004, WB Saunders.
4. Lake C, Hines R, Blitt C: *Clinical monitoring: practical applications for anesthesia and critical care*, Philadelphia, 2001, WB Saunders.

INDEX

A

D

NOTES

NOTES